Mother of Invention

Mother of Invention

HOW THE GOVERNMENT CREATED
FREE-MARKET HEALTH CARE

Robert I. Field

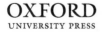

OXFORD
UNIVERSITY PRESS

OXFORD
UNIVERSITY PRESS

Oxford University Press is a department of the University of Oxford.
It furthers the University's objective of excellence in research, scholarship,
and education by publishing worldwide.

Oxford   New York
Auckland   Cape Town   Dar es Salaam   Hong Kong   Karachi
Kuala Lumpur   Madrid   Melbourne   Mexico City   Nairobi
New Delhi   Shanghai   Taipei   Toronto

With offices in
Argentina   Austria   Brazil   Chile   Czech Republic   France   Greece
Guatemala   Hungary   Italy   Japan   Poland   Portugal   Singapore
South Korea   Switzerland   Thailand   Turkey   Ukraine   Vietnam

Oxford is a registered trademark of Oxford University Press
in the UK and certain other countries.

Published in the United States of America by
Oxford University Press
198 Madison Avenue, New York, NY 10016

Library of Congress Cataloging-in-Publication Data
Field, Robert I., author.
Mother of invention : how the government created free-market health care / Robert I. Field.
p. ; cm.
Includes bibliographical references.
ISBN 978-0-19-974675-0 (alk. paper)
I. Title. [DNLM: 1. Health Care Sector—United States.   2. Government—United
States.   3. Health Care Reform—United States.   4. Public-Private Sector Partnerships—United
States. W 74 AA1]
RA393
362.1—dc23
2013029712

9 8 7 6 5 4 3 2 1
Printed in the United States of America
on acid-free paper

To Mary, David and William

TABLE OF CONTENTS

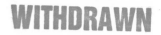

PREFACE

"Keep the government out of my health care." That and similar refrains have permeated health policy debates in the United States for more than a century. Opponents cried "socialized medicine" when reformers first tried to create government-financed health insurance plans in early part of the twentieth century. They raised the alarm again when President Harry Truman proposed universal coverage in the 1940s, when President Lyndon Johnson proposed Medicare in the 1960s, and when President Bill Clinton put forth his comprehensive reform plan in the 1990s. It is by now a familiar call, and it has often achieved notable success in defeating or forestalling reforms.

The rallying cry was proclaimed with special stridency in recent debates leading up to passage of the Affordable Care Act (ACA), the massive health reform law enacted in 2010. Opponents charged that the law amounted to a "government takeover" of the health care system. They argued that American health care is doing just fine and may even be the best in world. Why let the government in? It can only mess things up.

Underlying these concerns is an ongoing debate over the relative merits of the government and the private market in delivering and financing health care. Over the years, researchers in academia and think tanks have conducted countless studies and analyses to compare the efficiency, effectiveness, and compassion of both sectors. Often, they compare America's market-based system to those of Europe, where governments play a more pervasive role. What would happen, they wonder, if the government ran health care in the United States? How would things be different?

The problem with these debates is that they miss a key point. The speculations about government-run health care, both positive and negative, are largely for naught. There is no need to guess about the possible effects of letting the government take over the American health system because it already has.

Take any component of health care in the United States. Its most visible manifestation is likely to be a collection of private companies, many owned by outside investors, doing business with the public and earning profits in return. But look a bit closer and what appears to be a uniformly private sector is revealed as a mosaic of private and public elements. The government's hand is everywhere.

This book examines four such health system components, arguably the four most important. The first is the pharmaceutical industry, which is comprised almost entirely of private investor-owned companies. They create a stream of new products in response to market pressures in an environment that can be highly competitive. Their enterprise and initiative has made them among the most profitable in the country over the past two decades. Yet the ultimate source of innovation for these engines of profit is a massive federal program—the research funding of the National Institutes of Health (NIH). With a budget of almost $30 billion a year, it creates much of the raw intellectual fuel on which the industry thrives. That fuel takes the form of advances in basic biomedical science that makes virtually all of the industry's new products possible.

The second is the hospital industry. The government owns only a small minority of American hospitals. The majority operates as private corporations, some on a for-profit and some on a nonprofit basis. They represent a significant economic presence in cities and towns across the country and offer an ever-growing array of technologically advanced services. This sophisticated care is extremely expensive, so much so that it is out of the financial reach of most patients. Payment from insurance plans is the only viable source of funds, and the government administers the largest single plan in the form of Medicare. Without it, few hospitals in the United States could survive in their present state.

The third is the medical profession. America's complement of physicians is dominated by specialists who earn more than their colleagues almost anywhere else in the world. Once again, they have the Medicare program to thank. It not only reimburses practitioners for much of the high-end specialty care they deliver at generous levels but also helps to fund their training.

Finally, there is the private insurance industry. It has grown over the past several decades from a niche player into a major force in the financial sector, with huge national corporations playing dominant roles in many markets. They would not exist but for the guiding hand of federal policy. Government decisions shaped the industry in its formative years in the 1930s and 1940s, and government subsidies support it today to a considerable extent with a substantial tax break for coverage provided through employers. Government programs also account for a sizeable share of the industry's overall business by offering private insurers the opportunity to administer coverage under Medicare and Medicaid and by creating and subsidizing a huge market for individual policies sold through insurance exchanges under the ACA.

None of this is news to those who work in these components of the health care industry. Pharmaceutical researchers readily credit NIH funding as the backbone of the research enterprise that creates new drugs. Hospital executives carefully plan their service offerings and medical staff composition around the intricacies of Medicare reimbursement rules. Physicians in many specialties fill their practices with elderly patients who turn to Medicare to cover their bills. Insurance executives vie to market policies to employers that can then offer coverage to workers as a tax-free benefit.

However, the size and pervasiveness of the government's role is news to many, perhaps most, people outside the industry. They directly see the private face of health care in their routine interactions with the system, but the government foundation that lies beneath it remains opaque. As a result, they perceive a market-based system that operates apart from the public sphere. To be sure, few are oblivious to the substantial government role in regulating every component of American health care. The list of agencies is extensive, and the actions of many of them—such as the Food and Drug Administration, the Centers for Disease Control and Prevention, and state departments of health—routinely make the headlines. But regulation is commonly perceived as an external force that holds the private health care system in check, rarely as an integral, intricate part of that system.

This book aims to change that perception. It demonstrates how a system that seems so clearly rooted in the free market in fact rests on a huge partnership between the public and private spheres. The government does much more than simply oversee an industry built by private entrepreneurs. It is the primary source of guidance and funding on which almost every aspect of that system relies, and it has played that role for well over half a century. Without it, "free-market" health care as we know it today would not exist.

The notion that private markets grow from a foundation of government initiatives is not new. Observers have noted it for as long as there have been private markets to observe. The father of free-market economic theory, Adam Smith, commented in the late eighteenth century on the key role of several kinds of government infrastructure in enabling markets to function. More recently, economist Joseph Steiglitz described the importance of public support in underpinning much commercial activity. Even Milton Friedman, the champion of laissez-faire economic policy, noted that private firms need some forms of public intervention in order to thrive.

The phenomenon of public support for private markets is widespread and hardly limited to health care. In fact, it pervades the entire economy. This book begins by noting the connection between government programs and the growth of four major industries. The Internet enabled personal computing to grow from a curiosity into a mainstay of the entire economy. Interstate highways transformed the automobile from a convenience to a necessity. The space program launched satellites on which the cable television industry relies to transmit content. Mortgage support programs led to an explosion in housing construction (although with less than auspicious results in recent years).

However, in no industry is the link between public initiatives and private enterprise as close as it is in health care. The government directly funds the provision of over half of all medical services in the United States. When indirect support through tax breaks and other means is considered, the total is closer to two-thirds. And the portion continues to grow. Those funding programs carry with them innumerable conditions that determine the shape of American health care at all levels—from the structure of giant corporations like pharmaceutical firms and for-profit hospital chains to the nature of private physician–patient encounters. Without the government, the health care industry in the United States would be unrecognizable.

This book tells this story through statistics on growth trends and through case studies of prominent private health care players. All of the sectors that it considers predate government involvement, in some cases by thousands of years. However, the size and shape they take today emerged from a crucible of public policy and financial support. Each is now dominated by huge private enterprises that owe their prosperity, and often their very existence, to a partnership with the government of one kind or another.

Government intervention in support of private markets can take different forms. It can, for example, provide funding through subsidies, both directly with grants and indirectly with tax breaks. It can facilitate commercial activity by building and maintaining essential infrastructure. It can encourage business relationships by establishing and enforcing regulatory standards that enhance consumer trust and set the ground rules for fair competition. And every level of government can initiate such efforts—federal, state, and local. However, regardless of the form, it is public policy that is driving private initiative, and this book considers the government's role broadly to reflect its range of incarnations as they apply across American health care.

The tale of each sector ends with a thought experiment that considers what that industry segment would look like had the government not intervened. The answers are, of course, conjectures that are highly speculative. We can never know with certainty what form an alternative health care world would have taken. However, we can wonder what other player could have provided the resources and national perspective needed to create modern health care. And, for each sector, such a player is hard to imagine. We would be hard-pressed to find models of any major industry that reached its present size and vitality without a government initiative of some sort, and there is no basis to believe that health care could have been an exception.

Of course, to identify the driving force behind our system is not to uncritically praise it. The American health care system leaves much to be desired, and many of its shortcomings can be traced to the very government programs that created it. The system falls short on each of the key determinants by which policy analysts measure effectiveness. Quality is inconsistent, with wide variations in practice across regions and an epidemic of errors that are a constant cause of patient harm. Costs perennially rise at an unsustainable rate, now eating up more than 17 percent of the nation's overall economic output. And access is limited for tens of millions of people who lack insurance coverage, many of whom remain uninsured even under the ACA.

Aside from these obvious shortcomings, government initiatives by their nature also create substantial inefficiencies. In particular, the private industries they have nurtured use their substantial government-granted resources to lobby their sponsor for ever-growing levels of support. Once an industry gains sufficient size, it can translate its wealth into political influence, and the government often finds it impossible to control what it has wrought. A clear example is the behavior of providers that rely on Medicare for their financial stability. Hospitals, home health agencies, outpatient clinics, and numerous medical specialties, among countless others, continuously lobby Congress to maintain the flow of reimbursement. They do not obtain their objective every time, but they succeed often enough to add substantial costs to the system for services that sometimes offer little benefit. The effects can be seen in a surfeit of hospital capacity, an imbalance in the composition of the medical profession in favor of specialty care, and excessive use of sophisticated technology.

The government's oversight of health care is also subject to what political scientists term "regulatory capture." This occurs when the entities subject to regulation gain enough power to control their own overseers. They use this power to soften regulatory supervision and to tilt its focus away from safeguarding public well-being and toward protection of their economic interests, for example by shielding existing firms from new sources of competition. And, of course, government regulators can also be susceptible to outright corruption.

Economists describe the effects of these inefficiencies as "rents," a term that denotes the excess price that a producer can extract by holding a favorable economic position. Health care providers are able to extract rents in several contexts. For example, restrictive licensing laws that limit entry into many forms of clinical practice make it easier for established practitioners to raise their fees. Public reimbursement programs that guarantee payment for services, such as Mediare, enable some facilities to charge for providing excessive amounts of care. When rents are extracted, resources are diverted from more productive uses.

Free-market advocates often hold up this inefficiency as proof of the inherent inability of the government to effectively guide private enterprise. They point to the massive waste of resources and redirection of effort away from public goals to argue that government intervention in markets, however well meaning its original intent, invariably harms societal well-being. Left alone, they argue, markets deliver needed goods and services in the most efficient way possible.

From the other side, critics of private health care markets charge that they are wasteful and inefficient. They point to the large profits many firms generate that are paid as dividends to investors and as high executive compensation. These substantial sums represent overhead expenses that leak from the system. They inflate costs without adding anything to the amount or quality of care that patients receive. Critics have dubbed the economic engine that generates these expenses the "medical-industrial complex" to denote the capture of our health care system by corporate interests, focused more on financial gain than on patient well-being.

The purpose of this book is not to debate the relative merits of private markets and government programs in providing Americans with health care. Rather, it makes a very different point. Free markets and government regulation do not represent a dichotomy of opposing forces that contend one against the other but are rather manifestations of the same underlying dynamic. In a broad sense, free-market entrepreneurs and government regulators are partners in a common enterprise. To be sure, businesses and their government overseers regularly spar with one another, and their relationship is commonly characterized by intense antagonism. But these contests generally center on short-term concerns. Across a range of major industries including health care, in the longer term, one side could not exist without the other.

Private health care markets do not arise on the scale they have reached in the United States in the absence of some form of government support. They arise because the government played an active role in creating them. Free-market advocates may be correct in their observation of inherent and pervasive government inefficiency; however, the antidote of dramatically less government involvement is misguided. If the government stepped aside, the private health care industry would not find itself in a world of expanding horizons. It would encounter a world in which it would be difficult or impossible to even survive. To speak metaphorically, the government tills the field in which the private market takes root and blossoms. Without it, we might still have plant life, but we would have less of it and it might not be of a kind we want.

Much of the nurturance that tends the field for private enterprise takes the form of basic infrastructure that makes commercial activity possible. This book describes several forms that this infrastructure takes in health care. Basic biomedical research, for example, is a public good with benefits that are available to all. It also serves as an essential ingredient in pharmaceutical innovation, but no private firm could afford to invest in its production on a broad enough scale to meet its own needs because the payoff is too speculative and the results too difficult to shield from competitors. Health insurance for the elderly is difficult for private insurers to provide because the risk of expensive claims is too high, yet without it hospitals would have no means of payment for a large portion of their patients. Medical education provides us with a steady supply of new physicians, yet the cost would be prohibitive without some form of external support. And reassurance of the public in the quality of the drugs they take, the hospitals in which they receive care, and the physicians who treat them requires an external objective source of oversight that only the government can provide.

The critics of government are correct that such elements of publicly created infrastructure can be extraordinarily inefficient and susceptible to undue influences. The partnership with private industry that created American health care is riddled with examples of each. Yet, removing the government from the equation is not a realistic solution. Meaningful improvement requires that we craft reforms with sensitivity to the corrupting influences that can misdirect elements of the system, and build on our ingrained public–private partnership to implement them.

The last chapter of the book considers some specific steps along these lines. It does not contain a manifesto for change along an explicit path but rather an approach to reform that takes into account the intricate nature of the system as it actually exists. More than anything, the book is intended as a resource for advancing the discussion over what that change should be by explaining how we got the health system that we have and how we can realistically understand possibilities for reform.

The intricacy of our public–private system and the difficulty of remediating its shortcomings are demonstrated with particular poignancy by the arduous gestation and complex framework of the ACA. Dubbed "Obamacare" by its opponents, it serves as an easy target for their criticisms because of its massive size and mind-numbing complexity. However, for all of the dramatic changes that the law implements, it represents anything but a break from the established paradigm of American health care. To the contrary, it is entirely consistent.

Before considering possibilities for further reform, the final chapter considers the Act's place within health care's underlying paradigm. The overriding goal of the law is to expand coverage so that they everyone is guaranteed access to insurance regardless of health status. It does not achieve universal coverage, but it substantially reduces the number of Americans who are uninsured. The most straightforward way to accomplish this goal would have been to create a government program that provides coverage directly. Advocates of a single payer financing system have been promoting that approach for decades. However, we have gone too far down the road toward a public–private structure for such an approach to succeed politically. Instead, the Act channels substantial new government involvement along the same lines that it has for decades by creating a foundation that enables the private sector to do the job. It accomplishes this by establishing insurance exchanges through which private insurance companies sell policies to individuals and through an expanded Medicaid program, much of which is administered by private insurance plans.

The ultimate lesson to be drawn from America's public–private health care partnership that led up to and that includes the ACA is that the two sectors do not compete in a zero-sum game. Growth in the size of one does not necessarily detract from the size of the other. When the government expands its role, private activity is not crowded out. Rather, expansion of either sector creates more room for the other. Historically, more government involvement in health care has invariably broadened the range of opportunities for the private sphere. And, by the same token, a smaller government role would cause the private sector's prospects to decline.

The United States does not have either a free-market or a government-based health care system and should not endeavor through reform to try to create either one. The government is the only viable source of direction and funding for key segments of health care, and private enterprise provides a key source of essential innovation and vitality. The notion that there is an incompatibility between the free market and the government in the health care system's orientation distorts public debates and misdirects policy analysis. To ignore this dynamic is to ignore the true nature of American health care and to fundamentally misunderstand the opportunities for reform.

On a broader level, political debates are misguided when they pit the virtues of the free market against those of government oversight. Regulatory programs represent more than an ongoing contest between opposing forces, and public policy does not have to choose sides. Most private industries would not approach their present size or take their present form without the government initiatives that created the infrastructures on which they rest. For its part, the government could not operate these industries on its own without creating massive new inefficiencies.

An understanding of the true nature of this relationship can lead to more accurate perceptions of what truly drives America's health care system and of how policymakers can productively address its serious challenges. In doing so, it may add a new element of rationality to policy debates. At the least, it can refute the rallying cry of keeping the government out of our health care, which has distorted public discourse for far too long. Perhaps it can also put an end to reckless scare stories that "death panels" and "rationing" lurk within government initiatives, which poisoned debates over the Obama health reform plan. To achieve meaningful results, further reform of American health care must focus on ways of improving government policies, not of eliminating them. If we were to get the government out of health care, we might find that we do not have much of a health care system at all. This book endeavors to explain why.

ACKNOWLEDGMENTS

A book of this scope is possible only as a collaboration, and this one is no exception. I am indebted to a number of people who contributed in many important ways. I was fortunate to have help in the early stages from several able research assistants—Majesh Abraham, Nicole Martin, Joseph Pecora, Jonathan Richina, and Natasha Zaveri. In the later stages, Joanna Suder assisted with several aspects of the research. I am especially grateful to Erica Cohen for her tireless and meticulous research assistance as the book neared completion. To call it invaluable would be an understatement.

I benefitted from insightful reviews of drafts of the manuscript from several people. Tim Harper provided editorial assistance. Several experts in health law, health policy, and economics contributed technical expertise. Andrew Fichter, Stephen Metraux, and Mark Stehr reviewed major portions of the manuscript. Barry Furrow and Sandra Johnson read it through in its entirety and broadened my perspective on many points. I was extremely fortunate to have the input of two such prominent authorities in the field. Chad Zimmerman at Oxford University Press was a source of steady guidance in moving the manuscript through the publication process. Of course, any errors that may remain are mine alone.

I also owe thanks to Dean Roger Dennis of the Earle Mack School of Law for his support throughout the project. Finally, I gratefully acknowledge the support of the Brocher Foundation in Hermance, Switzerland (www.brocher.ch), which provided an idyllic setting in which to complete much of the writing.

Earlier versions of portions of the book have appeared in the following journal articles: "Government as the Crucible for Free Market Health Care: Regulation, Reimbursement, and Reform," *University of Pennsylvania Law Review* 159, no. 6 (2011): 1669–726; "Regulation, Reform and the Creation of Free Market Health Care," *Hamline Journal of Public Law & Policy* 32, no. 2 (2011): 301–31; and "How the Government Created and Sustains the Private Pharmaceutical Industry," *St. Louis University Journal of Health Law & Policy* 6, no.1 (2012): 11–68.

1

What's Private About the Free Market?

> The third and last duty of the sovereign or commonwealth is that of
> erecting and maintaining those public institutions and those public
> works, which, though they may be in the highest degree advantageous to
> a great society, are, however, of such a nature, that the profit could never
> repay the expence to any individual or small number of individuals.
>
> —ADAM SMITH, *THE WEALTH OF NATIONS*[1]

In 2011, the patent for Lipitor, the best selling drug in history,[2] expired. Over the
course of the 15 years since it was introduced, it had dominated the market for
statins, a class of medications taken by 25 million people worldwide to treat high
cholesterol. Lipitor generated $125 billion in sales for Pfizer, its manufacturer and
the largest pharmaceutical company in the world. Even in the year that Lipitor
first faced generic competition, Pfizer's net income reached $10 billion and its total
revenue $67.4 billion. It employed a workforce of 110,600, and, in 2012, its market
capitalization stood at $180.5 billion.[3]

The same year, Hospital Corporation of America (HCA), the largest for-profit
hospital chain in the country, reported profits of $1.9 billion on revenue of $7.8
billion. The company operated 163 hospitals nationwide and employed 170,000
people to work in them. In 2012, it enjoyed a market capitalization of $14.4 billion.[4]

The largest health insurer in America, United Health, generated profits of $8.5
billion that year, and it brought in total revenue of $102 billion. The company
employed 99,000 workers and provided coverage to 26 million customers. Its market capitalization stood at $54 billion in 2012, as it looked ahead to the promise
of dramatic growth in its customer base with full implementation of the massive
health reform law passed in 2010.[5]

Health care professionals also reaped substantial financial rewards in 2011.
The United States had 954,000 practicing physicians, who generated over $500 bil-
lion dollars in reimbursement.[6] A few specialties did especially well. The nation's
23,662 cardiologists, for one, enjoyed an average income of $314,000,[7] with the top
earners reaching $3 million.

Overall, the American health care system generated $2.5 trillion dollars of
economic activity in 2011. That sum is more than one-sixth of the output of the
entire economy. It employed 10 percent of the nation's nonfarm workforce. This
gargantuan enterprise is one of the largest commercial endeavors in the world.

Pfizer, HCA, United Health, and thousands of physicians owe their considerable financial success to their place as part of that enterprise, as do thousands of other health care businesses and individual practitioners. Their good fortune stems from the alignment of many factors. There is the hard work of thousands of dedicated professionals. There is the creative genius of countless innovators. There is the risk-taking of entrepreneurs and investors. But there is also a silent partner behind every success story in the private health care sector. It laid the foundation and provides the ongoing sustenance that makes all of these market-driven enterprises possible. That partner is the government.

It is taken as a truism that America's health care system is rooted in the free market. No other developed country looks to private enterprise to drive the provision and financing of care to the same extent. Entrepreneurs devise new products and services, corporate payers set prices, and independent practitioners offer services. With the tremendous growth of the health care sector in America over the past several decades and the ever-expanding array of medical miracles that it offers patients, it would be easy to hold out American health care as an example of the fruits of a robust market-based system.

The problem with this conclusion is that it misses an essential aspect of the arrangement. It overlooks the omnipresent support and guidance of the central, indispensable player that makes the market-based system possible. The government funds, directs, and nurtures American health care on a fundamental level. Its role is so pervasive and of such longstanding importance that it can be credited with creating health care as we know it today. The private health care sector in the United States, the largest in the world, emerged from a series of government programs that launched its key sectors and continue to shape it today. Every major aspect of the system grew out of a public initiative. What is more, governments at both the federal and state levels continue to pump more money, directly and indirectly, into the system than all private players combined.

The Government's Hand in Health Care

Direct government funding of health care reached $1 trillion in 2008 through programs such as Medicare, Medicaid, and veterans' health.[8] In that year, the overall system cost slightly more than $2 trillion.[9] But the government's trillion dollars represented only direct spending, the appropriations that appear in formal budgets for the world to see. An additional $250 billion was spent indirectly, in ways that are less obviously apparent but no less forceful in their effect.

The bulk of indirect government funding of health care is accomplished through tax exemptions that permit substantial portions of the industry and their customers to avoid assessments on a range of activities. The largest of these is the tax break for health insurance premiums when the coverage is obtained through employment. That benefit alone was worth $240 billion in 2010.[10] The government also grants tax exemptions to hospitals and other health care institutions that operate on a nonprofit basis, which represent the majority of them. That benefit is worth more than $12 billion a year.[11] Add to that the premiums that the federal and state governments pay for the more than 2 million workers in their employ and their dependents, and the tab grows even larger. According to one thorough estimate, direct and indirect government payments cover the cost of almost 60 percent of the American health care system.[12]

Who receives the fruits of this largess? The most apparent beneficiaries are the millions of patients whose care is financed and whose insurance premiums are subsidized. But considering them alone only scratches the surface. More than one-sixth of the American economy receives an injection of revenues through the government's payments for health care.[13] Within this gigantic economic sector are hospitals, outpatient clinics, physicians, allied health professionals, insurance companies, and pharmaceutical firms, to name only a few. In addition to those components that directly contribute to the actual provision of care, thousands of scientists are funded to uncover the secrets of biomedical science, paving the way for new advances that keep the industry vibrant and innovative going forward.

Each of these players owes a significant portion of its income to government programs. For some of them, that portion approaches 100 percent.[14] But their debt runs even deeper than that. Not one of them would exist in anything close to its present form had the government not created the economic structure within which it operates. A series of programs, most enacted during the middle of the twentieth century, established regulatory structures and massive funding commitments that shape every major aspect of the health care system as we know it today.

In essence, the government created American health care and maintains it in its present form. What appears on its surface to be a market-based system is actually a huge public-private partnership in which the two sides form a symbiotic pair.[15] Private markets lend energy and vitality to the health care enterprise. Competition drives innovation throughout the industry. The flexibility of private enterprise permits experimentation and risk-taking that is essential to health care's vibrancy and renewal. But private organizations and professionals could not function as they do if they did not have government-imposed structure and funding. In its absence, the industry would be much smaller overall, and the range of medical services available to Americans would be much more limited.[16] Health care would not consume anything close to its present share of the economy.

Government programs that support private health care markets are initiated and maintained at all levels of government—federal, state, and local. They take a range of different forms. Some lend financial support, either with direct subsidies for patients, providers, and payers or with indirect assistance through tax breaks. Others create and maintain basic infrastructure that enables private markets to function. Still others enhance trust in the system through oversight of quality and regulation of market competition. Regardless of the form, they all extend the public role in support of private initiative.

The largest and most visible source of government involvement in American health care is the funding of care administered by the Medicare and Medicaid programs, which together account for more than 70 percent of federal health care spending.[17] They provide financial support and regulatory oversight to facilitate the work of thousands of private providers. The Veterans Health Administration, which serves military veterans through government-owned hospitals and clinics and government-employed physicians, contributes another 4 percent of the federal investment in health care.[18] Beyond these initiatives, dozens of other programs spend additional billions of dollars and exert effects that, although less direct and obvious, are no less fundamental to the system's vitality.

To be sure, this government largess has produced a system with a plentiful share of shortcomings. Most notably, it is a major reason why the United States has the most expensive health care system in the world by far. The generosity of public programs enables many private health care businesses to charge exorbitant prices and to render unnecessary services, enriching themselves substantially in the process. They then devote some of their government-granted riches to lobbying to protect and extend their lucrative position. However, none of this is to deny the importance of public programs in nurturing America's private health care industry. Rather, it is to vividly illustrate their pervasive influence.

Does America, therefore, have a free-market or a government-run health care system? The answer is that it has both and it has neither. Both are extreme characterizations that reflect a superficial description of reality. Neither kind of system has ever existed in this country or probably ever could. Without a mix of public initiative and private enterprise, our health care system would bear little resemblance to anything we think of as American health care today. The chapters that follow show how these efforts work in concert to form the foundation on which all of our health care system rests.

The Government's Hand in American Industry

In a larger context, a mix of government and market forces drives much of the American economy. In fact, there are few large American industries that do not owe their size and shape to a government foundation. At times, the government extends its influence indirectly, in ways that go largely unseen, but with no less dramatic effects. A look at the government's role in shaping key aspects of the larger economy illustrates how public involvement in health care, although it may be distinctive in its magnitude, is hardly unique in its foundational importance.

The government's role as creator and nurturer of private markets is not new. In fact, its origins date back to the dawn of the country's industrialization. More than 150 years ago, government support underlay one of the seminal elements in America's economic modernization. In the mid- and late-nineteenth century, the federal government partnered with several large corporations to create the intercontinental railroad and a network of rail lines that spanned the country. The collaboration built a massive transportation infrastructure that formed the backbone for industrial growth.

The government's primary contribution to the railroad enterprise was the grant of large tracts of public land on which the system was built, the first of which was authorized by Congress in 1850. Over the course of the rest of the nineteenth century, the size of the grants grew steadily, as did the fortunes of the companies that received them. By the turn of the twentieth century, the railroad industry had grown into one of the wealthiest and most powerful in the United States.[19]

The government and the railroad companies each had its own set of goals in entering into the partnership, all of which were amply realized. The government sought to stimulate economic development, raise revenue for public works, and encourage settlement of the West. The companies sought new avenues for profits. The coincidence of interests ultimately transformed the economy and the social fabric of the country. It created new forms of commerce to an extent its early proponents likely never dreamed of and helped to propel America to economic prominence in the world. It also set the pattern for similar ventures that today pervade almost every aspect of the economy.[20]

In supporting railroad construction, the government did more than simply offer assistance to a nascent industry. It initiated a joint venture that guided the industry over the course of its existence. As the partnership grew, it sent not just ripples but tidal waves across all of American society.[21]

Of course, none of this is to say that America would not have developed a railway system had Congress not initiated the land grant program. Private companies might eventually have found the resources they needed through other avenues, or the government might have contributed to the industry's development in some other way. No advanced economy entered the late nineteenth century without an extensive rail network, and it is unlikely that America would have followed a different course. It is also not to say that the land grant program produced the optimal result. The railroad industry that it created consolidated into regional monopolies that stifled competition, to the detriment of many consumers. Nevertheless, regardless of whether government support was administered as wisely as it might have been, it is difficult to imagine that private entities could have developed as extensive a rail system without substantial public support in some form to supply their most essential asset, huge tracts of land.

Contrary to widely held views of the effect of public intervention in private markets, the government did not throw a dead weight on the formative phases of the railroad industry. To the contrary, it served as a seminal force. Rather than preempting the private market, government intrusion into the burgeoning field of rail travel built its foundation. In doing so, it also set the course for the country's industrialization and the emergence of incalculable numbers of other private enterprises along the way.

A look at some more recent examples of the government's foundational role in key industries offers a framework for analyzing health care. Four large industrial sectors serve as examples of pillars of the economy that would bear little resemblance to their present states in the absence of major government programs that created an infrastructure on which they rest. The programs took different forms and reflect varying approaches to government support for private markets. In some cases, they produced unintended effects that created new sets of policy concerns. But they were undeniably instrumental in launching and sustaining important new forms of commerce.

For each sector, we can ask a question that is posed in subsequent chapters about key segments of the private health care market. What would they look like had the government not intervened? Or, to ask the question more directly, could they have taken their present size and shape in the absence of critical government support?

To start, what would the computer industry look like without the Internet, a creation of the United States military that was expanded for commercial applications in the 1990s? The Internet was originally designed for defense applications, and its effect on private computing was inadvertent. After giving it a start, the government left much of its operation to private entities. Yet, anticipated or not, the Internet initiated a flood of market-based activity that turned it into the foundation for the large and growing high-technology industry. It exemplifies a government infrastructure initiative that launched a new industrial sector.

What would the automobile industry look like without the interstate highway system? Unlike the Internet, this huge public works project was intended from the start to enhance private commerce. However, once built, it went even further and transformed the country's economic and social structure in ways that enshrined automobile manufacturing as a lynchpin of the economy. The interstate highway system exemplifies an initiative that reinforced and directed industrial growth.

Where would the telecommunications industry be without satellites launched by the space program? Space-based transmission of video and audio signals created vast new capabilities for companies that transmit entertainment and information. It changed the nature of everything from television programs to e-mail by making instantaneous global communication possible. It reflects an initiative to transform a promising industry in size and structure.

And where would the construction industry be without a set of financing programs that ease the process of obtaining home mortgages? Government guarantees for mortgages supported a spurt of home buying starting in the years following World War II, which created tremendous opportunities for builders to meet the demand. In lending financial support to the housing market, the government used subsidies to effectuate an explosion in size for an important sector of the economy.

In every case, the answer to the question is the same. All of these industries would still exist. Each is essential to the overall economy, and each would have emerged in some form on its own. However, they would all be much smaller, less diverse, and less innovative. They would also have a dramatically more circumscribed set of opportunities to devise products and services. The same can be said for almost every aspect of health care.

Of course, government support for private markets has not always been implemented wisely, and we might well be better off had it shaped these industries differently. An often-cited example is the flight of residents and business from inner cities to suburbs and the consequent abandonment of many urban cores that was engendered by the proliferation of automobiles. Growing reliance on automobiles also led to relentless increases in traffic, which perpetually spawn the need for even more new roads. Subsidized mortgages led to overbuilding in many regions. They also helped to create speculative secondary markets for mortgage debt that can implode, as they did in 2008, with disastrous results for the overall economy. Nevertheless, from the perspective of the industries involved and of the numerous investors who have made fortunes in them, government policy has been the engine of prosperity.

Information Technology and the Internet

Consider information technology. Personal computers first became commonplace in the early 1980s, as Apple and then IBM created machines that could sit on top of a desk. By the late 1980s, portable computers were introduced that could rest on a user's lap. Sophisticated applications evolved for word processing, spreadsheets, presentations, and database management, not to mention countless games and other diversions. Industry sales grew steadily for both computer hardware and for software to make it run. But a transformation began in 1994 that sent the industry into hyperdrive. In that year, the first web browser, an initial version of Netscape, was introduced to the public. It provided a set of keys that let the average computer user gain access to thousands of computers around the world that were connected through a network called the Internet. Anyone, even the most technologically naïve, could use it to literally explore the world from the comfort of home.

The Internet had existed for decades before the private sector entered the game. The concept of a network linking multiple remote computers was proposed in 1962, to enable the military to maintain control of missiles and bombers after a nuclear attack.[22] The Department of Defense launched it in 1968, with four computer hosts. The network's capabilities expanded when the first e-mail program was created in 1972, and the name "Internet" was first applied to the system in 1974. After numerous enhancements over the next several years, largely funded by the Department of Defense and the National Science Foundation, in 1983, researchers at the University of Wisconsin developed the domain name system that allowed users to access servers on the network with words rather than difficult to remember numbers. In 1993, researchers at the University of Illinois created the first graphical user interface, or web browser, which was the step that opened the network to a vast audience of computer users worldwide, including rank novices.

Soon after Netscape was released in 1994, Web traffic soared with the first significant commercial applications. These followed the lead of Pizza Hut, the first business to offer web ordering. At about the same time, Amazon developed its business plan to become the first broad-based Internet retailer. The next year, the National Science Foundation contracted with four private companies to provide public access to its backbone system and instituted the now-familiar system of domains.[23]

The growth of the Internet since then is a tale that hardly needs retelling. A few statistics capture the story. In December 1995, there were an estimated 16 million Internet users, representing 0.4 percent of the world's population.[24] By December 2000, that number had grown by more than 20-fold to 359 million, representing 5.9 percent of all people on the globe. As of June 2008, almost 1.5

billion people, representing more than 20 percent of the world's population, were online. In the United States today, the Internet pervades almost every aspect of life. New uses seem to arise almost daily, and it is the basis for a significant portion of overall economic activity.

In the wake of the Internet's commercialization, the nature and size of the computer industry experienced a transformation. Between 1986 and 1990, 28.1 million personal computers were sold in the United States at an aggregate value of $76.4 billion.[25] During the next five years, sales jumped to 64.3 million, bringing in $153 billion. During the period between 2001 and 2006, the numbers had reached 267 million units sold for an aggregate cost of $424 billion. Overall sales for the entire period between 1981 and 2006 were almost $1 trillion. Consumer spending on software rose from $500 million in 1990 to $17.8 billion in 2000 and on personal computers from $1.6 billion to $108.8 billion.[26] Countless related industries have also arisen and grown as offshoots.

Of course, the coincidence of growth in personal computer sales and in Internet use does not prove that one caused the other. Undoubtedly, other applications and overall enhancements in computer utility played important roles as well. Even in the absence of the Internet, these forces could have pushed computers onto the desks of large numbers of people over a relatively short period of time. However, it is undeniable that the Internet expanded the range of uses of personal computers to a tremendous degree and greatly increased the demand for these machines. It also increased demand for software to run on them; peripheral equipment, such as printers and monitors to expand their usefulness; and a large range of related products.

What would the personal computer industry look like if the government had not created the Internet? It would certainly still exist as an important and vital part of the economy, as it had for almost two decades before the Internet was commercialized. It also surely would have grown over the years as new applications were devised and old ones perfected. However, it would almost certainly be nothing like the ubiquitous presence it is today in all spheres of activity. Personal computers, via the Internet, now shape most aspects of our lives, from our social interactions to our financial transactions to our health care. A robust private sector manufacturers them in a vibrant market that the government, almost inadvertently, unleashed.

Automobiles and Interstate Highways

Consider the automobile industry. Americans took a shine to cars as soon as they were invented in the 1890s.[27] Automobile use climbed at an accelerating pace through the next several decades, as the speed and convenience of this mode of travel enticed growing numbers of people. After World War II, millions of returning servicemen took advantage of financial assistance offered through the GI bill to purchase homes, many in new suburban developments that sprouted around major cities. Suburban homes required transportation to reach jobs that remained in urban centers, and suburban communities were designed based on the assumption that cars would fill this need. Automobile sales responded by moving into even higher gear.[28]

By the early 1950s, automobiles had become entrenched in the American economy, but not yet entirely in the American way of life. Commuting and intercity travel were still accomplished largely on public forms of transit such as trains, airplanes, trolleys, subways, and buses. Car-based cities like Los Angeles, Phoenix, and Houston were the exception, as the country's population remained concentrated in older cities designed for communal transportation and walking.[29]

As early as the 1930s, the federal government considered the value of facilitating easier automobile travel through the creation of "super highways."[30] These were to be limited-access roads that spanned the country on either a north-south or east-west axis. In 1938, Congress passed the Federal Aid Highway Act that directed the Bureau of Public Roads to investigate the feasibility of building three such highways along each axis. In 1944, Congress added legislation designating a "National System of Interstate Highways" to contain up to 40,000 miles of roads. The first 37,000 of those miles were selected in 1947, and funding to build them was approved in 1952. The total length of the system was subsequently expanded to include 46,837 miles.[31]

A few states had begun building these wide, limited-access roads on their own just before and in the aftermath of World War II. The first leg of the Pennsylvania Turnpike was opened in 1940, and traffic started flowing on the New Jersey Turnpike in 1952. These were incorporated into the new interstate system. The first construction under the federal plan began in 1956 in Missouri.[32]

With the opening of interstate highways, automobiles quickly became even more valuable to travelers as a means of commuting and traversing long distances. Growth in automobile use in the United States over the next several decades far outpaced population expansion.[33] Again, a few statistics tell the story. Between 1956 and 2003, the number of citizens increased from 169 million to 294 million, a difference of slightly less than double. Over the same period, the number of miles driven grew from 628 million to almost 3 billion, a difference of almost fourfold. The number of all registered vehicles grew from 54 million to over 135 million, and the number of registered trucks, which are particularly heavy users of interstate highways, grew from slightly less than 11 million to almost 95 million. The number of buses, another major user of the Interstate system, grew from 272,000 in 1960 to almost 2 million in 1998.[34]

The new network of high-speed roads was clearly a popular amenity. Americans found that with them automobiles were an increasingly convenient and economical means of transportation. The attractiveness of cars meant that competing modes of travel saw shrinking demand, with passenger trains and mass transit claiming a diminishing share of the market. Commercial transportation also changed course, with long-haul trucking increasingly encroaching on railroads in the market for moving goods.[35]

Today, Americans take it for granted that they can travel long distances across the country at high speeds by car. Automobile travel outpaced trains as a preferred means for intercity transportation long ago. Trips in private cars of hundreds of miles or more have come to be considered routine. Commutes by car of dozens of miles every day are similarly commonplace.

The availability of interstate highway travel affected not only the number of cars sold in the United States but also the kinds of cars that reached the market. Automakers emphasized vehicles that could transport passengers long distances at high speeds in relative comfort. The American automobile market of the 1950s and 1960s was filled with cars that featured large amounts of horsepower and heavy chasses. In the 1980s, minivans were introduced that offered even larger enclosures. In the 1990s, the size and weight of the average American vehicle took another leap upward with the popularization of sport utility vehicles, commonly known as SUVs. Although all of these conveyances are used for suburban commuting and short-distance errands, they are particularly well suited for long-distance travel along interstate highways.[36]

Some would argue that the emergence of this kind of automobile market has not been for the best. Large cars use large amounts of gasoline and emit substantial levels of pollutants. Automobile travel also results in more accidents per mile traveled, including fatal ones, than transport by air or rail.[37] There are frequent calls to redirect funding from highways to rail and mass transit systems. For all of these reasons, the government policies that emphasized cars in shaping American transportation may not have been the wisest ones. However, their impact on the structure of the economy cannot be denied.

What would the American automobile industry look like without the interstate highway system? Clearly, the automobile industry would still be a major force in the economy. The private market would undoubtedly have produced a range of vehicles and served as an important source of technological innovation. However, the industry would just as surely look quite different in size and structure. By building interstate highways, the government shaped the private automobile market and offered it a huge platform on which to prosper.

Telecommunication and Satellites

Electronic telecommunication has grown through a series of technological leaps.[38] The technology was born in the 1830s, with the invention of the telegraph, which allowed patterns of pulses representing words to be sent nearly instantaneously over long distances. Wires were strung through cities and across the country to accommodate this technological marvel, and, in 1866, the first cable for telegraph communication was laid beneath the Atlantic Ocean. The total length of wires laid by Western Union expanded from 37,380 miles in 1866 to 187,981 in 1891, and the number of messages sent grew from 5.9 million in 1867 to almost 60 million in 1891.[39] In 1876, the telephone was invented, permitting the transmission of actual voices. Telephone poles began to sprout like weeds in most cities. Radio was first publicly demonstrated in 1901 with a transatlantic transmission, allowing voices to be heard across long distances without the need for wires.

Television, first publicly showcased in 1927 and popularized in the 1950s, built on the concept of radio transmitters to send moving pictures along with words and other sounds.

In the 1960s, the industry was healthy and its services were ubiquitous, but it was poised to take another quantum leap forward with an even more astonishing advance. This was again the result of a major government initiative, this time in the form of the space program. The technology that sent men to the moon by the end of that decade was put to more immediate use sending transponders into orbit that could bounce radio waves across vast distances. A signal that contained television images could travel into space from a transmitter on Earth and bounce off a satellite to a receiving station across a continent or across an ocean. From there, it could be retransmitted to another satellite in a different position to be bounced to another distant location. In this way, television signals could reach anywhere on the globe almost instantaneously, along with radio, telephone, and, decades later, computer data.

The first active communications satellite, Telstar, was propelled into space in 1962, as a collaboration between two private companies, AT&T and Bell Telephone Laboratories, and a number of government agencies in different countries.[40] In the United States, the lead agency was the National Aeronautics and Space Administration (NASA), and it was joined by the General Post Offices of Great Britain and France. NASA's installation in Cape Canaveral, Florida provided the facilities for the launch. A series of additional satellites entered the heavens over the next ten years, to be placed into geosynchronous orbits. This stationed them above key locations on the globe from which they could transmit a steady stream of communications between fixed points. Syncom 3 was placed above the Pacific Ocean in 1964, Intelsat 1 hovered above the Atlantic starting in 1965, and others took positions over North America and Europe in the 1970s.[41] Satcom 1, launched in 1975 and placed over the United States, served as the conduit for the initial development of national cable television networks.

Today, television viewers can watch programs from around the world, and television networks can show images live from almost anywhere on Earth. Telephone calls can be placed and computer data can flow worldwide over the Internet via satellites. Much private economic activity relies on satellites to transmit key information for business transactions, such as credit card verification at the point of sale and insurance authorization at pharmacies.

Growth in the broadcasting industry following the advent of satellite transmission was dramatic. Revenue from television rose from $3.6 billion 1970 to $16.1 billion in 1983.[42] For cable television, which relies heavily on satellites to transmit content, the growth over this period was from $300 million to $6 billion, a 20-fold increase. Over the period from 1975 to 1983, the revenue of satellite carriers grew by 350 percent, that of television broadcasters grew by 204 percent, and that of cable television operators grew by 650 percent. Rapid expansion continued in the decades that followed, although at a somewhat slower pace. Between 1991 and 1998, total revenue for television grew from $21.9 billion to $32.8 billion and for cable television from $25 billion to $49 billion.[43]

The prevalence of television and radio in daily life also continued to expand during this time. Television sets were found in 59 million American households in 1970 and in 97 million in 1997.[44] Cable television's presence grew over the same period from four million households to 64 million.

What would the telecommunications industry look like today had there been no space program? There would, of course, still be television, radio, telephones, and computer connections, but they would travel over cables using landlines. The result would be slower communication of information than we have today and probably less of it. The range of television programs available to viewers would be much smaller, and the content of news programs that rely on foreign correspondents would be more constrained. Telephone conversations across long distances would be less reliable and more expensive. Overall, the industry would be less reliant on instant data access, making impossible many kinds of transactions that are now taken for granted. By launching communications satellites, the government literally opened the heavens for the private market to exploit.

Home Building and Federal Mortgage Support

The vitality of the home building industry depends on the ability and willingness of families to purchase houses. Although many families want to own homes, few but the very wealthiest could afford the entire cost if they had to pay it all at once. Mortgages that are paid back over the course of decades make houses more affordable, but, even with this form of graduated payment, the financial demands of owning a home exceed the cash flow of many families. Painful experience has demonstrated that without a free flow of credit for housing, the entire real estate sector of the economy fails to function effectively.[45]

Several government programs have implemented an explicit policy to encourage home ownership. The Federal Housing Administration was established in the 1930s to insure 30-year loans, making banks more willing to offer them to a larger range of borrowers. It continues to provide loans today to home buyers who meet income and other limits. The Federal National Mortgage Association, commonly known as Fannie Mae, was established in 1938 as part of President Franklin Roosevelt's New Deal, to purchase mortgages for resale to other financial institutions.[46] In addition to reducing the risk to lenders, the resale of loans provides banks with infusions of cash with which to offer new ones. In 1968, Fannie Mae was restructured as a private shareholder-owned company to continue the same mission. As of the end of 2007, it held more than $723 billion in mortgages.[47] When combined with more than $2.4 trillion in other loans and guarantees, its book of business totaled more than $3 trillion.[48]

In 1970, Congress created the Federal Home Loan Mortgage Corporation, commonly known as Freddie Mac, to serve the same function and spun it off as a private company in order to inject an element of competition into the secondary mortgage market.[49] In the ten years between 1997 and 2007, this organization pumped $4.5 trillion into the housing market through loans and other kinds of investments that served more than 30 million homeowners.[50] In 2007 alone, almost half a trillion dollars was invested serving more than 2.6 million homeowners. In combination with Fannie Mae, the pool of money entering the housing sector, and thereby available to promote new construction, grew to an enormous size.[51]

The federal tax code also subsidizes home purchasers through a tax deduction for the interest they pay on their mortgages. The value of the subsidy varies greatly among families depending on their incomes. For some, it can make the difference between owning and renting a home, and for others it is the difference between owning an entry-level house and a more luxurious one. In either case, it further encourages the flow of money into the housing market. The cost of the subsidy to the federal government in lost revenue reached an estimated $76 billion in 2005.[52]

With more Americans able to afford homes, an estimated 37 million in 2005, and with a greater percentage able to purchase larger ones, demand for houses has grown over the years. Until the financial crisis that began in 2008, well over 1 million new private homes were built every year since 1960, and, in many years, the number was closer to 2 million.[53] The total number of housing units in the country grew from slightly less than 88 million in 1980 to slightly less than 129 million in 2007.[54]

Increased demand has meant greater opportunities for those who are in business to meet it. In this case, that includes home builders. The market for homes has fed a vibrant construction industry that has become an important engine for economic growth in many communities. In recent years, the value of residential construction in the country grew from $346 billion in 2000 to $613 billion in 2006 before the drop-off during the Great Recession and, of all construction, from $621 billion to $911 billion.[55] Despite a retrenchment in home building with the housing market crash of 2008, the construction industry remains an important part of the economy.

What would the home building industry look like without government programs to finance home ownership? In the absence of federal mortgage assistance, millions of Americans would still own homes, and home building would still generate considerable economic activity to meet the demand. Population growth alone would have contributed to a growing need for housing. However, the number of Americans seeking to purchase their own homes would be much smaller, as would the scale of the industry. With fewer private homes, the physical structure of many American communities would also be quite different and most likely much more compact. Whether or not this would be for the better, as some believe, it is undeniable that federal subsidies for the mortgage market have served as a substantial stimulus for an important economic sector.

The True Nature of Free Markets: Government Initiative and Private Innovation

Each of these examples describes an important American industry that has, over the course of many years, fostered innovation, provided jobs, and earned substantial profits. In each case, private markets have been the driving force behind a series of entrepreneurial explosions. It is difficult to imagine that government agencies alone could have displayed the energy and flexibility needed to build this set of economic powerhouses. Nevertheless, in each case, the private market owes its vibrancy to the government. All of these industries are essential to a thriving industrial economy, and they would have held important positions in some form or other under any circumstances. However, their size, shape, and influence would not have come close to matching what they are today had major government initiatives not provided crucial support.

The reality in these industries and in many others is that government initiatives and private enterprise have not been opposing forces continually at odds. Nor have the two sectors competed with one another in the sense that the success of one diminishes the well-being of the other. Instead, they have both served as essential aspects of the same endeavor. In essence, a government-facilitated market-based engine has generated innovation and growth.

Government needs the private, market-based sector to drive economic activity. There is no motivating force as powerful as the discipline of the market to direct producers to meet consumer demands. In each of these industries, this dynamic has had revolutionary results, and, for the most part, American consumers have reaped tremendous benefits in a continual parade of new and better products and services. But, to truly flourish, the private sector needs the government. No other entity has the resources or the legal authority to create the infrastructure that is necessary for robust free markets to achieve their potential. Computers need interconnectedness, cars need highways, communication devices need long-range links, and construction needs housing markets to maintain consumer demand. No single industry or even combination of industries has the ability to create these elements on a national scale.

The characterization of public policy as a contest between the market and regulation is a false one. The notion that public policy must choose between them raises a spurious issue that distorts policy debates, impairs accurate understanding, and impedes productive reform. To use an analogy, it is like asking whether the rules of organized football should favor the players or the referees. It should favor neither, because there would be no meaningful game without both.

The issue is not whether government regulation or private markets are better at achieving economic goals. They are inseparable. The real issue is how to use the power of government initiative to create the best infrastructure to enable private innovation to flourish. Economic growth requires that policymakers determine the ideal nature and extent of government intervention needed to build and reinforce markets, not whether public policy should be concerned with them at all. Leaving private markets entirely unfettered, even in the few cases where it is theoretically possible, would let key industries founder at the starting gate. Government promotes vibrant private markets not by letting them be but by crafting active policies to promote them.

What Is a "Free Market"?

Talk of the relationship between free markets and the government begs an important question. What does the term "free market" actually mean? Although it is a commonly used expression in economic and political debates, its definition in those debates can vary. Ambiguity as to its meaning lies at the heart of much public disagreement.

In political discussions, a "free market" commonly means one that is free of all government intervention. Under this understanding, a market is free when it has no, or minimal, regulation. The government imposes few constraints on the behavior of buyers and sellers and offers no subsidies or other incentives that distort naturally occurring market forces.

Some economists share this view. In a basic textbook, Karl Case, Ray Fair, and Sharon Oster explain that "[I]n a free market system, the basic economic questions are answered without the help of a central government plan or directives...the system is left to operate on its own without outside interference."[56] From this perspective, the phrase "free-market economy" is synonymous with "laissez-faire economy." It is a system in which the government lets private firms and people pursue their self-interest without restriction.

However, other economists define the term with a somewhat different emphasis. Greg Mankiw, who has a conservative orientation, defines a free-market economy as one that "allocates resources through the decentralized decisions of many firms and households as they interact in markets for goods and services."[57] Paul Krugman and Robin Wells, who are more liberal in their outlook, offer a definition of a "market economy" as one in which "decisions about production and consumption are made by individual producers and consumers."[58] The emphasis here is on the latitude of market participants to determine the consumption and production of goods and services rather than on any role that the government may or may not play.

Standard dictionary definitions tend to follow this latter approach. The Oxford English Dictionary defines a "free market" as "an economic system in which prices are determined by unrestricted competition between privately owned businesses."[59] The Merriam-Webster dictionary calls it "an economic market operating by free competition."[60]

The emphasis in the definition can have important implications. The absence of government intrusion does not necessarily make a market competitive or leave its participants free to set its course. In many instances, the lack of government intervention would make unfettered exchanges between buyers and sellers impossible.

On a fundamental level, the government facilitates markets by protecting property rights, which form the bedrock of all private enterprise. Without laws to determine who owns what, economic incentives to create goods and services evaporate, since firms have no assurance that they can claim ownership in what they produce. The nature of property protection can be quite complex, and government policies regarding it can create or doom whole industries. For example, rules concerning rights to intellectual property, which are especially relevant in health care, require intricate policy judgments regarding the kinds of inventions that merit protection from competition through patents and the types of artistic works for which reproduction should be restricted through copyrights. Rules regarding the right to own and use real estate rely on similarly complex policy judgments. Without the government foundation that property rules provide and the allocation of rights and responsibilities to enforce them, no private commercial activity would be possible.

Beyond this foundational role, the government can correct instances of what economists call "market failure," in which the allocation of goods and services is less than optimal for the overall economy. This can occur, for example, when either buyers or sellers lack sufficient information to make a reasoned judgment about whether to produce or consume a good or service. The government can correct the imbalance by facilitating information dissemination, either by requiring disclosure by private parties, as it does with the hazards of prescription drugs, or by providing information itself, as it does in publishing quality data on hospitals.

Market failure also arises when a transaction fails to account for effects on parties who are external to it, a phenomenon that economists call "externalities." Negative externalities arise when a third party suffers uncompensated harm, such as when a home located downwind of a power plant is damaged by smokestack emissions. The government can account for the cost in several ways, for example by regulating the permissible level of emissions and by allowing the homeowner to recover damages in a lawsuit. Positive externalities arise when a third party benefits, such as when a vaccine prevents someone from contracting and then spreading an infectious disease. The government can encourage transactions that lead to such outcomes by, among other approaches, subsidizing them, as it does with programs that cover the cost of vaccination.

Markets can also fail in the provision of a category of goods and services known as "public goods." Once created, they benefit everyone, and it is difficult to charge for their use by restricting access. City streets, outdoor lighting, and sanitation are a few of them. Markets may also fail to enable fair bargaining between buyers and sellers over essential goods and services, like lifesaving drugs, over which buyers have little negotiating leverage.

Absent government intervention, competitive markets can also breed collusion and degenerate into systems dominated by monopolies, oligopolies, and cartels. When a single seller or group of sellers controls supply, they are free to raise prices to levels that are many times the cost of production. This can lead to significant inefficiency by preventing buyers from purchasing desired quantities of a good or service that they could otherwise obtain. Economists use the term "rents" to describe the excess revenue that a firm can generate by leveraging a favorable position, such as a monopoly, and view them as a measure of the unproductive use of resources. The market may be free of distortion from governmental forces that are external to it, but internal dynamics can corrupt it just the same.

By the same token, competition can thrive in a market that is subject to extensive government intrusion. For example, regulations that prohibit false advertising and other deceptive practices remove obstacles to the flow of accurate information. Rules that establish and enforce minimum quality standards provide essential reassurance for buyers when the quality of a good or service is difficult to discern. Regulations that prevent the formation of monopolies and collusion among sellers help to permit competition to operate freely. And government programs can establish and maintain an infrastructure that makes the manufacture, distribution, and sale of goods possible at all. In each of these cases, it is the presence of government that permits effective market competition to take place.

In reality, no market is truly "free," regardless of how the term is defined. The government plays a role of some sort in all forms of economic activity, as it did in nurturing the computer, automobile, telecommunications, and construction industries. And in no market does competition take place on a truly level playing field. Corrupting forces are always present, whether they take the form of limits on buyer information, overbearing sales techniques, aggressive advertising, or any of countless other practices that impede fair bargaining between buyers and sellers.

Yet the term "free market" referring to a phenomenon possessing both of these attributes permeates public discourse. Often, those who use it pay scant attention to what they really mean. It represents an ideal of a system that brings together freedom and commerce, a compelling vision to be sure. Such an idealized system is governed by fair, unrestricted interchanges between buyers and sellers, with outside intruders like the government staying away. Unfortunately for all of us, this utopian dream has never actually existed in reality and probably never could.

So, what is meant by use of the phrase "free market" in the title and discussion in this book? Is a new definition proposed? The answer is no, and that is the point. The term "free market" is used with a sense of irony, to emphasize its distorting effect on public debates. It is often applied to our overall health care system and many of the sectors within it, but, in that context, it is so imprecise that it really has no meaning at all. The structure of that system as described in the chapters that follow demonstrates the need to move public debates to a more accurate frame of reference.

Our system can truthfully be characterized as one that relies heavily on enterprises that are "private" and "investor-owned." One can further describe much of it as "market-based" because it relies on exchanges between buyers and sellers. These terms are principally used in the chapters that follow to describe the health care system's nonpublic aspects. However, in no instance is this market of private participants either fully competitive or free of government involvement.

When observers bandy about the term "free market" in the context of health care, they are, perhaps unwittingly, applying it to an industry in which the government is anything but absent. In fact, it is one in which public programs play more of a foundational role than almost anywhere else in the economy. If that is the "free market," then the government is hardly its foe.

The real issue is not whether the government plays a role in the market but the nature of the role that it plays. Without question, some government programs can inhibit or even destroy competition and private enterprise. At the extreme, the government can preempt the private market by producing goods and services itself. It can also subject the market to central planning that determines the kinds of products that will be produced, the quantities that will be available, and the prices that will be charged. But government intervention can also have the opposite effect. It can be the force that creates and sustains private market-based industries.

As the examples discussed in this chapter show, government intervention has been critical in the creation and growth of whole industries and markets throughout the American economy. The result has been a constellation of vibrant and profitable private industries, including health care. Removing the government from the equation would not make these markets "free." It would shrink their size, reduce their level of competitiveness, and, in some instances, possibly force them out of existence.

For much of American industry then, the term "free market" in its strict sense has no real meaning. Markets do not fall into the categories of either "free" and "not free." Rather, there are differences of kind and of degree in the government's role and in the level of competitiveness and efficiency it engenders. To understand private markets, it is useless to ask whether the government has intruded and whether it should. The meaningful question is how.

How Others See Government in the Free Market

This is hardly the first analysis to draw attention to the foundational role of government in one form or another in the functioning of capitalist economies. Even Adam Smith, the eighteenth-century economist who wrote the seminal description of the workings of free markets, identified dozens of government functions that he saw as essential to private enterprise. In his most influential work, *The Wealth of Nations*, he extolled the virtues of unfettered markets but also explained that they could not reach their full potential without some forms of public support.[61] He saw particularly important roles for the government in creating and sustaining public infrastructure and in guarding against collusion and monopolization in the market.[62]

Among the specific roles that Smith believed government should play were enforcement of contracts, maintenance of national defense, and construction of public works such as roads, bridges, canals, and harbors. In his vision of free markets, private industry also relied on public support in such forms as regulation of banking to place limits on interest rates, rules governing the structure of corporations, public education, export taxes, and public health measures against "leprosy or any other loathsome and offensive disease."[63] The significance of the symbiotic relationship between private markets and at least some forms of government initiative does not seem to have escaped notice by the father of free-market theory.

Nor was the relationship lost on the framers of the US Constitution. Article I, section 8 enumerates the powers granted to Congress, including three that direct it to facilitate commercial activity.[64] These are the powers to regulate interstate commerce, to establish post offices and post roads, and to protect intellectual property rights "to promote the progress of science and useful arts." The framers thereby enmeshed the government's role in supporting American business into the legal fabric of the country.

A more modern market-oriented economist to acknowledge a key supporting role for the government in the private sector was Milton Friedman. As a general matter, he saw private enterprise at the core of economic prosperity and viewed most government market interventions as destructive. However, despite his deep antipathy toward most forms of public initiative, he believed that private markets could not function without some elements of it. To Friedman, the government was essential in setting the "rules of the game" for commerce and in interpreting and enforcing them.[65]

Another recent perspective is that of political scientist Daniel Carpenter. In his comprehensive history of the Food and Drug Administration (FDA), he argued that public esteem for government regulators translates into greater confidence in the industries they oversee.[66] In the context of pharmaceuticals, without an impartial external arbiter of safety, patients would be less likely to trust the quality of the drug supply. Uncertainty about pharmaceutical products would make patients less willing to take them and physicians less likely to prescribe them. Regulation builds public confidence in pharmaceutical products in a way that no amount of advertising or marketing could ever achieve. When the reputation of the FDA declines, the industry's standing and fortunes shrink along with it.

As a law professor, Senator Elizabeth Warren pointed to the importance to private business of the basic infrastructure that the government builds and maintains in forms such as roads, education, police, and fire protection.[67] She argued that business success always depends on some form of underlying public support. The relationship between entrepreneurial accomplishment and communal sustenance, in her view, creates a "social contract" with mutual obligations in which businesses rely on ubiquitous taxpayer-financed resources to build enterprises through which they, and the rest of society, can realize tremendous benefits.

However, the connection between public initiatives and private innovation goes even deeper than the relationships these observers describe. Certainly, the government builds and maintains the basic physical and economic infrastructure on which all commercial activity rests. But it also creates resources that specifically target the needs of narrower constituencies. The examples of industries built on government foundations reveal the power of focused initiatives that produced those resources—the Internet, interstate highways, communication satellites, and mortgage support—to engender huge industrial powerhouses capable of transforming the entire economy and even the fabric of our daily lives.

None of this is to say that all government programs are successful or wise. Quite to the contrary, many clearly are neither. Without question, numerous government programs are plagued by substantial waste and inefficiency. Perhaps America's major industries would be even more profitable and robust had the government programs behind them been designed differently. Undoubtedly, every program could be improved in one way or another. However, regardless of whether they have been optimally designed, the formative impact of government initiatives is always present.

The regulatory role of government rests on a theoretical foundation that recognizes the need for a corrective force against inherent failings of markets. In his survey of regulatory theory, Supreme Court Justice Stephen Breyer described particular failings in the imbalance between the power of buyers and sellers in situations involving differential access to information.[68] In such circumstances, he argued that government intervention must always be balanced against its potentially disruptive effect on commerce, even when it is necessary to protect the integrity of the market.

Regulation can certainly be disruptive. However, placing constraints on market behavior is not its only role. In a broader sense, it can also create markets.

Breyer describes the first major federal regulatory initiative as the creation of the Interstate Commerce Commission, which was established in 1887. Congress charged it with overseeing the carriage of goods and passengers on the country's newly constructed railways and later expanded its mission to include trucking and other modes of transport as they emerged. Since this first foray into the federal oversight of commerce, the number of agencies, laws, and regulations has expanded exponentially. At the same time, so has the size of the American economy, which has dwarfed that of every other country in the world for more than half a century. If regulation in the aggregate has stunted our economy's overall growth, it is difficult to tell. Regulatory programs over the decades since 1887 have responded to increasingly complex forms of market failure engendered by an increasingly complicated economy. Some of the programs, in turn, enable the economy to grow even further, creating the need for yet more new forms of corrective oversight. As they have evolved in this pattern, regulatory growth and private business expansion have not proceeded in isolation. Rather, they have been, and continue to be, part of a single dynamic system.

Without question, government agencies often act in ways that are contrary to the short-term interests of the individual enterprises they regulate. In fact, the relationships between most regulated industries and the government agencies that oversee them are commonly characterized by hostility. However, disagreements over specific practical concerns do not necessarily translate into differences over long-term goals. The Interstate Commerce Commission had no desire to put the railroads or trucking companies out of business. With no one to regulate, the agency would have met its demise along with them. And these industries benefitted from enhanced public trust engendered by the Commission's external oversight.

Similar tensions characterize interactions between private industries and many of the private funders with which they deal, which function as business regulators in their own right. Banks, financial underwriters, venture capital firms, and insurance companies impose stringent rules on the clients they support, and these rules often serve as a source of ongoing friction. Nevertheless, the long-term interests of all parties lie in the ultimate success of the industries' business plans. All players lose if an enterprise does not prosper, and they rely on one another to achieve this end. The lurking subtext of tension does nothing to change the dynamic of a collaborative effort toward a common goal.

Of course, to highlight the role of government in building key industries is not to propose that this half of the partnership could have created or operated them on its own. Private markets are almost always more efficient and productive than the government in actually producing goods and services. Imagining direct government production of computers, automobiles, telecommunication services, and houses is to envision an arrangement that could be a bureaucratic and political nightmare. Economist Joseph Stiglitz makes the point that when the government tries its hand at manufacturing, for example through ownership of steel mills, "they typically make a mess of it."[69] Nevertheless, he also observes that private control of such endeavors is problematic unless "preconditions" in the form of adequate government oversight have been satisfied.

However, public operation of industry is not the realistic alternative to unregulated private activity. To take this view would be to reduce economic structures to a set of absurd extremes. Creating an infrastructure that nurtures private markets is quite different from taking over those markets. In fact, it usually represents the exact opposite. It is, instead, a process of creating the sustenance on which private markets thrive.

The relationship between the government and these private enterprises is akin to that between an ecosystem and the species that inhabit it. Public programs coalesce into an environment that supports economic activity. The initiators of those programs may not even appreciate the full range of commercial possibilities they have created. Private businesses, facing competitive pressures to survive and expand, then devise ways of realizing those possibilities and of thriving as a result. They may design novel devices that serve as gateways to the Internet, build vehicles to operate on interstate highways, transmit information via satellites, construct homes that families can purchase with mortgage support, or find any number of other commercial niches. The success of the ecosystem and of its inhabitants is inextricably linked in these market-based industries, as they are in a natural system.

The fact is that major industries rarely, if ever, evolve entirely on their own. Every large enterprise requires a significant infrastructure, and the government has historically been the only source with the wherewithal to provide it. Understanding the complex interplay of the public and private sectors is a much more productive guide to understanding industry dynamics and to charting future public policy than reducing their underlying roles to that of hypothetical contestants.

Public–Private Markets and Health Care

The chapters that follow examine how this public–private dynamic has played out in health care to create the system that the United States has today. The private sector implements much of the system, but government programs inject essential structure and funding. In health care, the interrelated needs of a range of affected interests are particularly complex. Among them, patients need a source of financing when the economic burden of illness is too great to bear on their own. Private insurance markets need a mechanism to structure and pool risks. Researchers need funding when they quest for revolutions in knowledge that have no immediate commercial value. Professionals and institutions need a steady source of payment that adequately compensates them for the extensive training, equipment, and facilities they must have in order to render medical care. And numerous other groups of individuals and businesses that play important roles need sources of support as they interact with one another in countless ways.

In each of these instances, there is a major government program or combination of programs that provides needed structure and financial support. The initiatives that these programs represent have come to create the backbone of the health care system. They are the reason that companies like Pfizer, HCA, and United Healthcare thrive, to the delight of thousands of investors and employees.

At the same time, it is important to bear in mind another side to these business success stories. That is the power and influence that companies such as these are able to wield in the public sphere. The huge health care industry that the government created has grown into a substantial constituency to which its own sponsor is beholden. In some regards, this outcome can be described as the capture of regulators by the entities they oversee. Yet, it extends much further into a dynamic that permits the industry to shape the very public programs to which it responds.

Examples of industry influence abound across government initiatives. Three of the most significant of the last half-century demonstrate how health care industries whose stature the government had helped to create used that power to extract even greater amounts of public largess. In the first instance, hospitals campaigned successfully for inclusion of a generous reimbursement formula under Medicare when it was created in 1965. In the second, when the program underwent its largest expansion with the addition of a prescription drug benefit in 2006, the pharmaceutical industry secured inclusion of a provision that prohibited the government from directly negotiating with it over prices. In the third, private insurance companies successfully advocated for a mandate requiring all Americans to maintain coverage under the Affordable Care Act, when it was enacted in 2010 to expand access to care. In each instance, businesses that owed much of their prosperity to the government were able to translate their financial strength into political clout to expand the flow of public funds even further.

An important consequence of this dynamic is the constrained ability of the government to use its own power to limit the growth of costs in the system it built. Private firms across the health care industry leverage their influence to maintain generous levels of government reimbursement under various programs, essentially extracting economic "rents" as surely as marketplace monopolists. The relationship between the public and private sectors in health care is complex, and it affects every player in the system in varied, and often contradictory, ways. The intricacy that results makes it all the more important to comprehend the underlying role of the government in the overall health care enterprise.

The chapters that follow do not present a specific prescription for change so much as a resource for accurately understanding the system that we have. This grounding is the most basic ingredient for rational debate on possibilities for meaningful reform. Beneath the façade of a free market lies a complex web of interrelationships between the public and private spheres and a sometimes colorful history that led up to them. It is this interplay that sets the context for appreciating what truly drives American health care.

2

The Government and the Private
Market in Health Care

The development of medical care, like other institutions, takes
place within larger fields of power and social structure.
—PAUL STARR, *THE SOCIAL TRANSFORMATION OF AMERICAN MEDICINE*[1]

The collaboration between public initiative and private enterprise can claim no
greater accomplishment than the creation and sustenance of American health
care. Every core element of the system was fashioned and shaped in one way or
another by the government, but each operates largely through the private sector.
A market-based industry that is visible to all drives much of the day-to-day functioning, yet a government foundation operates behind the scenes to support the
overall enterprise.

Four core elements of health care demonstrate this structural dynamic most
clearly. These are pharmaceutical manufacturers, which create the key products in
the clinical armamentarium; hospitals, the central institutions in providing health
care services; the medical profession, which renders most technical services; and
private insurance, through which the single largest share of finance flows. In each
case, a government program or combination of programs filled an essential need
that the industry sector could not have addressed on its own and thereby created
the foundation that enabled the sector to take its present form.

This chapter presents in brief overview the elements of government intervention that shaped these sectors of American health care. The chapters that follow
present their stories in greater depth. Each sector has followed a distinctive course
and relies on government support in a different way, but a complex public–private
interaction lies at the core of them all.

The Pharmaceutical Industry

America's pharmaceutical industry perennially ranks as one of the most profitable.
Its rate of return regularly approaches 20 percent, over three times the average of
other American industries.[2] Its top-selling products, such as Lipitor, generate billions of dollars in revenue each year. The industry is populated with huge for-profit
companies. Yet beneath all of this financial success lies the pervasive hand of a

web of government agencies. None of them is more influential than the National Institutes of Health (NIH), one of the greatest success stories in the history of public policy. It is a financial engine that, since its founding in the 1930s, has powered a steady burst of lifesaving discoveries. More than 100 scientists have received Nobel Prizes based on NIH-funded research.[3]

THE NATIONAL INSTITUTES OF HEALTH AND THE FOUNDATIONS OF BIOMEDICAL RESEARCH

Congress created the NIH in 1930 to fund investigations into basic biomedical science across the country.[4] Its formation was the culmination of a decade-long effort to increase the money available for science, as medical breakthroughs in the early part of the twentieth century demonstrated the value of the results that could be achieved. In 1937, Congress established the National Cancer Institute, which became a component of the NIH, the first distinct institute to focus on a single kind of disease or physiological system. Additional institutes were added in the years immediately following World War II, along with substantial budget increases. Today, the agency operates through 27 such component agencies. In 1940, it acquired new capabilities to conduct intramural research, that is, experiments within its own walls by its own employed scientists, with the opening of its sprawling campus in Bethesda, Maryland.

The importance of the NIH to biomedical research today cannot be overestimated. It is by far the largest single source of financial support for basic science in the world. Its funding underpins the scientific enterprise not only in the United States but in many other countries as well. The annual NIH budget in 2012 stood at almost $31 billion.[5] This reflects a doubling in its size between 1998 and 2003.[6]

More than 80 percent of the NIH budget is awarded to researchers outside of the agency through a process of competitive grants.[7] More than 325,000 investigators at more than 3,000 universities and private research institutes receive this funding, and they are located in every state and in several foreign countries. The remainder of the budget supports 6,000 scientists who work in the agency's own facilities. Beyond the hundreds of thousands of established researchers whose careers are sustained by NIH funding, there are thousands of future researchers whose entry into the world of science is supported by NIH training grants, not to mention thousands of graduate students who work in the labs of NIH-funded investigators.

In addition to funding, the NIH also manages a regulatory apparatus that governs much of the biomedical research conducted in the United States. A particularly important part of this role is its administration of the Patent and Trademark Law Amendments Act of 1980, commonly known as the Bayh-Dole Act, which grants patent protection to institutions that host NIH-funded research for discoveries that ensue.[8] Another key regulatory responsibility is the protection of human subjects in biomedical research under the National Research Act of 1974. This is accomplished through Institutional Review Boards (IRBs) that are housed in each funded institution and overseen by NIH's Office for Protection from Research Risks.[9]

The rise of the NIH over the second half of the twentieth century paralleled breathtaking advances in medicine, most of which were achieved in whole or in part with its financial support.[10] A reflection of their value is the increase in overall life expectancy in the United States from 47 to 77 years from the start of the century to the end.[11] The agency also boasts that its sponsored research helped to bring about a decline in the death rate from heart disease by 40 percent and from stroke by more than 50 percent between 1975 and 2000. Among other health care triumphs to which it contributed, the five-year survival rate for childhood cancers rose from less than 60 percent in the 1970s to almost 80 percent in the 1990s. AIDS-related deaths fell by almost three-quarters between 1995 and 2001. Infant deaths caused by Sudden Infant Death Syndrome (SIDS) declined by more than 50 percent between 1994 and 2000. And a number of once-dreaded diseases, including rubella, whooping cough, and pneumococcal pneumonia, are disappearing from memory because of vaccines that the NIH helped to create.

As dramatic as the NIH's accomplishments have been, the role of the public sector in advancing medical science is only part of the story. The United States government does not manufacture pharmaceutical products or medical devices, nor does it employ most of the physicians who prescribe them or operate most of the hospitals within which they are used. Private industry plays that role, and this is where one of the most important partnerships in American health care takes shape. NIH-funded research, for the most part, represents basic science; that is, fundamental knowledge that advances overall understanding of biological processes. Applied research turns this basic knowledge into actual therapies, and it is, for the most part, conducted in the realm of private companies.

Research and development spending by the pharmaceutical industry more than doubled in the decade between 1994 and 2004 from slightly more than $15 billion to almost $40 billion,[12] and the figure stood at more than $49 million in 2011.[13] In 1999, the amount spent by private companies on pharmaceutical research surpassed the research spending of the NIH. There is a synergy between the research sponsored by each. Although some overlap exists, the preponderance of the $49 billion in private funding supports clinical trials and other applied investigations on products in development, whereas most of the NIH budget supports basic studies that expand basic knowledge.

These two funding sources thereby work in tandem to create medical innovation. The government carries the front end that generates conceptual support for new product ideas, and private industry brings up the back end by putting new concepts to work. In this way, the two halves of the research enterprise rely on one another to function.

Without basic research, the pharmaceutical industry would lack the intellectual fuel that drives its innovation. However, support for such investigations is not suited for the private market. By its nature, this enterprise is highly speculative. There is no way to predict whether a line of inquiry will lead to productive results or, if it does, how long it will take to do so. This is not a recipe for creating shareholder value. It is a venture best left to a different kind of player, which is where the government—through the NIH—steps in.

GOVERNMENT SUPPORT BEYOND BASIC SCIENCE

Beyond the apparatus of NIH funding, government initiatives support the private pharmaceutical industry in several other ways. Most notably, the government grants patent protection for new products. For a period of 20 years from the date it files a patent application, the company that discovers a new drug effectively holds a monopoly on its manufacture and sale. Although the timeframe for marketing is shortened by the lengthy process of US Food and Drug Administration (FDA) review, in most cases, various other laws make up for some of the shortfall by extending the period during which competition is prohibited. The result is a substantial period of exclusive marketing for virtually all new drugs, which is long enough to permit their manufacturers to reap substantial profits, sometimes in the billions of dollars.

Another source of support is provided through the Orphan Drug Act passed by Congress in 1983, which implemented a set of targeted incentives to induce companies to develop drugs for rare conditions, commonly referred to as "orphan diseases."[14] Many companies are ready and eager to develop therapies for conditions that afflict relatively few patients but could never recover the cost, let alone make a profit.[15] The Act provides a financial push to make it worth their while to risk entering these markets. In the 25 years following the law's enactment, more than 300 treatments for orphan diseases received FDA approval, compared with only 10 in the prior decade.[16]

Beyond government funding and financial incentives, the private pharmaceutical industry has benefited from a regulatory apparatus that reassures the public about the products that it sells. For all of the industry's complaints about the FDA's slowness and bureaucratic inefficiency, the oversight process creates an environment that enhances consumer trust.[17] This makes patients more willing to use its products and physicians more willing to prescribe them.[18]

Congress gave the FDA authority to oversee the safety and efficacy of drugs and devices in a series of steps over the course of 100 years. They include the Pure Food and Drug Act of 1906,[19] which created the FDA; the Food, Drug, and Cosmetic Act of 1938,[20] which mandated that the agency assess the safety of drugs before they reach the market; the Kefauver-Harris Amendments of 1962,[21] which added efficacy as a criterion in the review process; and the Food and Drug Administration Amendments Act of 2007, which enhanced post-market safety oversight.[22] Each of these laws was enacted to reassure the public in the wake of a scandal over drug safety, and each largely achieved that goal.[23]

The synergistic relationship between public support and private product development has engendered its share of controversy. Critics argue, for example, that for-profit corporations should contribute more to the cost of taxpayer-supported basic research from which they benefit. Another target of criticism is the granting of patent rights for products that flow from public research funding under the Bayh-Dole Act. Critics charge that funded entities receiving patents may drag their feet in bringing the fruits of their research to market where it can benefit patients. Another source of dispute is the length of patents, which some observers believe facilitates unreasonably high prices and excessive profits.

However, regardless of whether the relationship could be improved to achieve a fairer balance, it is unquestionably an essential contributor to spectacular medical progress and significant private sector financial rewards.

THE PHARMACEUTICAL INDUSTRY TODAY

How have the decades of government support in these various forms affected the pharmaceutical industry? Most notably, they have left it as one of the most profitable in the United States.[24] Between 1995 and 2002, it was the most profitable of all. Since then, it has ranked in the top three every year. Sales of prescription drugs now exceed $300 billion a year in the United States.[25] They exceed $837 billion worldwide.[26]

What would the pharmaceutical industry look like if the government had not stood behind it over the course of the past century? Without the NIH, there would be less funding to build the knowledge base on which drug discovery relies, leaving manufacturers with fewer scientific paths to explore. This would have narrowed the range of pharmaceutical products on the market and limited their therapeutic value. The industry as a whole would be smaller and less profitable.

And what would the pharmaceutical market look like if the FDA were not empowered to vigorously oversee the industry? There would be little but manufacturers' claims to verify the safety and efficacy of products. Without a neutral third party to vet drugs and devices before dangerous ones could injure patients, honest companies would see much greater competition from unscrupulous competitors that would be free to make claims without verification. Their questionable products would taint the entire market, leaving patients uncertain of which companies, if any, they could trust and therefore less likely to purchase drugs from any source.

If America had neither the NIH nor the FDA, the pharmaceutical industry would undoubtedly still exist. Medicinal drugs were manufactured and sold for thousands of years before these agencies came into existence. However, it would not come close to its present size, and the clinical advances it has made that have helped to create modern medicine would be far fewer. The products that did reach the market would be less effective, and medicine overall would function in a more primitive form.

The Hospital Industry

American hospitals trace their origins to the middle of the eighteenth century. At that time, patients with financial means could receive state-of-the-art medical care, such as it was, at home from a private physician. With a limited arsenal of treatments, most of this care simply provided comfort and support. For those without financial means, care at home was not feasible. More than anything, patients required a place of rest with staff to attend to their basic needs. In 1751, Benjamin Franklin and Dr. Thomas Bond helped to found the first hospital in North America, Pennsylvania Hospital in Philadelphia, as a successor to the almshouses that housed many of the poor. In 1771, New York Hospital was founded along the same model, and, in 1821, Massachusetts General Hospital was established in Boston.[27]

This picture hardly describes the hospitals of today. These modern-day centers of high-tech treatment bear little resemblance to their forebears of 200 years ago. Many factors fostered this transformation over the years, including the growth of the medical profession in the late nineteenth and early twentieth centuries and a series of medical advances that occurred at about the same time. These included anesthesia and antisepsis that made surgery possible and x-ray imaging that opened up new possibilities for diagnosis. Developments such as these advanced the nature of hospital care and the capacity of these institutions to render treatment beyond simple custodial care.

GOVERNMENT FUNDING FOR HOSPITAL EXPANSION

During the latter part of the twentieth century, the hospital industry, which had steadily advanced in technological sophistication, experienced a particularly dramatic growth spurt. Access to hospital services improved in many previously underserved regions, the capabilities of institutions expanded, and facilities were upgraded. These changes transformed and modernized the industry as a whole, and they were brought about by a set of major government programs that injected financing and new forms of regulatory guidance.

The first government program was the Hill-Burton Act, which Congress passed in 1946, to fund construction of new hospitals and expansion of existing facilities on a mass scale.[28] The primary purpose of the law was to improve access to hospital services in regions of the country where it was limited, with a focus on rural areas. Over the next 30 years, more than $3.7 billion was appropriated under this law, representing grants to more than half of the hospitals in the United States.[29] Hill-Burton funding added 344,000 inpatient beds to the nation's supply, which translated into more than 40 percent of all hospital beds in use in the United States today.[30]

Hill-Burton funding offered a lifeline for many rural hospitals and the regions that they served, but it came with many strings attached. Among them, the law required hospitals receiving funds to provide minimum amounts of indigent care, to maintain emergency rooms, and to refrain from discriminating against patients based on race.[31] Participation in Medicare and Medicaid was added as a retroactive requirement in the 1970s. The law also implemented a system of state-level planning to determine the allocation of funding. This system laid the groundwork for a more comprehensive planning process that was implemented in the 1960s to determine which clinical services and which facility improvements could be added at which hospitals.

The result of Hill-Burton's combination of funding and regulation was a blueprint for the shape of the American hospital industry. With one hand, the government determined through state health planning boards where hospitals would be located, and it enforced a business model that required care to be rendered to broad segments of the population. With the other hand, it fostered a tremendous expansion in the size and scope of the nation's overall hospital enterprise.

TRANSFORMATION THROUGH MEDICARE

The second major finance program that fostered the growth of the American hospital industry was Medicare, which covers the cost of care for almost 50 million elderly and disabled beneficiaries. Enacted in 1965, this reimbursement mechanism has grown relentlessly over the years. It provided more than $135 billion for inpatient care and more than $30 billion for hospital outpatient care in 2011, and the rate of growth continues to accelerate.[32] This is in addition to almost $400 billion that Medicare paid for other services, such as physician care, prescription drugs, and other kinds of institutional care.[33] Its companion program, Medicaid, injected almost another $400 billion into the system through coverage for several categories of the poor.[34] Of particular importance to the growth of the hospital industry is the mechanism that Medicare used in its early years to reimburse hospitals for part of the cost of capital expansion. In many instances, it paid for almost 50 percent of the cost of new facilities. It is not surprising that the first 20 years of the Medicare program corresponded with a major boom in hospital construction.[35]

As a third government financial boost, those hospitals that continue to operate on a nonprofit basis receive an indirect government subsidy through a tax exemption. It permits them not only to avoid paying tax on income that they earn, but also lets individuals deduct the value of donations from their own taxable income. In addition, it permits investors who purchase the hospitals' bonds to earn interest tax-free. This enables these institutions to pay lower rates than would otherwise be needed to attract private funding. Tax-exempt hospitals can also avoid many state and local levies.[36] In return for receiving a tax exemption, nonprofit hospitals must abide by a set of rigorous regulatory requirements through which the government further guides their operations.[37]

As hospital operations expanded during the decades following World War II, the value of this subsidy did, as well. Today, the federal government forgoes about $6 billion each year in taxes that nonprofit hospitals would otherwise pay, and state and local governments forgo an equivalent amount, for a total of more than $12 billion.[38] In this way, the government injects billions of dollars into the industry while using the leverage that comes with this funding to shape the underlying business model of the recipients.

The financial fortunes of the hospital industry grew in tandem with the rollout of these government programs. Total spending on hospital care in the United States rose from almost $92 million in 1980 to almost $534 million in 2004, an increase of just under sixfold.[39] Hospital construction in constant 1972 dollars grew from $3.1 billion during the years between 1945 and 1949 to $16.3 billion during the years between 1975 and 1979.[40] This growth reflected an increase in the percent of total nonresidential construction that hospitals accounted for from 10.0 to 16.8.[41] As a result, during this time, the hospital industry rapidly evolved into a major economic force.

Ironically, hospitals might have ballooned in size even further had it not been for another government program that held them in check. As part of the state planning process that Congress had mandated, each state was induced to enact a certificate-of-need law during the 1970s, which prohibited hospitals from adding new facilities or services unless they could demonstrate a community need.[42] In 1986, Congress allowed the mandate to lapse, letting states decide for themselves whether to continue the programs. About a third of the states opted not to continue them, and most of these states soon experienced large increases in hospital construction, taking advantage of the federal financing that was still in effect.[43]

THE HOSPITAL INDUSTRY TODAY

Had there been no Hill-Burton Act, Medicare program, or tax subsidy, would America still have a hospital industry? Of course it would. But would the industry look anything like it does today? Most likely, it would not. Over the course of the past 40 years, hospitals would have received more than $1 trillion less in government funding. There almost certainly would be far fewer institutions, most would be much smaller, and the range of services they offered would be more limited. Moreover, without the tax benefits of nonprofit status, the majority of facilities would likely have chosen to operate as profit-making enterprises, radically altering the character of the industry.

The Medical Profession

The medical profession was a somewhat disreputable often low-paid avocation until just over a hundred years ago. Physicians were as likely to be trained through apprenticeships as through formal education. Very few of them worked in or even had any contact with hospitals. Many earned more of their income selling potions and patent medicines than from rendering services. Patients could consider themselves lucky if these products were merely ineffective rather than outright dangerous. Many practitioners were itinerant physicians who earned a living traveling from town to town, sometimes one step ahead of angry patients.[44]

MEDICINE'S UPWARD MOBILITY

Members of the profession initiated their own standardization to reverse their uneven social and economic standing. The American Medical Association (AMA) was founded in 1847 to systematize the education that physicians received. Its efforts led to the passage of licensure laws in every state between 1874 and 1915, and to the establishment of a private accreditation process for medical schools. By 1920, medicine had emerged as a respected science-based enterprise with rigorous standards for new entrants.

The seminal step in the process of lifting the quality of medical education was a survey of medical schools initiated in 1904 by the AMA's Council on Medical Education and conducted by the Carnegie Foundation. Under the Foundation's auspices, a young educator named Abraham Flexner visited every school in the country to evaluate the quality of instruction and the adequacy of resources. The outcome was a report issued in 1910 that recommended closing about half of the schools.[45] The Flexner Report had the intended effect. The number of schools declined substantially in its wake. Those that remained emphasized rigorous scientific training coupled with intensive hands-on clinical experience in hospitals.

The centerpiece of the regulatory structure to oversee the medical profession that emerged was the process of licensing physicians in each state.[46] At the same time, the profession retained a role for itself in controlling the two pillars on which the licensing process rested—the accreditation of medical schools and the administration of examinations to test competence. This gave it tremendous authority both to enforce quality standards and to control the flow of new entrants who could compete with established practitioners. Once licensing laws were in place, the days of potions, patent medicines, and snake oil, along with the uneven standing of the medical profession, were over.

In the decades that followed, new sets of regulatory programs enabled the profession to further hone its standing. In the 1930s, the AMA first recognized specialties within medicine by fostering the creation of boards to certify that practitioners met additional standards that would qualify them to claim special expertise.[47] Today, there are boards in 24 fields that recognize skill and training in areas ranging from cardiology to neurology to nuclear medicine. Starting in 1965, the Medicare program required physicians to meet eligibility criteria to participate. In the 1980s, managed care grew in prominence as a reimbursement mechanism and imposed new requirements on physician members. All along, physicians have also needed permission from hospitals to admit patients and to render clinical services. Hospital credentialing committees vet applicants based on a range of criteria and review their professional conduct on an ongoing basis.

All of these regulatory efforts served to enhance public respect for the profession. By restricting entry into the field, some of these programs also helped to foster steady growth in income. However, the initial expansion in the number, specialization, and incomes of physicians that was engendered by these efforts was insignificant compared to the explosion that occurred during the last half of the twentieth century, and it was the hand of government that ignited the fuse.

THE PROFESSION'S GOVERNMENT-INDUCED GROWTH

The story of the federal government's contribution to the elevation of the medical profession in the late twentieth century began in 1965, when policymakers turned their attention to barriers that limited the access of many Americans to health care. A major source of concern was an anticipated shortage of physicians and a maldistribution of those already in practice. To increase the supply, Congress allocated significant funding to the creation of new medical schools and the expansion of existing ones.[48] In response, the number of medical schools grew from 88 when the program started to 126 in 1980, and the number of graduates grew from 7,409 to 15,135 over the same time period.[49] More tellingly, the ratio of physicians to population increased from 148 per 100,000 to 202 between 1960 and 1980. In 2004, the United States had 780,000 physicians in active practice, about two-thirds of whom were specialists.[50] By 2010, the number had grown further to more than 850,000 active physicians, three-quarters of whom practiced in specialties.[51]

Management of the physician workforce did not eliminate cost and distribution concerns, but it did help to transform the nature of the profession. By the time funding for the expansion boom had ended, America had twice as many physicians. Medical education had also doubled in size as an enterprise, which served to solidify the standing of medical schools as research-based institutions. Advances in technology, many developed at newly invigorated medical schools, helped physicians to find new services to offer and new ways to specialize. By funding an explosion in the number of physicians, the government had conferred on the profession new prestige and new revenue-generating opportunities.[52]

MEDICARE'S TRANSFORMATIVE ROLE

However, management of the physician workforce was only the start. The most powerful force in transforming the medical profession during the late twentieth century was, once again, the Medicare program. The spigot of funding and the regulatory structure that it implemented brought medicine to a level few had envisioned. Medicare offered huge amounts of money for physician services, permitting demand for them to grow dramatically. Part B of the program, which provides reimbursement for outpatient care, began with a budget of $2.2 billion in 1966 and went on to spend 100 times that amount, more than $230 billion, in 2011,[53] while the pool of beneficiaries grew from 19.5 million to more than 47 million.[54]

Medicare worked in tandem with government funding for physician training to promote growth in the size of the medical profession during the late twentieth century. But the story does not end there. New physicians have tended to cluster in the most lucrative aspect of the profession, specialty practice. The 30-year-long expansion of the profession that the government fostered included an increase in the number of physicians in general practice from 46,347 to 73,234, for a growth rate of about 58 percent.[55] The number of office-based specialists, on the other hand, increased from 166,987 to 456,330, for a rate of 173 percent. Specialties that focus on conditions that primarily afflict the elderly experienced some of the greatest rates of growth, with the number of cardiologists more than tripling from 5,046 to 17,252; the number of neurologists growing almost fivefold, from 1,862 to 9,632; and the number treating pulmonary diseases growing almost sevenfold, from 1,166 to 7,072. In other words, the expansion of the medical profession over this period focused on those components for which Medicare provides the most funding.

Beyond its huge financial outlays, the Medicare program took two significant steps during the late twentieth century to craft the shape of the expanding physician workforce. The first was through payments for clinical training of new physicians. After completing medical school, new doctors usually spend the next three to five years as residents in hospitals, where they learn as apprentices in a specialty. These physicians-in-training play an important role in the clinical care that their hospitals provide, but they require a considerable amount of supervision, which detracts from the hospital's overall productivity. To compensate for this cost, Medicare adds a supplement to the amount paid for patient care to teaching hospitals that operate physician training programs, up to a predetermined number of eligible slots. By controlling the number of slots, Medicare plays an important role in determining the quantity of new physicians who can enter the workforce.[56]

The second way that Medicare crafts the composition of the medical profession is through the structure of its payment mechanism for physicians in practice. When the program began operation in 1966, hospital services were reimbursed according to the actual costs incurred in rendering care, and physician services were reimbursed according to the prevailing rates in each community. By the late 1970s, it had become evident that this system encouraged overuse of services and excessive cost. Both components of reimbursement were subsequently changed in ways that altered the structure of the profession.

In 1983, the hospital payment process was changed to a prospective system that based reimbursement on the patient's diagnosis.[57] This new payment arrangement dramatically altered the financial incentives that facilities faced. They found that some diagnoses could be treated efficiently, and so the care of patients who had them could be quite profitable. Others required resources that were disproportionate to the economic reward and could be a monetary drain. Many hospitals responded by structuring their medical staffs to include more practitioners who performed profitable procedures and fewer of those whose work was less remunerative. They also pushed some kinds of procedures to outpatient clinics to avoid the prospective payment constraints. Outpatient surgery and radiology clinics now dot the landscape of many parts of the country, and they offer substantial income potential for the physicians who practice in them. This, in turn, enhanced the attractiveness to new physicians of the specialties involved.[58]

In 1992, Congress changed the method of reimbursing physicians to a fee schedule formally known as the Resource-Based Relative Value Scale (RBRVS).[59] Its payment rates were initially more rewarding for primary care physicians and less so for surgeons and other procedure-oriented practitioners than those in the prevailing market in most communities. However, the pendulum soon swung the other way, with higher relative payments for providing procedures than general primary care. The result once again was a reshaping of the economic incentives that guide physician practice through the hand of government policy.[60]

Physician incomes reflected Medicare's shifts. During the decade of the 1980s, while hospital prospective payment was being introduced, overall physician earnings rose by about 25 percent in constant dollars. This is a considerable rise, but when examined more closely, the story is more interesting. Surgeons saw the greatest increase, at almost 50 percent, and other medical specialists enjoyed a boost of more than a third. General and family practice physicians, who treat a much smaller share of Medicare patients, gained only about 10 percent.[61]

THE MEDICAL PROFESSION TODAY

By crafting the reimbursement incentives of the largest single health care payment program in the country, this series of government actions was instrumental in determining the present size, shape, and economic structure of the medical profession. In important ways, the effects of this structure may have been less than ideal. A surfeit of specialists has encouraged reliance on aggressive treatments based on procedures and tests as mainstays of our health care system in lieu of prevention, which is the hallmark of primary care. This can result in overtreatment, which is a major contributor to American health care's excessive cost. However, for the majority of American physicians who render those services, this cost funds wide-ranging and extremely lucrative practice opportunities that did not exist a half century ago. And from the perspective of patients, these programs have generated an abundance of physicians, particularly specialists, who are available to treat a wide range of ailments.

Would there still be a vital and robust profession if none of these public initiatives had intervened? Of course there would. Physicians have practiced for thousands of years, since the time of Hippocrates and even before. But would the profession's structure resemble what it does today? It is difficult to imagine that it would. There would almost certainly be fewer physicians, practicing in a more limited range of specialties, and earning lower salaries. Without the government as its partner, medicine in the United States would have evolved very differently.

The Health Insurance Industry

Before passage of the Affordable Care Act (ACA), the massive health reform program of President Barak Obama, the United States was the only major industrialized country without a universal health care system guaranteeing coverage to all citizens. Even with the Act, it is estimated that as many as 20–30 million Americans will remain without coverage.[62] This fact is the starting point for numerous debates over the shortcomings of American health care. However, this gap in the country's safety net does not mean that government involvement has historically been absent from the health insurance market. To the contrary, it has intervened to shape this sector of health care as pervasively as it has for all the others.

The government's most visible role in the financing of health care has been to directly cover three segments of the population that are most difficult for private companies to insure: the elderly and totally disabled under Medicare and the poor under Medicaid. However, it has also shaped, overseen, and funded much of the private health insurance market for well over half a century. Private health insurance in its present form would not exist in the United States were it not for a sustained government role, and its further evolution will be guided even more substantially by the government under the ACA.

GOVERNMENT ACCOMMODATION AND THE CREATION OF HEALTH INSURANCE

The first private health insurance plans were created at the start of the Great Depression. Money was scarce, even for a need as basic as health care. One idea to address the dilemma was to ask potential patients to pay a small fee in advance in lieu of much larger costs if they became sick. Baylor University Hospital in Houston was the first organization to put the idea into practice when it launched a financing plan using this approach in 1929. It offered a group of 1,500 school-teachers up to 21 days of hospital care each year for the sum of six dollars. The concept proved popular and soon spread to other states. In the early 1930s, plans were developed in California and New Jersey to provide care at multiple institutions, and this arrangement spread, as well. The model was formalized on a national basis under the name "Blue Cross." In 1939, a similar concept was applied to physician services in Sacramento, California. The force behind it was, again, the providers seeking a steady source of payment, in this case physicians. The mechanism again proved popular and spread from state to state under the name "Blue Shield."[63]

For these newcomers to the world of finance, operating under the same structure as established for-profit insurance companies presented challenges. They could not raise and maintain the same level of financial reserves that state regulators generally required of insurance companies to guarantee the ability to pay claims. New York was the first state to address this imbalance in 1934, when it enacted an enabling statute that conferred special regulatory status on the new health insurance mechanisms. Under New York's approach, if Blue Cross plans agreed to maintain their operations on a nonprofit basis and remain under the control of member hospitals, they would be exempted from the reserve requirements that applied to the rest of the insurance industry. Similar statutes were enacted in 25 other states over the next five years. Blue Shield plans later received similar favorable treatment.[64]

EMPLOYMENT-BASED COVERAGE TAKES CENTER STAGE

Through this form of regulatory leniency, state governments enabled the first health insurance plans to take shape. However, a set of more significant government interventions launched them on a path to tremendous growth and established their central role in health care finance. These steps also transformed the business model under which they functioned.

The government catalyst for the expansion of the health insurance market was a byproduct of World War II. As the country ramped up the production of war supplies, and as millions of young men headed overseas to fight, the economy faced the threat of rampant inflation from a constricted supply of goods and of workers to make them. In response, the federal government imposed a freeze on prices and wages, outlawing any increases unless approved by a federal board. In 1943, to accommodate the needs of employers facing difficulty in attracting workers, the War Labor Board permitted "fringe benefits," such as health insurance, to be added to compensation by exempting them from the definition of wages. Companies were quick to take advantage of this recruiting tool. Enrollment in Blue Cross plans, which were widely offered through employment as a result of this ruling, increased almost fourfold during the war from 7 million to 28 million.[65]

This regulatory action led to an even more influential government step in the post-war years. The 1943 ruling by the War Labor Board had established the precedent that sums paid by employers for health insurance were not considered part of a worker's pay. In keeping with this reasoning, the Internal Revenue Service (IRS) determined that they were therefore not subject to income tax. In 1954, as part of a comprehensive overhaul of the country's tax laws, Congress ratified this position in legislation.[66] Since then, employer-sponsored health insurance has been provided to workers tax-free.

While employment-based health insurance enjoyed this substantial financial boost, coverage obtained directly by individuals from insurance companies did not. This meant that money used to pay premiums for these policies comes from income that has been fully subject to taxation. This differential tax treatment has encouraged the market to gravitate toward employer-sponsored plans. As a result, many of those without access to this form of coverage, including those who are unemployed, self-employed, or who work for firms that do not offer health benefits, can have tremendous difficulty finding insurance. They have historically comprised a large portion of the ranks of the uninsured.

This governmental largess that favors one route of obtaining insurance over another helped to tilt the market toward employment-based coverage. This engendered a system of health care finance with employers at its center. Insurance sold directly to individuals came to represent a tiny portion of the market, in the range of about 5 percent.[67]

The amounts lost to government coffers by exempting employer-paid health insurance from taxation represent a subsidy for those who are willing and able to take advantage of this form of coverage. Over the years, the amount of this subsidy has grown to a gigantic size.[68] In 2010, the total amount lost to federal and state governments by exempting employer-paid health insurance premiums from income tax was estimated at more than $250 billion.[69] This makes the tax subsidy for private insurance the third largest government health care financing program, behind Medicare and Medicaid. It covers more than one-third of the aggregate amount that Americans pay for private employer-sponsored coverage each year.[70]

The magnitude of government financial support for private health insurance means that this product is sold through a market that is not fully private, but rather one that is heavily shaped and funded by the government. By paying Americans more than $250 billion each year to obtain health coverage at work, the public–private partnership that began with special regulatory treatment for the first Blue Cross plans now guides the entire structure of private health insurance. It also covers a significant portion of its cost.

FURTHER REGULATORY SUPPORT FOR PRIVATE MARKETS

This partnership took another major step in 1974, when Congress granted employer-sponsored coverage a set of additional regulatory exemptions in the form of the Employee Retirement Income Security Act (ERISA), which upended the existing regulatory structure for employment benefits.[71] The regulatory scheme that ERISA implements for health benefits is extremely complex, but at its core is an exemption for employer-sponsored health plans that places them beyond the reach of many state laws. Among the more important of these laws are statutes that limit unfair insurance practices and case law that permits aggrieved beneficiaries to sue insurance companies for damages in state courts. With these oversight measures out of the way, insurers can exercise greater leeway in claims handling and other business practices.[72]

Beyond this, ERISA is particularly kind to plans that employers fund themselves without the use of insurance companies. In these self-funded plans, the employer pays claims directly rather than purchasing coverage for its workers. ERISA placed these arrangements beyond the reach of almost all state insurance regulation, a benefit conferred on no other form of insurance, and one that is not granted to policies purchased directly by individuals. By easing regulatory strictures, ERISA added another inducement for companies to offer coverage and for insurance companies to market policies through employers.

THE MANAGED CARE REVOLUTION

As important as these transformative government policies were, an even more significant initiative was yet to come. That was the set of steps that altered the underlying nature of health insurance from a passive reimbursement vehicle to an active participant in the process of delivering care. The new paradigm for coverage was the model of managed care.

The managed care approach to health care finance initially took the form of health maintenance organizations, known popularly as the HMOs, entities that arrange both the provision of and payment for care. The concept originated in the late 1960s, in a proposal by Paul Ellwood, a Minneapolis family physician, who looked to the model of what were then known as prepaid plans, health plans that collected a premium in return for direct access to services.[73] Prepaid plans operated clinics where members could obtain physician services, and they either owned or contracted with hospitals for inpatient care. They did not reimburse providers or patients for the cost of services rendered but provided, or arranged for the provision of, those services directly. By steering patients to participating facilities, they were able to offer coverage at lower cost than conventional insurance.

Prepaid plans originated in the 1930s and 1940s, under the auspices of large employers and labor unions. Kaiser Aluminum launched the Kaiser-Permanente plan in the 1940s to cover its shipyard workers on the West Coast during World War II. Its success led to the spin-off of the health plan after the war into an independent nonprofit organization open to employees of other companies. The International Ladies Garment Workers Union created the Health Insurance Plan in New York in the 1930s, to cover union members and their dependents, and it also opened it to a wider market after the war. Similar plans to arise during this time included the Group Health Association in Washington, DC and the Group Health Cooperative of Puget Sound in Seattle, Washington.[74]

Dr. Ellwood saw in these plans a way to finance the full range of care while keeping a tight rein on costs. By directly employing physicians and owning or managing the facilities in which they worked, prepaid plans had strong tools with which to enforce cost control. Of particular importance in this regard was their incentive structure. They paid physicians a salary that generally remained fixed regardless of the number of services provided or procedures performed. This eliminated the financial incentive to overtreat because doing so no longer engendered additional payments.

The concept behind HMOs is to craft a prepaid plan without the bricks and mortar of actual clinics. Physicians remain in their own practices and continue to render services in their own offices but under a new payment structure. Primary care physicians are paid based on a system known as "capitation," under which they are responsible for a panel of patients who can see them as often as necessary. In return, they are paid a set monthly fee for each patient, regardless of how often the patient is actually seen or the number of services actually provided. Beyond capitation, HMOs also use an additional set of tools to limit the number of expensive specialist visits, procedures, and tests that patients receive, as well as the length of hospital stays. Dr. Ellwood believed that this structure would mimic the outcomes of prepaid plans in terms of costs and quality of care but would do so with dispersed networks of providers that were more convenient to patients than centralized clinics.

Policymakers in Washington, particularly those in the Nixon administration, which was in office when Dr. Ellwood first promoted his idea, liked the idea as a private, market-based approach to health reform.[75] They sought a way to give HMOs an initial push to introduce them into the market. The push took the form of the federal Health Maintenance Organization Act, which was passed by Congress in 1973.[76] It gave HMOs a powerful tool to force their way into local markets and implemented a regulatory structure that determined the shape this new concept would take.

The HMO Act gave these new financing vehicles the right to demand inclusion in employer benefit offerings if the company provided health coverage. To be eligible to request inclusion, the HMO had to meet a set of standards that defined it as "federally qualified." As further encouragement, the Act also provided loans and grants to new HMOs to help with start-up costs. Once established, HMOs were subject to regulation of their operations by each state.

Starting about ten years later, the government gave managed care another huge boost by creating a public market for HMOs and serving as a major purchaser of their services.[77] In the 1980s, a few states experimented with the use of private HMOs to provide services under contract for Medicaid, with an eye to harnessing their cost control techniques. The experience was considered successful, and the approach to administering benefits became an established practice. It spread from state to state so that, by the end of the 1990s, all of them were using managed care for a portion of their Medicaid populations. With this model in mind, the Medicare program tested the waters starting a few years later. After initial trials seemed promising, managed care was formally integrated into the program as a beneficiary option under the Balanced Budget Act of 1997.[78] It was originally named "Medicare + Choice," and then expanded and renamed "Medicare Advantage" by the Medicare Prescription Drug, Improvement, and Modernization Act of 2003.[79]

The opening of these two huge public markets enabled many managed care organizations to grow their scope of operations significantly, and the horizons of established companies expanded well beyond their original expectations.[80] Many smaller companies sprang up throughout the country, often to be acquired by larger ones seeking to meet the growing market demand. What had been a largely local industry in the 1970s expanded to include many national players starting in the 1990s, which grew through mergers, consolidations, and acquisitions to become financial powerhouses.[81]

As markets and companies expanded, managed care companies began to innovate, as well. The original HMO model of stringent oversight of all aspects of care was modified with variations that permitted more patient choice. These took the form of preferred provider organizations (PPOs) and point of service (POS) plans that retained many elements of the management of care while permitting patients to obtain some services with less oversight and from providers outside of predetermined networks. These alternatives eventually surpassed HMOs in market share. With these changes, employers could select from among a range of insurance products to offer their workers, with different levels of restriction and corresponding variations in premiums, all under the paradigm of integrating the financing and provision of health care. This is not to say that employees were always happy with the choices, but they often did see significant moderations in premiums.

The growth of managed care since the government first served as the market catalyst has been tremendous. Today, it is the dominant form of health insurance coverage in the United States. In 1988, only 27 percent of insured Americans were covered by managed care, but, over the course of the next 12 years, the percentage grew dramatically. It reached 54 percent in 1993, 73 percent in 1996, and 92 percent in 2000. In 2007, more than 97 percent of insured workers were covered under a managed care arrangement of some sort, with 21 percent of them in traditional HMOs.[82] Many Americans today have never experienced health insurance in any other form.

During the 1990s, as large national managed care companies swallowed smaller local ones, the bargaining clout of these behemoths drove down fees paid to hospitals and physicians in many markets. This, in turn, led many providers to seek greater negotiating power by consolidating into health systems, hospital chains, and large physician group practices. By the end of the 1990s, much of American health care had emerged as a more centralized enterprise. In effect, the rise of managed care had revised the structure of health care provision and, with it, the actual care that millions of people receive.

THE PRIVATE HEALTH INSURANCE INDUSTRY TODAY

What would the private health insurance market look like without the tax subsidy and regulatory benefits that the government has bestowed on it? Undoubtedly, there would still be insurance. As health care grew in complexity and cost over the years, private companies would undoubtedly have found ways to offer financing mechanisms for it. However, it is unlikely that the mechanisms would be linked to employment to the same extent as health insurance is today. Of greater significance, without the tax subsidy to lower the real cost of coverage, premiums would have to be considerably lower to be affordable. This, in turn, would leave insurers with a smaller pool of money for reimbursing providers, leading to lower reimbursement rates. The result would be smaller incomes for many physicians and less revenue for hospitals.

And what would managed care look like had the government not catalyzed its creation and growth? Would this form of health care finance even exist? The original prepaid plans predated the HMO movement by several decades, and, undoubtedly, they would have remained a part of American health care. However, without the government initiatives that fostered managed care's growth, it is difficult to imagine that they would have engendered a transformation of health care finance. Government programs gave managed care its initial push, granted it special favorable regulatory treatment, and expanded its reach into the largest public health care programs. The shape of American health insurance has not been the same since.

Health Care as a Pillar of the American Economy

As these examples illustrate, the government, through numerous means, has served as the driving force that shaped and guided health care over the course of the twentieth century. The inventiveness of private entrepreneurs, as important as it has been, did not create and does not sustain our system on its own. A long list of public initiatives that harnessed private enterprise has been the crucible for the private markets that provide most of the health care services and products that Americans receive today. Yet, the ramifications of the government's role in inventing American health care go even deeper than the molding of a single industry, as important as that industry is to the life and well-being of every citizen. In creating health care as we know it today, the government established a pillar of the entire economy. The health care industry represents more than one-sixth of America's gross domestic product.[83] That portion is widely expected to reach one-fifth over the next 10 years.[84]

In occupying such a central economic role, health care has also become one of the country's most important engines for creating jobs, accounting for almost 1 out of every 10 nationwide.[85] In some regions, the portion is even higher. Many towns depend on a single hospital or other health care institution as the foundation of the local economy. Several major cities rely on health care as a crucial economic pillar, among them Boston, Philadelphia, San Francisco, and Nashville. Cities such as these, and the states in which they are located, are home to major teaching hospitals, medical schools, and pharmaceutical companies that employ significant fractions of their workforces. And government money pours into these regions to provide the lion's share of the industry's funding. The direct contribution of just one federal agency, NIH, is illustrative. In 2005, it sent more than $2 billion in grants to Massachusetts, almost $1.5 billion to Pennsylvania, and more than $3 billion to California.[86]

When a region relies on health care for economic vitality, it builds on the public–private paradigm that created American medicine. Hospitals, medical schools, and pharmaceutical companies are private enterprises, some for-profit and some nonprofit. Their coffers are filled with capital from debt or equity markets and, in the case of nonprofits, with private donations as well. Yet, all the while, underlying the revenue base that generates their cash flow is government funding. Hospitals receive reimbursement from Medicare and Medicaid, and the payments they collect from private insurers are heavily subsidized by a tax preference that inflates the size of the premiums that insurers can charge. Medical schools receive direct government support from a range of programs and large amounts of research funding from NIH. Pharmaceutical companies sell substantial portions of their products to patients who are covered by public programs and by tax-subsidized private insurance. Health care, in other words, functions as a gigantic machine that takes in government money and oversight at one end and generates private sector activity at the other.

From the perspective of the overall economy, the health care industry, flush with these resources, exerts the same effect as a huge government jobs program. The substantial portion of overall employment that it represents tells only part of the story. Between 2001 and 2006, a period of generally moderate growth, health care accounted for the creation of 1.7 million new jobs.[87] No other industry came close. Without health care, national employment during this time would actually have contracted. Looking ahead, over the next 25 years, health care is projected to account for more than 30 percent of all new jobs. It could be on its way to becoming the single most important industry in the economy.

More recently, health care was one of the only industries that continued to thrive during the Great Recession. It seems almost recession-proof. It was one of only three sectors of the economy that added jobs during that time. The others were universities, which also rely heavily on government support, and the federal government itself.[88]

Could either the government or private sector have brought health care to such a vaunted status on its own? Although any answer is, of course, speculative, it is difficult to imagine that anything remotely resembling this economic powerhouse could have emerged. And the symbiotic relationship between the two sectors stands to be reinforced going forward. As discussed in Chapter 8, the ACA will further expand the country's health care sector by building on the same public–private paradigm.

Moreover, the robustness of the public–private partnership that underlies health care stands to be reinforced even further by a revolution in the nature of medical care that lies on the horizon. A transformed health care system based on genomics, information technology, and standardization of clinical practices is already changing the landscape of the industry. These new technologies will permeate almost every aspect of clinical care. However, as discussed in Chapter 8, they cannot reach fruition through the efforts of either the government or the private sphere alone. The resources needed and societal ramifications they produce are too large for either one to handle on its own. To revolutionize health care, the public and private sectors will have to work hand in hand, as they have in the past, to bring the industry into this new clinical terrain.

The examples of government-created health care industry segments presented in this chapter and elaborated on in the chapters that follow are certainly not exhaustive. Numerous others readily come to mind. Home health and hospice care owe their existence to their eligibility for Medicare reimbursement. Many allied health professions, such as physical therapy and occupational therapy, have similarly flourished in recent years courtesy of the same program. Obviously, prescription drug plans that administer benefits under Medicare Part D would not exist at all if that program did not. And other examples too numerous to list abound. One would have to search far and wide to find a segment of American health care that did not emerge from a government crucible or that does not look to the public sector for essential sustenance.

Public Support and Private Influence

American health care has perennially faced challenges, but recent trends are magnifying them to near crisis proportions. The system's cost is on its way to devouring one-fifth of the nation's entire economy. Even under the ACA, at least 20 million people still lack a means of financial access. Tens of thousands die each year from preventable medical errors, and standard medical practice continues to vary markedly from region to region, without clinical justification. This is a crucial time to visit the system's past for lessons on ways to address these large and growing concerns that threaten to shake health care at its core.

As discussed in more depth in Chapter 8, the public–private structure that underlies the system is not likely to change. We are too far down the road to turn back. The most likely alternative would be a system of direct government control over health care delivery or finance, but such an arrangement would have difficulty garnering substantial public support. As the history of health reform teaches, efforts to replace private health care finance with a direct government plan perennially face tremendous political resistance. Truman got nowhere in his efforts to create one. Johnson brought Medicare to fruition only by weaving a role for private insurers into its structure. Clinton failed even though his proposal relied heavily on some components of the private market. And Obama succeeded in gaining passage for the ACA only by crafting a plan that promoted the interests of several large private industry sectors.[89]

The private health care sector that the government created is today a force to be reckoned with. It applies the significant financial resources that it accumulated, largely at public expense, to gaining influence in the political process. That influence is then used to induce lawmakers to maintain and expand the programs that feed it and to structure those programs in ways that are favorable to their interests.

Advocates of purely public financing mechanisms, such as those that exist in many European countries, have lacked the means to mount an effective response. The more the private health care sector grows, the more difficult it is for reforms to dislodge it. The public–private paradigm of American health care, therefore, is likely to remain in place for some time to come.

Lessons for Public Policy

What are the consequences that our system has wrought? On the positive side, America leads the world in access to many kinds of high-technology care. Our hospitals draw patients from around the globe for numerous high-end services. And, according to the World Health Organization, once in American facilities, patients are likely to be treated with more respect and better amenities than anywhere else.[90]

On the negative side, our system is by far the most expensive in the world. The cost of health care places a crushing burden on many employers, with ripple effects felt throughout the entire economy. It is a major contributor to the federal budget deficit and to budget woes for a large number of states. Health care expenditures are rising around the developed world, but nowhere more so than in the United States.

Yet, for all of this spending, the quality of care is uneven. Researchers at Dartmouth Medical School have found wide variations in medical practice across different regions of the country.[91] Treatment decisions are often guided more by local custom and reimbursement concerns than by evidence of what is most effective. Beyond the variability of medical practice, the care that Americans receive is often prone to errors. Lapses in hospitals are common, and they lead to the deaths of tens of thousands of patients each year.[92] And care often lacks coordination. America trails much of the developed world in treating chronic diseases that require the services of multiple practitioners in different disciplines. Physicians who care for the same patient often fail to communicate with one another, a phenomenon that can lead to inconsistent treatments, often with harmful effects.[93]

These system features, both positive and negative, flow from the underlying nature of the public–private partnership that guides it, which creates a distinctive set of incentives that direct the behavior of all participants. Americans enjoy relatively good access to technologically complex care because physicians receive higher levels of reimbursement for rendering it than for counseling patients in primary care settings. They receive better amenities as inpatients because hospitals in competitive markets use comfort and convenience as inducements to attract patients. The partnership raises overall costs by enabling the private sector to use its resources to pressure the government to maintain reimbursement arrangements that are generous, often to the point of excess. It leaves room for errors by imposing relatively few financial penalties on hospitals that allow them to be committed within their walls.[94] Mistakes rarely reduce reimbursement, and studies show that fewer than one in ten affected patients brings a legal claim in response.[95]

They discourage coordination of care by rewarding most providers for rendering services themselves, rather than in concert with others.

But it does not have to be this way. Inefficient and counterproductive financial incentives are not an inevitable part of a public–private health care system. As discussed in Chapter 8, although constraints imposed by the American political system make it difficult to change the underlying structure, opportunities abound for public policy to guide the partnership toward better results.

The single most important change would be to abandon the prevailing paradigm for provider reimbursement in which a separate fee is paid for each service rendered. The incentives this system creates favor the provision of excess and wasteful care, negligible reliance on national practice standards, and minimal coordination among providers. Experiments have proliferated in the public and private sectors to test alternative arrangements, like combining payments for a range of related services into a single bundled amount and paying alliances of providers as a group for treating all aspects of a patient's condition. Provisions to facilitate experiments along these lines are contained in the ACA.[96] The public–private partnership could build on those experiments that have successful outcomes to restructure the prevailing payment paradigm while leaving the underlying nature of public–private interaction intact.

Similar changes are possible with regard to other system failings. Reimbursement arrangements could encourage adherence to established best clinical practices. They could also impose financial penalties for errors that harm patients. And payment amounts for goods and services could be based on clinical utility rather than on the cost to produce them. In each case, the government and private sector can continue to play their historical roles, but their joint efforts could be directed along more productive lines.

We have seen how public policy can create huge private enterprises. Those enterprises have laid the foundation for major industries across the economy, including health care. The government continues to foster health care's growth and evolution with a continual parade of major new programs and initiatives. In recent years, it has multiplied the size of the market for private insurance with a massive health reform plan, laid the foundation for a new era in pharmaceuticals by deciphering the human genome, and promoted the widespread adoption of computerized information systems with a set of financial inducements. Initiatives like these are essential to the continued development of American health care. Without them, the system would stagnate, and medicine would fail to advance.

However, decades of history have also shown where the system can go astray. Showering financial rewards on private businesses and individuals, as public policy has done for most of the past century, can induce innovation and efficiency, but it can also produce waste and substandard care. If the government has the power to create new industries and expand the horizons for existing ones, it can use that power to direct them toward desired outcomes, like efficiency and fairness. To that end, programs can be designed more prudently. More health care is not always better health care. Government policy can launch juggernauts that transform care, like the huge research enterprise supported by the NIH, but it can also create monsters that devour resources to no useful end, like the surfeit of technological equipment that is overused in many hospitals. The force that created American health care, if harnessed wisely, could make it truly the best in the world in all regards.

Health Care and American Society

Debates over proposals to reform the health care system are always highly emotional. They were that way in the early twentieth century when several states entertained the first plans for government-sponsored universal coverage, and they were no different a hundred years later when Congress considered the Obama administration's massive reform legislation. They brought out equally strong sentiments when numerous other measures were introduced in the years in between. What other issue could inspire unfounded widespread fears that government-run "death panels" will decide the fate of elderly citizens, which were stoked in the debates over the Obama plan? The government has intervened in almost every American industry in one way or another, but nothing inspires political passions in the same way as health care.

Why does health care stir us so? It is because it affects the lives and well-being, both of ourselves and of those around us, more directly than any other endeavor. Access to care is literally a matter of life and death. We can do without the goods and services produced by many other industries but not those of health care. Changes in government policy could disrupt patterns of care that we have come to depend on in ways that are often difficult to predict, and nothing is more frightening than the unknown. Since the health care system is bewilderingly complex, reforms can seem particularly confusing. This leaves ample opportunities for opponents to characterize them as threats.

Good health is also an essential ingredient in the strength of our economy. It is a fundamental driver of the nation's productivity because ill health can severely impair worker efficiency. Our financial fortunes can depend on the health care system as much as does our physical well-being.

Debates over health reform also bring out deep-seated philosophical differences over the role of government. Should the public sector directly provide for our physical, social, and economic security? Or, should it stand back and let the private market tend to these needs? In many respects, debates over health care serve as a surrogate for discord over these broader questions. They force us to revisit long-standing disagreements over the political and economic foundation of the country.

Discussions of health reform also take on an important ethical dimension. Advocates for a larger public role tend to see health care as a fundamental right that the government is obliged to protect. From this perspective, access to care takes on the character of a moral imperative for which the larger community bears responsibility. Supporters of private markets view health care as more of a commodity that should be allocated through unconstrained exchanges between buyers and sellers. Although it may be appropriate for the government to supply a basic safety net for those with limited financial means, for everyone else, the task of obtaining health care services should be a matter of personal responsibility.

These special characteristics of health care make it all the more important to understand the true nature of our system. When we debate health reform, whether it is the Obama plan or future initiatives, what are we really arguing about? The answer is some of the most fundamental concerns over our physical well-being, economic strength, and character of our political system. With so much at stake, misunderstandings over the role of government and of private markets can be especially pernicious.

The Story Behind the Creation of Health Care

This overview illustrates the nature of the public–private symbiosis in broad sweep. Behind the public programs and secular trends lay countless stories of industry constituents that were created, grew, and prospered though this paradigm. The chapters that follow explore in greater depth how the government created the major segments of American health care and examine how the interplay of public initiative and private enterprise engendered the system that is so often termed a "free market." They illustrate how superficial that characterization actually is.

Beyond telling the historical story, each chapter presents examples of individual private health care enterprises that grew and flourished through government intervention and largess. With this perspective in mind, the future path of American health care will come into clearer focus. Of more immediate relevance, it places the transformations wrought by the ACA in their larger context as part of a decades-long sweep of political and economic forces.

3

How the Government Created the Pharmaceutical Industry

> If the American government is retreating on research, it's bad for everybody.
>
> — HAROLD VARMUS, FORMER HEAD, NATIONAL CANCER INSTITUTE[1]

> I think adequate funding for the NIH is critical for the health of the nation. The relationship between industry and government funded research is symbiotic.
>
> — MACE ROTHENBERG, SENIOR VICE PRESIDENT OF CLINICAL DEVELOPMENT, PFIZER[2]

Year after year, the private pharmaceutical industry is one of the most profitable in the United States. It employs hundreds of thousands of people and consistently rewards comparable numbers of investors. Its success is built on a cascade of products, some of which generate billions of dollars in sales each year. New ones continually enter the market to replenish the supply.

This economic powerhouse is a prime example of private enterprise in action. Private investors own the corporations that develop and manufacture prescription drugs. Their management answers to shareholders. They compete for business in a market-based environment that is often characterized as a "free market." However, the pharmaceutical industry does not function in a private-sector bubble. It has an indispensable outside partner through the entire drug development process—the government.

New drugs emerge from many different sources. Some come from research that applies basic biological knowledge. Some emerge from trial and error. Others materialize from serendipity when they are least expected. It is a long and expensive path from the initial conjecture that a substance may have clinical potential to its ultimate entry into the market. The path has countless twists and turns, and many journeys do not succeed. When one does, a single player rarely travels the entire road alone. Whatever the initial source of discovery, multiple partners usually join the effort, and they come from both the public and private spheres.

Few would dispute the value of government-funded research as the foundation of drug discovery. Even the most ardent admirers of private innovation concede the importance of the government in promoting the underlying science on which it rests.[3] Debates may rage over the relative amount of credit each side deserves, but the necessity of both sectors to the advancement of pharmaceutical science is rarely questioned.

Most of the drugs in wide use today resulted not from industry inventiveness alone but from public–private collaborations. Of the 21 drugs with the highest therapeutic impact, 14 stemmed directly from an enabling discovery that the government had supported.[4] Often, public and private research continues to interact even after a new drug therapy has reached the market. Such ongoing interchanges have produced major breakthroughs, such as better understanding of the mechanism of action of azidothymidine (AZT) as a treatment for HIV infection.

Moreover, the public–private partnership does not end with a handoff from government-backed basic scientists to applied investigators in corporate settings. The public sector contributes to drug development throughout the lifecycle of new drugs in many ways.[5] Perhaps most significantly, it creates vast markets for drugs through public health insurance programs. Medicare, which insures the elderly, spends more than $55 billion a year on outpatient prescriptions and more than $10 billion a year on drugs administered by physicians.[6] Medicaid, which insures the poor, devotes more than $26 billion a year to these costs.[7] In addition, the government purchases drugs for veterans through the Veterans Health Administration and through the Department of Defense for military personnel and their dependents.

Government intervention also shapes the pharmaceutical industry through regulation. The primary agency involved is the Food and Drug Administration (FDA), which serves as a gatekeeper to determine which drugs may reach the market. To pass through the gate, new products must undergo years of clinical testing that assess safety and effectiveness. After approval, the FDA continues to monitor drugs for safety and to impose restrictions on marketing and promotion. The FDA-imposed testing process accounts for the lion's share of the cost of drug development and sets parameters for the kinds of drugs that ultimately reach patients. Although manufacturers may complain about bureaucratic inefficiency and delays on the agency's part, this vetting process is largely responsible for the public's confidence in their products.

Beyond the FDA, patent laws, administered by the federal Patent and Trademark Office (PTO) circumscribe the commercialization and marketing process. Patent rules determine the nature and length of the monopoly granted to new drugs, which is what makes them profitable to develop. These rules are supplemented by a number of related laws that further refine the contours of the pharmaceutical market. These include the Drug Price Competition and Patent Term Restoration Act,[8] commonly known as the Hatch-Waxman Act, which structures the market for generic competition, and the Food and Drug Administration Modernization Act (FDAMA),[9] which extends monopoly protection for drugs that are tested on children.

Of course, the industry has its share of critics.[10] Pharmaceutical companies are often lambasted for using their patent-created monopolies to charge exorbitant prices that contribute to America's health care cost burden. Some biotechnology drugs that treat life-threatening illnesses are priced at more than $100,000 a year.[11]

The industry is also often accused of resorting to deceptive sales practices, such as promoting drugs for unapproved uses and boosting sales with lavish gifts to prescribing physicians.

Moreover, the pharmaceutical industry is as skilled as any at using its financial resources for political gain. It used its influence to incorporate key favorable features into the Medicare prescription drug benefit when it was enacted in 2003, most notably a prohibition on direct negotiation over prices by the federal government. It was also able to extract key concessions from the Obama administration in the maneuvering that preceded passage of the Affordable Care Act (ACA) in 2010 in return for its support. Among other concessions, the administration agreed to retain the ban on direct government price negotiations over drug prices and to refrain from permitting patients to reimport drugs from Canada, where prices are lower.

Nevertheless, whether the industry's actions are cheered or condemned, they are undeniably central to the functioning of American health care and would not be possible without an underpinning of government support. On its surface, the pharmaceutical sector of the health care system would appear to be the most private of any. All of its major constituents are private corporations that function on a for-profit basis. A superficial glance might suggest that its fortunes rest predominantly on the behavior of these investor-owned entities. Yet beneath this façade lie all of these elements of a government role that is as active and indispensable as any in American industry.

America's Robust Drug Companies

PERENNIAL PROFITABILITY

Over the past 20 years, no American industry has outperformed pharmaceutical manufacturing in terms of profitability. According to the most widely used measures, drug companies earned three times the median of all Fortune 500 companies in 2004 and over five times the median in 2001. Between 1995 and 2002, pharmaceutical manufacturing was the most profitable industry in the United States, and, since then, it has remained in the top three every year. The rate of return on investment consistently hovers near 20 percent, a figure that most other industries can only dream of.[12]

Sales of prescription drugs in the United States now exceed $300 billion a year.[13] Even during the recession year of 2009, sales remained robust, growing at a rate of 5.1 percent from the year before. Global sales for 2009 stood at $837 billion after rising seven percent from a year earlier.[14] Both domestically and globally, these rates continue to accelerate.

THE FINANCIAL ENGINE: RESEARCH AND DEVELOPMENT

Several factors account for the pharmaceutical industry's consistent good fortune.[15] For one, demand for health-enhancing and life-saving products will never diminish, so the industry's output will always be needed. For another, most consumers today have assistance from third parties in paying for pharmaceutical products through some form of insurance, either public or private.

The pharmaceutical industry is also able to charge high prices for many of its products because they are insulated from market competition through patents. Although patents do not last indefinitely, they, along with various other legal protections, offer most prescription drugs between 10 and 15 years of market exclusivity after they first reach consumers.

The exclusive sale of life-saving products is certainly a recipe for financial success, but only if one more ingredient is present. As patents expire, competitive pricing by manufacturers of generic copies drives down profit margins, so a steady supply of new drugs is needed. The industry must devote a tremendous amount of its attention and resources to that end. To maintain profitability, fresh products must continually flow through each company's "pipeline."

The never-ending search for new products has shaped the pharmaceutical industry into the most research-intensive in the United States. It devotes more private resources to scientific investigation than any other.[16] In 2002, this investment equaled 18 percent of sales, which is roughly five times the average for American manufacturing firms.[17] Since 1992, this percentage has been higher even than that devoted by the computer industry.[18]

The exact magnitude of pharmaceutical research and development spending is subject to some dispute.[19] The industry's trade association, the Pharmaceutical Research and Manufacturers of America (PhRMA) uses a broad definition that includes spending on post-market monitoring of drugs after their final approval by the FDA. By this measure, research spending grew from $6 billion to $39 billion between 1980 and 2004 in constant 2005 dollars, reflecting an average rate of increase of about 8 percent. PhRMA puts the 2009 figure at $65.3 billion.[20] The National Science Foundation (NSF) calculated the value of industry research at the premarket phases only and found an increase from $5.5 billion to $17 billion over the same period, for an average rate of growth of 5 percent. Nevertheless, under either analysis, it is clear that the industry has steadily and dramatically expanded its commitment to research over a considerable period of time.[21]

Of course, not all of this scientific activity actually creates new drugs that are truly innovative. About two-thirds of the new drug applications submitted to the FDA each year do not involve a new molecular entity (NME). Instead, they represent reformulations or minor modifications of existing drugs or requests for approval for new uses.[22] Many of these applications are for drugs that use the same chemical mechanism of action but with a slightly altered active ingredient as existing drugs. These are commonly known as "me-too" drugs because they follow an established therapeutic approach. In most years, the FDA approves only about 20 drugs that are based on new NMEs.

However, regardless of the originality of the drugs being introduced, the steady flow of new products is a hallmark of the pharmaceutical industry. One can debate how much clinical value is actually contributed when new drugs mimic existing ones, but it is undeniable that the industry as we know it today thrives on a massive research and development apparatus. It is in this regard that the government provides it with the biggest boost.

The Cornerstone of Public Biomedical Research: The National Institutes of Health

How does the industry find the new drugs it needs to refresh its inventory? For two-thirds of its products, the answer is easy because they are me-too drugs based on established products. For the one-third of new drugs that represent true innovation, the answer is more complex. These are medications that are truly new and that emerge from advances in scientific understanding, the kind of knowledge that the government is uniquely suited to help build. It is the only entity with the resources and national perspective needed to take the decades-long perspective that is necessary to produce products with a universal payoff. What it generates is, in essence, a public good.

A MISSION TO UNDERWRITE BIOMEDICAL SCIENCE

The National Institutes of Health (NIH), the agency that carries on the government's foundational role in promoting biomedical research, is a massive organization. It functions as a component of the Department of Health and Human Services and spends about $30 billion a year to enhance the fundamental understanding of biology and medicine.[23] That amount has more than doubled since the mid-1990s.

The division of research roles between industry and government is not a simple split between applied and basic science. The NIH performs some applied clinical studies of new drugs, and private industry conducts some basic research. The relationship between the private and public spheres is further blurred by a range of other government programs that promote the translation of NIH-funded research into commercial uses. However, in all of these endeavors, the two sectors follow a similar pattern of partnership to produce new medicines.

The importance of government-sponsored research to pharmaceutical industry vitality cannot be overstated. One analysis estimated that every 1 percent increase in public research funding produces an increase of between 2 and 2.4 percent in the number of commercially available new compounds.[24] Another projected the rate of return from public funding of biomedical research at up to 30 percent a year.[25] Without question, government-funded science is an essential ingredient underlying the industry's business model.

THE NIH'S GROWTH FROM HUMBLE ORIGINS

The huge scientific enterprise that the NIH represents today began as a modest endeavor in the late nineteenth century in Staten Island, New York. Dr. Joseph J. Kinyoun set up a laboratory in a marine hospital there in 1887 to study bacteria that cause common infectious diseases. He succeeded in identifying the organism that causes cholera, the *Vibrio cholera* bacillus, which aided physicians in diagnosing suspicious cases of this deadly disease. Successes such as this led the government to move his laboratory in 1891 to Washington, D.C. and to give it a new name, the Hygienic Laboratory. Ten years later, Congress authorized $35,000 for a new building to house it.[26]

The Hygienic Laboratory gained new responsibilities and prominence in 1902, when Congress created a Division of Pathology and Bacteriology within the federal Marine Hospital Service to house its research. At that time, the lab also added PhD-trained researchers to the physicians in its workforce. Among its new responsibilities was setting standards and issuing licenses for the manufacture of vaccines and antitoxins by private companies, a role that was included in the Biologics Control Act passed that year. This responsibility was eventually transferred to the FDA in 1972. Along with this new regulatory authority came an expanded mission of research to support it.[27]

Another round of important scientific discoveries emerged from the laboratory in the years leading up to World War I. These included such practical findings as the link between pellagra and a dietary deficiency and between unsanitary conditions around military bases and disease outbreaks. In recognition of its growing contributions, scientists who worked in the lab were accepted for the first time as members of the executive branch of government. In 1912, the agency housing the lab was renamed the Public Health Service.[28]

As the value of biomedical science became increasingly apparent, efforts were launched after the war to expand its reach. Most notably, a group of scientists from a wartime agency, the Chemical War Service, sought industry funding to support research into applications of chemistry to medicine. However, several years of trying yielded no success in attracting private sponsors.[29]

In 1926, the scientists gave up their quest to find funding in the private sector and turned to Congress instead. They found a champion in Senator Joseph E. Ransdell of Louisiana, who, in 1930, successfully sponsored legislation to fund fellowships for basic research within the Hygienic Laboratory.[30] The Ransdell Act also changed the name of the Laboratory to the National Institute of Health. Initial funding was modest, but it marked the start of a new approach to the sponsorship of research under government auspices. Funding grew significantly over the years along with the Institute's mission, and the name was pluralized in 1948 to recognize a more diverse role.[31]

EXPANSION INTO A RESEARCH POWERHOUSE

The NIH today contains 27 component institutes that focus on specific categories of disease or types of therapy. The model for this structure originated in 1937, with the establishment of the National Cancer Institute (NCI). Originally organized as an independent agency, it was formally incorporated into the NIH in 1944. Each institute employs scientists to work in-house in its own laboratories but spends most of its resources funding researchers outside of the government in universities and research institutes.

The intramural research component of NIH's mission gained a major boost in 1940, when the agency opened its sprawling campus in Bethesda, Maryland. Today, it houses one of the largest collections of scientific research buildings in the world. In 1953, a large hospital, the Warren Grant Magnuson Clinical Center, was added to the site. When he dedicated the complex, President Franklin Roosevelt emphasized the significance of the enterprise to national security on the eve of America's entry into World War II by observing, "We must recruit not only men and materials but also knowledge and science in the service of national strength and that is what we are doing here."[32]

If anyone doubted the value of biomedical science to military strength at the time, World War II would have removed any uncertainty. As one observer noted, the war effort "had mobilized a concerted government effort—unprecedented to date—in applying research to practical use."[33] America's success in the war owed a huge debt to a long list of medical advances developed at that time, most of which continue to protect us today. These include penicillin for previously untreatable infections, sulfonamide drugs for wounds and burns, blood derivatives such as gamma globulin for measles and hepatitis, cortisone for inflammations, synthetic quinine for malaria, vaccines to prevent typhus and yellow fever, and DDT for delousing clothing.[34]

The importance of these medical advances was not lost on the public or on politicians. As the war ended, the NIH received significant new authority to maintain its research role. Initially, it received responsibility for phasing out war-time research contracts with universities, but Congress soon changed course and decided that many of these arrangements should remain in place. The agency continued to administer them, and it received additional funding and staff to pursue this mission. The Public Health Service Act of 1944, which had merged NCI into NIH, provided for the creation of additional component institutes, and it set in motion a series of dramatic budget increases that have continued ever since.[35] An NIH budget of $4 million in 1947 grew to $100 million in 1957, to $1 billion in 1974, to more than $27 billion in 2004, and to $30 billion in 2009.[36]

NIH AS THE BACKBONE OF BIOMEDICAL SCIENCE

From the perspective of public policy, the most significant aspect of the steady NIH budget increases is the portion directed to private researchers. About 80 percent of the agency's budget supports studies at universities, research institutes, and similar organizations. Scientists in these settings propose the actual structure of the studies they wish to conduct and the research questions they will pursue. The agency then constitutes committees of experts from outside of the government to determine which of these proposals merit funding. This arrangement shapes the huge research enterprise that the agency supports as a public–private partnership on a massive scale. In the words of one observer: "Never in the nation's history had public funds in such amounts been placed at the disposal of individuals working in support of their own objectives outside the framework of federal institutions."[37]

Over the years since World War II, the nation has looked to the NIH time and again as the first line of attack to address pressing health needs. In 1971, President Richard Nixon launched a "war on cancer" by asking Congress to expand funding for NCI. In the early 1980s, advocates for patients with AIDS lobbied Congress to increase support for NIH research into the disease's cause and potential treatments. In the late 1990s, advocates for patients with Parkinson's disease successfully lobbied for additional NIH funding for research into this condition.[38]

As the nature of medicine has changed, the focus of NIH-sponsored research has evolved along with it. In 1992, the agency added the National Center for Complementary and Alternative Medicine and, in 1993, the National Center on Minority Health and Health Disparities. With all of these changes in funding priorities and focus, the goal of Congress and the desire of much of the public has been to keep the government in the lead in moving American medicine forward.

The influence of the NIH on biomedical science in America extends well beyond its support for individual studies to a role in shaping a key foundation of the research enterprise—building and maintaining the pipeline of new scientists.[39] The agency funds the education of most doctoral students in biomedical sciences, along with the additional postdoctoral training that many of them receive. Before the NIH provided this support, PhDs in biomedical science were relatively rare. Today, those holding these degrees form the workforce that conducts most of the research that leads to new pharmaceutical products. In the words of one observer: "there is no question that the American pharmaceutical and biotechnology industries (which lead the world) could not exist, let alone thrive, without those thousands of trained people."[40]

NIH AS THE INSTIGATOR OF DRUG DEVELOPMENT COLLABORATIONS

When a finding in basic science holds therapeutic promise, the NIH does not have to wait passively for a private company to express interest. It is empowered to proactively seek out a corporate partner to help bring a product to market. This explicit path to collaborative drug development has led to the creation of numerous important medications, some of which have revolutionized medical practice and brought sizeable financial rewards to the private partners involved. Among recent successes along these lines are the development of Thyrogen, a form of thyroid-stimulating hormone commercialized by Genzyme; Prezista, a treatment for HIV infection commercialized by Tibotec; and Gardasil (sold by Merck), a vaccine against the human papilloma virus (HPV), which can cause cervical cancer.[41]

Congress facilitated the process of forming explicit government–industry collaborations such as these through several legislative enactments. It first focused on this area in 1980, the year that a ruling by the Supreme Court permitted the award of patents for artificially engineered life forms. The Court's decision in *Diamond v. Chakrabarty* formed the legal foundation for the rise of the biotechnology industry by offering investors a route to profit from genetically based inventions.[42]

Biotechnology companies seek to commercialize the fruits of academic, government, and industry research; however, the task of coordinating the contributions of each of these sectors can be daunting. They function in separate worlds with vastly different modes of operation. As the nascent industry began to take shape, barriers between them threatened to disrupt potential synergies that could help it to take off.

Congress used several strategies to encourage the growth of the biotechnology industry and the commercialization of biomedical discoveries. A simple one was to offer tax credits to companies that conduct research. These have proven quite valuable to the industry over time.

A more complex strategy with greater far-reaching impact was to create a framework for building explicit partnerships between the federal government and industry. The most important of the laws designed to accomplish this is the Patent and Trademark Law Amendments Act of 1980, commonly known as the Bayh-Dole Act.[43] It gives organizations that receive NIH research grants the right to patent inventions that flow from the fruits of that research. The goal is to give universities and research institutes an incentive to attempt to commercialize research conducted under their auspices.[44]

Despite this incentive, private firms are often reluctant to invest in the initial basic research that is needed before actual product development can begin. To address this gap, Congress developed a mechanism to formalize arrangements between government agencies and private entities to work jointly on the commercialization of breakthrough technologies. This is accomplished through a type of understanding known as a Cooperative Research and Development Agreement, or CRADA. These are partnerships that allow for joint development with a negotiated set of contributions, responsibilities, and remuneration for each party.

CRADAs are based on a series of laws that Congress enacted during the 1980s to encourage the transfer of technology from government labs to private firms that can commercialize them. The primary law is the Stevenson-Wydler Technology Innovation Act of 1980, which established a set of offices to coordinate technology transfer within each federal agency that conducts research.[45] In the NIH, the office is known as the Office of Technology Transfer.[46] An amendment to the law enacted in 1986 as part of the Technology Transfer Act mandated that the federal government actively seek opportunities to transfer technology to industry, academia, or state and local governments, rather than passively waiting for them to arise.[47] This mandate works in tandem with the Bayh-Dole Act, which permits private parties to obtain patent rights to the fruits of these efforts.

Under a CRADA, the government and the private partner share costs in their joint research and development effort. Both may contribute personnel, services, and property, but only the private party may contribute money to avoid triggering federal procurement statutes. The government can grant a license to the ultimate product to the industry partner, or it can simply waive its right of ownership. To reassure companies concerned about trade secrets, the government partner can protect confidential information developed under a CRADA from public disclosure for up to five years.

THE NIH'S ROLE IN CREATING THE FUTURE OF MEDICINE

The NIH began to take an even more active leadership role in advancing medicine in the final years of the twentieth century. In the late 1980s, it began working on several fronts to clear a path for a fundamental transformation of biomedical science based on the emerging field of genomics. Its explicit goal was an ambitious one—to promote a revolution in the understanding of human biology that will lead to products that can be commercialized by private companies. The initiatives that it launched demonstrate more poignantly than any of the agency's past efforts the indispensable role that it plays in fostering the vibrancy of the private health care sector. It is literally creating the future of the pharmaceutical industry. Two endeavors are particularly important in nurturing the private market to realize this transformation of medical science: the Human Genome Project and the National Center for Advancing Translational Sciences.

THE HUMAN GENOME PROJECT

Of all the NIH efforts to advance the scientific foundations of medicine, no initiative comes close in size or significance to the immense endeavor to map the entire set of human genes, known as the Human Genome Project (HGP). This massive enterprise is not only transforming health care at the most fundamental level but also the foundations of biology and even the ways we view ourselves as people. These changes will sweep the pharmaceutical industry along with them in ways we are only beginning to comprehend.

The Quest to Map the Human Genome

The molecular foundation of all living creatures was discovered in 1953, when James Watson and Francis Crick delineated the structure of deoxyribonucleic acid (DNA), the chemical building block of genes. It was a path-breaking finding that earned the two scientists Nobel Prizes. However, applications of this knowledge were relatively slow to advance in the first decades after its discovery. That started to change in the 1970s, when methods were developed to manipulate the genetic structure of microorganisms. With these new techniques, the era of custom-designed life forms began. The door to commercialization of these creations was opened in 1980, with the Supreme Court's ruling in *Diamond v. Chakrabarty*[48] that artificially created life forms could be patented. With legal protection for its inventions assured, the biotechnology industry was born.[49]

Designer microorganisms found an array of uses, but the real promise of genetic science lay in its applications to human health. Many diseases have been found to have genetic causes, making treatment and prevention by conventional means difficult or impossible. By understanding the genetic basis for these conditions, scientists foresaw the possibility of curing or preventing them by manipulating the actual composition of genes. At the least, tests could be devised to determine the extent to which individual patients were susceptible.

During the 1980s, researchers were able to pinpoint the genetic mechanisms behind several devastating conditions and, in some cases, to develop tests to diagnose them. A major breakthrough along these lines was the creation in 1986 of a test for susceptibility to Huntington's disease, a devastating brain affliction caused entirely by genetic factors.[50] However, humans have thousands of genes, and interactions between them can be as important in shaping physiological effects as their individual composition. The full potential of genomic medicine could only be realized if the full set of human genes, known as the human genome, were delineated.

Mapping the entire human genome required a massive effort. However, although the possibilities for improving health were enormous, the specific applications to which it might lead were speculative. This was a prime example of basic research with an indeterminate payoff. Once the map of the genome had been created, it would be a public good that could facilitate research to benefit everyone. Private companies could then develop actual applications based on it to diagnose, treat, and prevent disease. As with other basic research, the natural sponsor for such a venture was the government.

Recognizing the potential need, Congress authorized initial funding in 1988 for a joint effort of the federal Department of Energy and the NIH to map the human genome. In 1990, NIH formally launched the HGP within a new National Human Genome Research Institute. The DOE's role was to promote research into the effects of radiation on genetic mutations. The effort relied both on scientists within the government and on researchers at numerous external organizations.[51]

The HGP's Fruits

The HGP produced a first draft of the genome's map containing 90 percent of its contents in 2001 and a final version in 2002, with the entire set of genes, several years ahead of schedule. The speed was due in part to an implicit, and unexpected, collaboration with the private sector. To pique the interest of private scientists and to encourage them to join the effort, the HGP in 1996 began placing all findings in a public database within 24 hours of their disclosure, with no limits on their use. In 1998, a private company, Celera Corporation, took up the challenge of using this information by initiating an effort to develop a map of its own. A friendly competition ensued, and it ended with HGP and Celera officials jointly announcing in 2000 that they had completed an initial analysis of the genome's sequence.[52]

The HGP's accomplishment in mapping the entire human genome has been called "one of the remarkable achievements in the history of science."[53] It is a singular accomplishment of government-funded science that promises to revolutionize medical care and, with it, the entire pharmaceutical industry. In achieving this milestone, NIH laid the foundation for yet another level of pharmaceutical productivity.

Of course, mapping the genome is only the first step in bringing the promise of genomic medicine to fruition. The next step is to devise applications for this new knowledge. With this step, as with the previous one, a shared enterprise between the government and the private sector led the way.

The enterprise started to take shape almost a decade before the genome map had been completed. As early as 1993, as the first individual genes were identified, NIH scientists began to investigate the function of each and its role in human health and disease. Soon thereafter, several private companies began doing the same. As the overall map started to emerge, several hundred diagnostic tests were developed and initial experiments at actual gene therapy were launched in which new genes were inserted to replace defective ones in patients. The pace of development and of experimentation has continued unabated since ever since.

Genomics today is fast becoming a standard part of medical practice in several areas. Its effect is especially pronounced in the field of oncology. In a particularly important advance, scientists discovered in the 1990s that mutations in two genes that were labeled *BRCA1* and *BRCA2* significantly increase a woman's chance of developing breast and ovarian cancer. A test for these mutations was devised and is now routinely used by clinicians to advise women of their cancer risk. A private company, Myriad Genetics, has administered the test since its was introduced, and it enjoyed market exclusivity until June 2013 when patents that it held on the underlying genes were invalidated by Supreme Court. However, even without patent protection, Myriad's strong market position is likely to continue.[54] Its business of testing for *BRCA* mutations has proven extremely profitable and has attracted considerable interest from investors.[55]

By the time the HGP was completed, it had cost $3.8 billion, $2.8 billion of which came from the NIH. However, the biggest financial payoff from this investment has been in the private sector.[56] An estimate by the Battelle Memorial Institute put the amount of economic activity generated by the HGP at $67 billion a year, including the steady creation of tens of thousands of jobs. Genomics-related industries now employ about 310,000 workers. Battelle pegged the total amount of economic output driven by the HGP as of 2011 at $796 billion and the total amount of personal income generated by this output at $244 billion. This financial growth has returned an estimated $9 billion to the government in increased tax revenue, $3.7 billion of which was generated in 2010 alone.[57]

The Dawn of Personalized Medicine

As remarkable as the HGP's contribution to the private sector has been, its most significant returns are yet to come. Based on their understanding of the human genome, scientists are learning how to customize drugs to the genetic makeup of individual patients. This will enable clinicians to avoid using drugs that are destined to be ineffective or to produce significant adverse reactions in some of those who receive them. Many in the pharmaceutical industry see the dawn of an era of personalized medicine, in which products can be tailored to each patient's metabolic needs. The clinical potential of this new approach to medication is enormous.

As with much of genomics overall, the initial focus of personalized medicine in pharmaceuticals has been in oncology. Drugs that treat cancer are notorious for the variability of their effectiveness. Chemotherapy agents that achieve miracle remissions in some patients leave others with no improvement. Physicians have long suspected that the genetic makeup of patients, and of their tumors, is crucial in determining how they will respond. With a genetic profile in hand, they can predict responsiveness before a drug is administered. Several targeted medications have been developed for use with companion diagnostic tests in patients with specific sequences of genes, including Herceptin for metastatic breast cancer, Erbitux for metastatic colorectal cancer, and Gleevec for gastrointestinal tumors.[58]

Based on the HGP's map of the genome, new treatments tailored to genetic profiles will continue to emerge. Eventually, they will replace many of the conventional medicines in use today. Their introduction will transform the scientific and economic foundations of the pharmaceutical industry, thanks to a major initiative, the HGP, launched and funded by the government.

NATIONAL CENTER FOR ADVANCING TRANSLATIONAL SCIENCES

Although there have been many success stories, the bridge between basic research and commercial applications can sometimes be difficult to cross. With drugs taking up to a decade and hundreds of millions of dollars to bring from concept to market and a failure rate of more than 95 percent, pharmaceutical companies often hesitate to commit the needed resources when the end result is uncertain. This reluctance is most often displayed when a drug represents a novel approach to treatment that does not yet have a track record, a category that includes most genomic drugs. As a result, companies have been slower to delve into genetic drug development than many medical experts had initially hoped.

The pipelines of conventional drugs wending their way through the testing and development process began to shrink in the 1990, and, consequently, the rate of FDA approvals for new drugs based on novel therapeutic approaches began to decline.[59] Rather than taking the chance of achieving breakthroughs in genomics, many companies became risk averse and took the opposite course of reducing investments in research.[60] At the same time, venture capital firms started to hesitate in providing investment capital to small biotechnology companies for risky forays into genetics. Progress toward realizing the full promise of genetic medicine slowed dramatically as the industry grappled with the confines of its traditional economic model.

For the NIH, the hesitation of private industry to commercialize the fruits of government-funded basic research represented a threat to its underlying mission. Historically, the agency has been able to rely on the profit potential of new drugs to motivate industry to move drugs from concepts to clinical applications. If companies are unable or unwilling to do so, then the growing array of NIH- funded scientific discoveries will lie fallow.

The NIH as a Proactive Partner

In the reluctance of private companies to commercialize genomics and personalized medicine, the agency saw the need to move proactively. If industry were not in a position to create its future on its own, the government would have to do it. For several years, NIH considered ways in which it could take the lead in turning genetic discoveries into marketable products. In its view, the gap between basic and clinical research required a new form of investigation that would translate scientific findings into potential applications. This scientific endeavor has come to be called "translational research."

The job of stimulating this new kind of scientific inquiry called for novel approaches. Starting in the early 2000s, the NIH began identifying and implementing several of them with the goal of attacking the problem from different angles. The focus of its efforts was on enticing researchers into the new field and providing them with appropriate training. To that end, the NIH funded "pioneer awards" to support creative problem solving. It also devoted funding to facilities and to training of investigators. It promoted the creation of new resources, such as clinical trial networks, biospecimen repositories, and molecular screening libraries, and considered ways of restructuring itself to better accommodate its emerging translational role. The first step in this process was to launch a new funding program known as "Clinical and Translational Science Awards" to promote the development of academic centers to support translational work.[61]

The NIH's bureaucratic reshaping took a dramatic turn in 2010, with a proposal for a new center within the agency devoted explicitly to translating genomic science into clinical applications. The National Center for Advancing Translational Sciences was conceived that year and implemented in 2011. Its mission is to identify and remedy "bottlenecks" that stand between scientific discovery and clinical applications. In the view of the NIH director who initiated the proposal, Dr. Francis Collins, these arise in large part from the novelty of the paradigm for genetic drug development.[62] Genomics, he believed, involves a new scientific model such that "the entire framework of medical taxonomy requires rethinking."[63]

The biggest bottlenecks lie between the discovery of genes that can cause diseases and the initiation of research to test ways to control them. Without an established drug development road to follow, companies are reluctant to forge ahead on new ones. In a market-based economy, each company looks to its own interests. For many pharmaceutical firms that are peering ahead at a dramatically altered economic landscape, that means limiting exposure to financial risk. The safest course is to stand aside and let others test the waters. This leaves the government as the only entity with the mission of protecting larger national interests and the resources to do so.

The Center focuses its efforts on the initial steps in the drug development process: the time when drug testing begins and when the process is least attractive for private investors because the chances of success are most uncertain and the expected cost is greatest. It carries the ball for new drugs through as much of this phase as necessary until a private company feels comfortable taking over. It starts with preclinical studies both in laboratories and in animals and will follow this with testing in humans if a drug candidate seems promising. If the drug fails, the government will have borne the cost. If it succeeds through this phase, the chance that it will eventually reach the market is greatly enhanced. At that point, the Center will actively seek a private partner.

The new Center does not actually try to bring new drugs to market. The NIH is not interested in moving into the commercial sphere. The goal is, instead, to create the conditions that enable the competitive market to work in bringing genomic therapies to patients as it has with traditional drugs. As the pillar that has supported private pharmaceutical innovation for the better part of the past century, the NIH stands eager to extend that mission into this new terrain.

It seems that the more scientists learn about the way genes function, the more they find they have to learn to apply discoveries to the needs of patients. That requires a robust private sector to commercialize new products. However, the investment in basic knowledge that is required is still too great to entice most pharmaceutical firms to make the leap. The scientific infrastructure does not yet exist to translate the new paradigm of biomedical research into a market-based business. Industry needs the government to create that business, and, as it has in so many other ways, the NIH has taken up the challenge.

Government Support for the Pharmaceutical Industry Beyond NIH

Although the role of NIH is invaluable in generating the essential intellectual fuel on which the pharmaceutical research engine runs, it is far from being the only major government program that supports and maintains the industry. Drug companies depend on a range of other public initiatives, both directly and indirectly, for much of their economic viability. A few of them add particularly significant support.

Prescription drugs are sold in the United States largely through a private market, but it is one that has come to rely almost entirely on third-party payment by insurance plans. In 1960, insurance covered 4 percent of prescription drug spending in the United States.[64] In 2008, that portion was almost 80 percent. The most dramatic change occurred during the 1990s, when the share increased from 44.5 to 72.3 percent. As the rate of coverage has grown, the fraction of insurance represented by private and by public sources has remained about the same.

In 2010, government programs picked up the tab for more than $79 billion of the $259 billion that Americans spent on outpatient prescription drugs. The two largest contributors were Medicare at more than $59 billion and Medicaid at more than $20 billion.[65] In addition to drugs taken on an outpatient basis, these programs also pay billions of dollars a year for drugs administered in physicians' offices and to hospital inpatients.

Medicare first covered outpatient drugs in 2006, when Part D of the program was launched. In 2010, this benefit represented 11 percent of the program's overall budget.[66] Medicare covers prescription drugs administered in a physician's office through Part B and has done so since the program's inception in 1966. Additional drug spending comes through payments to hospitals for inpatient care under Part A and also through several other aspects of the program's coverage, including reimbursement for nursing care and for hospital outpatient services.

Medicaid covers outpatient prescription drugs in all states.[67] In 2008, this expenditure represented about 10 percent of the program's budget nationally. In many states, it also represents the fastest growing category of spending.

Some patients need thousands of dollars a year in prescription drugs. These customers would be locked out of the market for these life-saving products were coverage by a third-party payer not available.[68] By providing the financial means to help patients such as these purchase drugs, insurance increases both the size of the potential market for pharmaceutical companies and the amounts they can charge for their products.

Not surprisingly, growth in insurance coverage for prescription drugs has tracked growth in overall national drug spending. During the 1990s, when the rate of coverage almost doubled, overall prescription expenditures also experienced their highest level of increase, almost tripling from $40.3 billion to $120.6 billion. The trend continued during the early 2000s, when Medicare prescription spending rose from $2 billion in 2000 to over $39 billion in 2006 with the launch of Part D. During these six years, overall national prescription drug expenditures almost doubled, from $120.6 billion to $217 billion.[69]

The pharmaceutical industry was robust and profitable long before Medicare and Medicaid began covering its products. It undoubtedly still would have been a major economic presence even without them. It is also possible that some patients who rely on these programs might have been able to find alternative insurance in the private market or to pay more of the cost out of their own pockets. However, it is unlikely that Americans would have been able to come up with $79 billion a year for prescriptions on their own. Beyond funding the creation of new drugs through NIH, the government has positioned itself as the most important consumer in the private market through which these drugs are sold.

QUALITY ASSURANCE THROUGH THE FDA

It is difficult to sell a product if the public has no confidence in it. That is all the more true if the product can cause serious injury or death. This is the position the pharmaceutical industry is in when it sells medicines that can achieve miraculous benefits in some cases but that, under some circumstances, can produce significant harm.

Americans, by and large, trust the safety of the drugs their doctors prescribe. There have certainly been instances in which hazardous products have reached the market, but, most of the time, a vast apparatus of quality oversight keeps that from happening. The public reassurance that this engenders is crucial to sustaining the industry. If patients worried that they could be injured every time they filled a prescription, many would balk at filling them and many doctors at writing them.

THE GROWTH OF FDA AUTHORITY THROUGH SCANDALS

The source of public trust on which the pharmaceutical market relies was almost entirely created and is almost entirely maintained by the government. It begins with oversight of the professions most directly involved in bringing drugs to patients. Physicians who decide what drugs a patient should take do so under licenses granted by the state in which they practice. Pharmacists who dispense the prescriptions are also licensed by their state. Licensure provides for a review of basic qualifications before these professionals begin practice and ongoing supervision of their quality.[70]

However, the greatest source of reassurance for patients is in the quality of the drugs themselves, which is provided by the FDA. The agency came into being in 1906, at a time when pharmaceutical manufacturing could hardly be called an industry. Drugs were as likely to be sold by a physician or compounded by a pharmacist as to be centrally manufactured. The range of available drugs and their capabilities were extremely limited. Most of the products that are commonly used today, including almost all antibiotics, had yet to be invented. The law that created the FDA, the Pure Food and Drug Act, was passed after scandals involving two popular cold remedies were described in the popular press.[71] Those revelations, along with publication in 1906 of *The Jungle* by Upton Sinclair, which exposed dangerous and unsanitary conditions in the meatpacking industry, had undermined public confidence in the food and drug supply.[72]

Congress expanded the FDA's authority and created the basic regulatory structure that oversees the nation's drug supply today about 30 years later, after another major scandal revealed a serious flaw in the 1906 legislation. The old law had given the FDA authority to pull drugs from the market if they were found to be dangerous and to prevent further sale of them. It also permitted the agency to block manufacturers from making false claims about the composition of their products. However, before the FDA could act, the product and the claims about it had to have already reached the public.

In 1937, a dangerous antibiotic preparation entered the market without sufficient testing of its safety. Elixir of sulfanilamide contained a mixture of an antibiotic and a sweet-tasting solvent that made it appealing to children. The solvent turned out to be highly toxic, with a chemical structure that was similar to antifreeze. By December of that year, it had caused 107 deaths in 15 states, mostly of children. The FDA banned the manufacturer from selling any more of it, but was only empowered under existing law to act after the harm had already been done.[73]

In response, Congress tightened the restrictions on drug marketing in 1938 to require that the FDA review the safety of new drugs before they could reach patients. Under new authority granted to it by the Food, Drug and Cosmetic Act, the agency implemented a regulatory scheme under which new drugs must undergo years of testing before they may be sold.[74] The process starts with preclinical laboratory studies of drug effects including tests in animals and continues with three phases of clinical trials in human subjects.

These studies can take eight years or more to complete. All of the results must be submitted to the FDA for review before a drug can be approved. When manufacturing of the drug begins, the agency inspects the plants where it will be made for compliance with standards for safety and cleanliness. It also monitors ongoing use of the drug for signs of adverse effects.

This new regulatory arrangement averted a public health catastrophe about 20 years later. FDA approval was sought for a new drug known as thalidomide that was thought to be helpful when taken by pregnant women in preventing miscarriages and that also worked as a sleeping pill. It had already been approved and was widely prescribed in Europe. However, as use of it spread, so did reports of severe birth defects in the children of women who had taken it. By 1962, there had been more than 5,000 such reports worldwide. In response, the FDA slowed its review process to allow more time for information to accumulate. The link between thalidomide and birth defects eventually became clear and was widely reported in the press. Before the agency had made a final determination, the application for approval was withdrawn.[75]

Had the 1938 law not been in effect at the time, the FDA would have lacked authority to keep thalidomide off the market while it considered the news from Europe of devastating adverse effects. There is no way to know how many tragic birth defects would have occurred in the United States before the agency could have gathered enough evidence to pull it from the market, but it is likely that the number would have been considerable. In response to this near miss, Congress strengthened the FDA's authority yet again in 1962, with passage of the Harris-Kefauver Amendments.[76] These require that manufacturers establish a drug's efficacy in addition to its safety before the FDA can permit patients to receive it.

Additional refinements and enhancements of the FDA's authority have been enacted over the years. However, prior review of safety and efficacy remain the primary basis on which it approves new drugs. Pharmaceutical firms maintain a massive premarket testing apparatus to generate data to meet the agency's demands for information with which to conduct these assessments.

THE FDA TODAY

The FDA regulatory apparatus as it exists today is far from perfect. A number of drugs have been pulled from the market or subjected to heightened warnings years after approval when new safety hazards have come to light.[77] Moreover, the drug safety oversight process can also be prone to political influence. The pharmaceutical industry spends more than $100 million a year on lobbying, the highest amount of any industry.[78] These funds are spent on attempts to mold government policy on a range of issues, including the conduct of drug safety reviews. For example, the industry has fought vigorously to block the reimportation of drugs into the United States from foreign countries, framing it as a safety hazard. It has also campaigned through lobbying and through lawsuits to loosen restrictions that the FDA has imposed on marketing, such as limitations on television advertising of prescription medications and on promotion of drugs for uses that have not been approved.

Critics also charge that the industry insinuates itself into individual FDA review proceedings by forging ties with scientific experts on whom the agency relies for advice. The FDA often convenes an advisory committee composed of prominent researchers as part of its review of a new drug. It is quite common for members of these committees to have financial relationships with the manufacturer of a drug they are evaluating. For example, they may have served as consultants or accepted funding for their research. The agency maintains rules to limit such conflicts of interest, but the rules do not eliminate all conflicts, and studies have shown that experts with financial ties to a manufacturer tend to view its products favorably.[79]

For its part, the industry often complains that the process is stacked against it.[80] The clinical trials manufacturers must conduct to gain approval can sometimes take a decade or more to conduct. The FDA can protract the timeframe even further with requests for additional data. Once the trials have been completed, the agency can take up to two years to make a final decision. From the perspective of many pharmaceutical companies, the agency is a bureaucratic maze that favors excessive caution over promoting medical innovation. And, all the while it spends deliberating, the clock is ticking on the patent that protects the manufacturer from competition.

Without question, regulatory agencies such as the FDA can face considerable political pressures.[81] That is the nature of governmental oversight in a democracy. As a result, the process of drug safety review perennially invites calls for reform.

However, incidents of drugs entering the market with unknown and devastating side effects are relatively rare. Countless drug candidates have been blocked before reaching the public because of safety concerns that arise during the years of premarket clinical testing. At the least, the public knows that a tremendous amount of attention has been directed toward the safety of the drugs that are prescribed. Application of consistent regulatory standards also adds stability to the market by reassuring private companies and investors that products will be judged through an established scientific process.[82]

The FDA today is one of the most trusted agencies of the federal government. In a 2004 poll, 70 percent of the respondents reported having either a great deal or a moderate amount of confidence in it.[83] Although consumer advocates may complain about undue industry influence, and the industry may complain about bureaucratic inefficiency, the agency still inspires a basic level of confidence in the drug supply.[84] It does this by offering a stamp of approval for the industry's products that only an outside impartial force like the government can provide.

Direct Government Market Support

The government also acts affirmatively to shape the private market for pharmaceuticals by developing and sustaining key sectors that might otherwise not exist. These efforts guide the market in directions it would not have taken on its own. A few of them have been particularly influential.

FACILITATING A MARKET FOR GENERICS

Most importantly, the government has fashioned the competitive dynamics of the pharmaceutical market by facilitating the entry of generic drugs. These products include the same active ingredient as an existing drug, and they may be sold once the patent on that molecule has expired. Generic copies usually sell at much lower prices than the original drug and thereby bring an important element of competition to the market that can help control costs.

The Hatch-Waxman Act speeds the regulatory approval of generics by permitting their manufacturers to piggyback on the results of clinical trials for the original patented product. Rather than repeating all phases of testing, they only have to show that their version is comparable to the original in the amount that the body absorbs. This means that testing can be completed more quickly and cheaply than it would if a full set of trials for safety and efficacy were required. To speed the process further, testing of a generic copy can begin while the original drug's patent is still in force. With this head start, the generic company can have its product approved and ready to be sold as soon as the patent expires.[85]

The Hatch-Waxman Act has dramatically reshaped the market for generic drugs. In 1984, the year it was passed, generics represented just 18.6 percent of American pharmaceutical sales. By 1997, that share had grown to 44.3 percent. Today, most prescriptions filled in the United States are for generics.[86] The ripples of this turnaround have changed the landscape for brand name drugs as well. With the threat of vigorous generic competition looming once a patent expires, large pharmaceutical companies cannot rely on a stock of established products to generate profits indefinitely. They must continuously fill their pipelines with new drugs that have fresh patent clocks. This is a competitive force that the market would lack were it not for yet another form of active government intervention.

CREATING A MARKET FOR ORPHAN DRUGS

In 1983, Congress authorized the FDA to aid drug companies in producing medications for rare diseases when it passed the Orphan Drug Act.[87] These uncommon ailments are known as "orphan diseases" because the small number of patients who suffer from them leaves potential treatments with a meager potential market that is insufficient to generate profits. They include numerous conditions that are debilitating and even life-threatening, such as Huntington's disease, myoclonus, Lou Gehrig's disease, Tourette's syndrome, and muscular dystrophy.[88]

The Act authorized grants, tax credits, and seven years of additional market exclusivity beyond a patent's expiration for drugs that are designed to treat conditions afflicting fewer than 200,000 people in the United States. The FDA also gives these products special consideration in the approval process. With this government boost, more than 300 treatments for orphan diseases received FDA approval in the 25 years following the law's enactment, compared with only 10 during the previous 10 years.[89]

CREATING A MARKET FOR PEDIATRIC PHARMACEUTICALS

Another significant gap in the private pharmaceutical market has been in the attention paid by major companies to the needs of children. Clinical testing for pediatric drugs can be difficult and risky. Children often react differently than adults to medications, and adverse effects can be much more severe. To avoid the risks, most clinical trials include only adults as subjects. As a result, the safety and efficacy of new drugs when used to treat children are rarely known when the drugs are first approved.

Although pediatric testing may not make financial sense for private companies, there is still a significant need to determine how children will react to new drugs. To remedy this gap in market incentives, Congress in 1997 authorized special incentives to encourage companies to conduct clinical trials in children in the form of FDAMA.[90] That law offered companies a reward of six months of additional market exclusivity after a patent expires for drugs that have undergone pediatric testing. Two subsequent laws passed in 2002 and 2003 expanded the agency's authority to push companies to study and develop drugs for children.[91] These laws are credited with inducing manufacturers to conduct a substantial number of pediatric studies, thereby expanding the market for many new pharmaceutical products.[92]

THE FDA AND THE FUTURE OF GENOMIC MEDICINE

A final government initiative to expand the pharmaceutical market arose not from a program enacted by Congress but from the FDA acting on its own. In 2010, without waiting for new legislation, the agency took the initiative to prod the market to respond to the challenge of commercializing genomic medicine when it entered into a partnership with the NIH to facilitate the advance of translational science.[93] Under this arrangement, the NIH promotes research and training, while the FDA encourages companies to integrate genomics into their drug development processes. To that end, it tries to coordinate the review of genetic diagnostic tests that predict responsiveness to drugs with reviews of the drugs themselves. The goal is to facilitate the development of diagnostic-therapeutic combination approaches that aid clinicians, along with a review process that reassures companies that new technologies in which they invest will receive priority review.

The NIH-FDA partnership builds on the NIH's initiatives in translational medicine to extend the government infrastructure on which the nascent market for genomic medicine rests. In doing so, it will help to promote an even larger and more robust private pharmaceutical industry. The agencies acted on the belief that the market will not grow on its own but rather requires assistance from its indispensable partner, the government. In a joint statement, the heads of the agencies described the model they created as a logical extension of the paradigm on which so much of American industry is built:

> When the federal government created the national highway system, it did not tell people where to drive—it built the roads and set the standards for safety.

Those investments supported a revolution in transportation, commerce, and personal mobility. We are now building a national highway system for personalized medicine, with substantial investments in infrastructure and standards.[94]

More Government Subsidies Through Tax Breaks

In addition to all of these forms of support, the government also lends drug companies assistance of a more direct kind. It gives them money in the form of tax credits. This financial boost lets pharmaceutical firms lower their tax bills, and thereby keep more of their income, by devoting resources to research. Although the nature of the credits has changed over time with amendments to the federal tax code, the underlying mechanism of paying private companies to conduct research has remained.[95]

Three kinds of tax credit are available to companies. A research and experimentation credit allows them to lower their taxes in return for increasing the amount they spend on in-house research. A basic research credit encourages companies to fund scientific investigations at universities. The orphan drug credit rewards the development of drugs for rare diseases as part of the Orphan Drug Act. These inducements, worth a total of about $5 billion a year, do not significantly alter the nature of the industry, and the benefits tend to accrue mainly to larger companies. However, they help to encourage the overall growth of the private research enterprise.[96]

The Most Essential Government Support of All: Patents

Beneath the billions of dollars and intricate web of laws and regulations that comprise the government's active intervention to create and sustain the private pharmaceutical market lies an even more fundamental pillar: the protection that patent laws confer on its products. Without these laws, the industry could not exist in anything close to its present form.

Patents grant inventors 20 years from the date of filing to prevent anyone else from manufacturing, distributing, or selling their inventions. In effect, inventors enjoy a monopoly during this time and can take advantage of the lack of competition to set prices above those that an unrestricted market would sustain. The actual amount of time during which drugs can be marketed exclusively under a patent is less than the full 20 years in practice because clinical testing and FDA review can eat up as much as half of the full patent term. However, the time remaining once marketing has begun has been more than sufficient to support ample profits for most products. Moreover, the exclusive sales period is often extended by other laws, such as the Hatch-Waxman Act and FDAMA.

The exclusive marketing protection granted by patents is vital to the pharmaceutical industry.[97] Companies rely on patent protection as the bedrock of their economic model. Monopoly prices allow them to recoup research and development costs for patented products, amass funding to investigate new products that may not make it to market, and generate substantial financial returns. These prices provide the economic underpinning for the emergence of blockbuster drugs that bring companies billions of dollars in sales each year.

The law of patents is rooted in the US Constitution, which authorizes Congress to protect property rights in inventions.[98] The patent system that Congress established to effect this constitutional directive is administered by the Patent and Trademark Office (PTO), which decides whether inventions meet the criteria for patentability. Patents were not included in the Constitution or implemented by Congress with the pharmaceutical industry specifically in mind. They form a key underpinning of our entire economic system. Nevertheless, their application to drugs forms an indispensable part of the infrastructure that supports private pharmaceutical companies. Without this government foundation, the industry would take on a very different, and less profitable, form.

Government Support in Action: Case Studies of Medical Miracles

Whether they realize it or not, everyone who has taken a prescription drug during the past 50 years has experienced the effects of public–private collaborations firsthand. It would be difficult to identify a medication developed during that time that did not emerge from a base of at least some government-funded research. Medications for high blood pressure, high cholesterol, cancer, depression, and Parkinson's disease, to name just a few, grew out of government-funded research findings. A significant early example is penicillin, the first broadly effective antibiotic and progenitor of a revolution in the treatment of infections, which emerged from a collaborative enterprise in which the government played a critical role.[99] Along with the success of these drugs have ridden the financial fortunes of many major pharmaceutical firms.

Prime examples of successful public–private drug development sit inside the medicine cabinets of millions of Americans. Some reflect the importance of the implicit partnership between NIH-funded discoveries and industry commercialization under collaborations that evolved over time. Others emerged from an explicit effort by the NIH to identify and work with a corporate ally. Whatever the approach, in conventional drug development, private industry takes the laboring oar in vetting drug candidates after government-funded based research has pointed it in promising directions.

THE TRADITIONAL MODEL: AN AD HOC GIVE AND TAKE

The implicit model of drug development collaboration is illustrated by one of the most ubiquitous medications in the world—statins. Since the first one was introduced in 1987, these drugs have revolutionized cardiac treatment and created an entirely new approach to preventive care.[100] They have also come to represent a financial bonanza for several manufacturers.

The Story of Statins

Statins are among the most important pharmacological therapies in medical practice. They are used by millions of people worldwide to reduce blood cholesterol
levels and have proven extremely effective at preventing heart attacks, strokes, and
other heart-related ailments. Heart disease is the most common cause of death in
the United States and around the world, and much of it results from the buildup
of cholesterol plaque in the arteries.[101] In preventing heart-related ailments, statins
have saved millions of lives.

Because of their effectiveness at forestalling the most common deadly condition on Earth, statins have also come to represent a powerful financial force
in the pharmaceutical industry. Lipitor is the prime example as the most widely
prescribed drug in the United States for several years. In 2005, it generated $16
billion in sales derived from 144.5 million prescriptions. In 2006, physicians wrote
an average of 13.1 million Lipitor prescriptions each month.[102]

The Link Between Cholesterol and Heart Disease

The link between cholesterol and heart disease was first noted more than 100 years
ago. Dr. Rudolph Virchow, a German pathologist, observed on autopsy that
patients who died of vascular conditions in which the arteries were narrowed,
like heart attacks, often had thickened and irregular arterial walls.[103] He found
that the arteries in these patients were coated with a yellowish fatty substance,
which he identified as cholesterol. Dr. Virchow was not able to explain the role
of cholesterol in the pathological changes he observed or how it got there, but
he raised the intriguing possibility that this kind of fat could be connected with
heart disease.

The first clear evidence of a causal relationship between high levels of blood
cholesterol and the buildup of plaque in artery walls came from a large long-
term epidemiological investigation of risk factors for heart disease known as the
Framingham Heart Study. That research, funded by the NIH, involved a massive
effort to follow more than 10,000 residents of Framingham, Massachusetts, starting in 1948, to observe changes in a range of physiological markers and health
outcomes over time. In the 1960s, results of the research began pointing to high
levels of serum cholesterol as a key culprit in the narrowing of arteries that could
be a precursor to heart attacks.[104]

The Framingham Heart Study was the most extensive epidemiological investigation up to that time. The thousands of study participants received thorough
physical examinations and extensive blood testing on an annual basis over the
course of decades, with a cost that reached tens of millions of dollars. When the
project began, the benefits of this huge investment were largely speculative because
it was not possible to predict what the study would actually find. With no obvious commercial application, this was an ideal project for government sponsorship
through the NIH.[105]

The government's support for the study paid off handsomely. The most widely
known result is the identification of high cholesterol as a major cause of cardiac
disease, but it also identified over ten other risk factors, including salt intake and

smoking. Much of what is known today about heart disease and its prevention stems from this seminal research.[106]

The Hunt for a Way to Lower Blood Cholesterol

Once the Framingham Heart Study had identified cholesterol as a potential killer, basic research into its molecular composition began in earnest. Scientists were particularly interested in figuring out how it is synthesized in the body. Blood cholesterol can come from both external and internal sources. It enters the body from the outside through dietary intake of fatty foods. It is produced internally through synthesis in the liver. Dietary changes alone are often effective in reducing a patient's blood level, but when they are not, controlling cholesterol's internal manufacture represents the most likely alternative approach.

Research to explore the body's mechanisms of cholesterol synthesis was conducted by scientists during the 1960s at several universities and research institutes, including Harvard, the University of California at Los Angeles, the Max Planck Institute in Munich, and the National Institute for Medical Research in London. The NIH funded most of the research that was carried out in the United States. The results of this work delineated the steps that lead to the liver's manufacture of cholesterol and identified a way to disrupt the process by blocking the action of a key enzyme known as HMG-CoA reductase.[107] These findings set the stage for a search for drugs that might serve this function.[108]

The first challenge in finding a drug candidate was to locate a reliable source of the enzyme to use in tests. In 1960, a method was devised for isolating it from baker's yeast, along with a test to determine whether a drug candidate was effective at inhibiting its activity. These techniques were based on technologies that had been developed in the 1950s with support from the NIH and the National Science Foundation (NSF), another federal agency that funds basic science research.[109]

With the technology in place to conduct the search, the hunt began for inhibitor molecules. In the early 1970s, it peaked the interest of private pharmaceutical firms. One company in particular, Sankyo Pharmaceuticals in Japan, devised a method for evaluating molecular candidates in molds.[110] In 1976, it found one in a species related to the strain of mold that produces penicillin and gave it the name compactin. However, to test it on a large scale, sufficient quantities had to be produced. This was accomplished with technologies that had, again, been developed with support from the NIH and the NSF. These included x-ray crystallography and infrared and nuclear magnetic resonance (NMR) spectroscopy, which are used in a range of different kinds of basic and applied research.[111]

A Private Manufacturer Tests the Waters

The final step was to identify a molecule based on compactin that could be ingested as a drug to block the liver's synthesis of cholesterol and then to refine techniques to produce it in large quantities. That required a pharmaceutical company that would see the process through and try to bring a product to market. The first to take up the challenge was Merck. However, even in this commercial endeavor, it was only by collaborating with the government that success was achieved.

In 1979, scientists at Merck isolated an inhibitor molecule that seemed a likely drug candidate, a substance known as lovastatin that is similar to compactin. The company soon initiated clinical trials to examine its safety and effectiveness. Unfortunately for the effort, at about this time, the World Health Organization reported results of a clinical trial of another new lipid-lowering drug, and they were extremely disappointing. There was actually a higher mortality rate for patients on the drug than for those on a placebo. Then, in 1980, Merck received reports suggesting that compactin could cause cancer in dogs. The company's CEO, P. Roy Vagelos, who had strongly championed the quest for a cholesterol synthesis blocker, decided to terminate the clinical trials.[112]

With the private sector faltering in the quest for what promised to be a miracle drug, the government decided to step back in. Officials at FDA began working with Merck to help it to restart its efforts. Although some see the agency as a barrier that slows the process of drug development, in this case, it was the instigator that kept the process going. The FDA convinced Merck to make lovastatin available to researchers at Oregon Health Sciences University and at the University of Texas. Once these supplies were in the hands of academic researchers, the agency granted them permission to conduct new trials on human subjects. Merck also agreed to grant the investigators access to the drug's master file, the collection of public and proprietary information on it that the company had accumulated and that the FDA maintained.[113]

In 1984, the gloom surrounding the prospects for statins started to lift with encouraging news on two fronts. Results of a large clinical trial released that year showed that cholesterol lowering by any means, whether dietary changes or medications, could produce a significant drop in heart disease and death. And new genetic research on patients with high cholesterol succeeded in elucidating the means by which the most dangerous kind of cholesterol, low density lipoprotein (LDL), is disposed of by the liver.[114] The scientists who made that discovery, Dr. Michael Brown and Dr. Joseph Goldstein, were awarded the Nobel Prize the following year.[115]

With prospects looking up for lowering cholesterol pharmacologically stemming from the university-based research, Merck revived its own work on lovastatin in 1984. It was not long before the company had accumulated enough data to submit an application to the FDA for approval to market the drug. The agency took only nine months to act on lovastatin, one of the shortest approval times up to that point in the agency's history. Once the FDA had acted, Merck began marketing lovastatin under the brand name Zocor in 1987. It brought another statin, mevinolin, to the market at about the same time under the name Mevacor. By 1998, sales of Zocor had reached $4.7 billion worldwide.[116]

Other drug companies soon got into the act, and, over the next few years, several additional statins entered the market. These included Lipitor, from the Parke-Davis division of Warner-Lambert, now a part of Pfizer; Pravacol from Sankyo and Bristol-Myers Squibb; and Lescol from Novartis. Most of these products became blockbuster drugs, generating more than $1 billion in annual sales and serving as financial anchors for the companies that sold them.[117]

The Next Generation of Statins

Even with this remarkable clinical and economic success, work to improve the effectiveness of statins continued. Scientists were especially interested in finding new inhibitors of cholesterol synthesis that might be easier to produce in large quantities. The work relied heavily on computer graphics programs developed at the University of California at San Diego that permitted researchers to visualize and manipulate the three-dimensional structure of molecules. Previous methods of testing new drug candidates had required that they actually be synthesized, a much more expensive and time-consuming process. Computer graphics allowed molecules to be vetted based on computational models. The software behind this capability grew out of research funded by the NSF and the Department of Defense. It led to the creation of new statins that were simpler in structure and substantially cheaper to produce, including fluvastatin by Sandoz and atorvastatin by the ParkeDavis division of Warner-Lambert.[118]

Statins today are a mainstay of cardiac care and prevention. Over one-quarter of all Americans over the age of 45 take them.[119] They generate more than $30 billion in sales worldwide.[120] Lipitor has not only been the top selling drug in the world for several years but is also the world's all-time best-selling prescription drug, with cumulative sales of more than $130 billion.[121]

Aside from their staggering economic success, statins are remarkable drugs clinically. They substantially reduce the risk of serious cardiac events, including heart attacks, an accomplishment that had only been dreamed of in the years before they became available. Their development after decades of public–private collaboration saved countless lives, prevented untold suffering, and avoided incalculable treatment costs.

THE FORMAL APPROACH

Statins emerged from accumulations of basic research that built up over time and increasingly pointed to clinical applications. Collaborations between the public and private sectors that produced the final products evolved as the discoveries emerged. The arrangements in statin development were sometimes implicit and occasionally spontaneous. Other drugs develop along a different path. They emerge from explicit partnerships between the government and private companies, most commonly in the form of CRADAs.

A Miracle in the Woods and the Development of Taxol

Perhaps the most prominent example of success from an explicit collaboration is the development of Taxol, the best-selling cancer drug in history. It has extended the lives of thousands of woman suffering from ovarian and breast cancer and brought billions of dollars in revenue to several private companies. And it never would have been invented but for decades of effort by government scientists and millions of dollars of investment by government agencies.

Search the Forest

In 1960, Arthur Barclay, a botanist working for the United States Department of Agriculture (USDA), began an innovative field project in the Gifford Pinchot

National Forest near the town Packwood, Washington, close to Mount St. Helens. His work was part of an effort to explore the region's flora for medicinal properties. The investigations led him to focus on the bark of the Pacific yew tree, which he suspected of having a range of biological effects.[122]

Acting on his suspicions, Barclay collected and dried samples of the yew tree's bark and, in 1962, sent some to a laboratory of the US Department of Agriculture (USDA) located in Maryland. Researchers there and at the NCI, one of the NIH's component agencies, had become interested in screening naturally occurring chemicals as agents to fight cancer, and the agencies had entered into an agreement a few years earlier to cooperate in vetting plant samples. The scientists tested Barclay's samples for a range of possible effects, and the results confirmed his initial conjecture concerning the value of yew bark. One of the tests revealed significant activity in inhibiting cancer cell cultures.

Over the next several decades, Barclay's finding came to revolutionize treatment for certain types of breast and ovarian cancer. Today, the fruits of his work take the form of the drug paclitaxel, which is sold under the brand name Taxol.[123] Many consider it a wonder drug, and it is a life-saver for thousands of cancer patients. It was later discovered also to have another, quite different medical use as the coating for cardiac stents that hold open clogged arteries in patients with heart disease.[124]

Public–Private Collaboration to Produce a Drug

The story of Taxol is a tale of different sectors of the country's scientific enterprise working together under the structure that Congress had developed to promote such cooperation. After the USDA's initial finding of Taxol's potential anticarcinogenic effects, efforts began in earnest to isolate the active compound involved. Research was conducted within the USDA, at the NCI, and at several universities and private research institutes supported by NIH grants. In 1971, after almost a decade of effort, Drs. Monroe Wall and M. D. Wani of Research Triangle Institute announced that they had identified the chemical structure of the seemingly miraculous substance. In 1979, researchers at the Albert Einstein College of Medicine in New York delineated the mechanism through which it works.[125]

The NCI received permission from the FDA to begin clinical trials of the drug in 1982.[126] As these studies progressed through the 1980s, they increasingly pointed to effectiveness in treating the disease. Final results of the second phase of the clinical trials were released in 1988 and showed a response rate of 30 percent among patients with the most virulent form of ovarian cancer.[127] In some tests, the rate was as high as 60 percent. Such positive findings were unprecedented for an anticancer agent.

Not surprisingly, Taxol's success led to a surge in demand for it. However, sufficient supplies were difficult to come by. The original process for extracting Taxol required between 10,000 and 30,000 pounds of dried bark to produce 1 kilogram of the drug. The NCI estimated that in order to treat all the ovarian cancer patients who needed Taxol, 360,000 yew trees would have to be harvested every year, which made its use impractical.[128]

The answer was to create a synthetic version, and scientists in the United States, Asia, and Europe labored through the 1980s toward this goal. They achieved success in 1989, when researchers at Florida State University (FSU), funded by the NIH, developed a process for Taxol's semisynthesis. Their technique did not permit manufacture to be completed from scratch, but it enabled partial synthesis of the active ingredient. Of particular importance for ensuring future supplies, the raw material for the process came from a different type of yew tree that grew in greater abundance than the one that had originally been used.

The decades of effort had been well worth it. By 1989, the government, through the USDA and the NCI, had discovered paclitaxel in the forests of the Northwest, isolated it, and established its clinical utility. An academic partner, FSU, had found a way to manufacture it without causing massive deforestation. With this much accomplished, the NCI saw its role dwindling. It had spent over $25 million and did not have the resources for the next step, which was to produce the synthetic compound in sufficient quantities to be brought to market for large numbers of patients. The government needed a partner with the wherewithal to meet this challenge.

Bringing a Product to Market

In 1989, soon after FSU's successful semisynthesis of paclitaxel, the NCI solicited interest from pharmaceutical companies to enter into a CRADA to commercialize it. Of the four companies that responded, one stood out as the most prepared for the task, Bristol-Myers Squibb (BMS). In addition to extensive experience with oncology products, BMS had a track record of successful collaboration with the federal government in the development of an early treatment for AIDS. To NCI, the company seemed the natural choice, and, in 1991, it selected BMS for a CRADA to market paclitaxel.[129] The CRADA turned out to be one of the first to result in wide availability of a breakthrough drug.[130]

Soon after the NCI announced its search for a CRADA partner, but before the agreement had been finalized, BMS began to explore Taxol's potential. It obtained a license to use FSU's technique for semisynthesis of the drug the following year. The license also applied prospectively to any refinements of the technology that FSU might produce, and, in 1992, BMS gained the right to use a greatly improved semisynthesis technique that yielded a much larger quantity of Taxol's active ingredient. This corporate-academic partnership came to benefit both parties handsomely. BMS gained the ability to market an extremely lucrative drug, and FSU received more than $200 million in royalties, among the largest financial paybacks that any university has received from a technology transfer agreement up to that time.[131]

During the early years of testing, the NIH performed or funded most of the clinical trials on Taxol. BMS supplied the drug, which had been in short supply, to NIH researchers to facilitate the trials. Over the course of the CRADA, the number of research subjects participating rose from about 500 to 28,882 at more than 40 treatment centers. This led to faster-paced testing, which enabled BMS to speed the process. The company received approval from the FDA to market Taxol for treating ovarian cancer in December 1992, and the drug began reaching patients the following month.[132]

The NIH through the NCI and other component agencies invested considerable resources in the development and testing of Taxol both during the CRADA and after it had expired. The value of its clinical testing efforts is estimated at $183 million.[133] In the five years after the CRADA expired in 1997, it spent an additional $301 million, placing the total NIH investment at $484 million. BMS provided a partial offset by supplying NIH with supplies of the drug valued at $92 million for use in the trials.

BMS estimates that, for its part, it spent about $1 billion developing Taxol. The return on this investment was more than adequate. By 1994, the drug had reached the market in 50 countries. In 1998, sales stood at $1.2 billion, and, in 2000, they peaked at $1.6 billion. Through 2002, cumulative sales topped $11 billion after rising by an average of 38 percent a year. These rewards reflected both the large demand and the high price that BMS was able to charge. In 1993, a single gram of Taxol cost $5,846.[134]

BMS owed the NIH a royalty of 0.5 percent of its revenues based on a license agreement that had been reached in 1996. The resulting payments totaled $35 million. Although this was a tiny amount compared to BMS's overall return on the drug, it was enough to repay a sizeable share of the government's investment.[135]

BMS also owed some of its return on Taxol to another government source.[136] Public insurance in the form of Medicare covered the drug's cost for most elderly patients. Its reimbursement totaled $687 million by 1999, the year that a generic version of Taxol was first approved. This amount represented over one-fifth of the drug's domestic sales.

Public–Private Bargaining over Finances

BMS had entered the negotiations that led to the Taxol CRADA in a strong bargaining position. The NIH needed an industry partner that could bring an adequate supply of Taxol to market. When the CRADA was created in 1991, the drug was in short supply, which made clinical testing difficult. None of the other companies that had responded to NIH's solicitation of interest ranked close to BMS in its capability to supply the drug. The agency could have sought multiple partners because CRADAs do not have to be exclusive, but this would have made the arrangement much less attractive to private partners. The NIH also wanted to act quickly because the drug promised life-saving benefits to dying patients.

The NIH's bargaining position was further limited by its inability to transfer rights to an actual patent.[137] Taxol did not qualify for patent protection because, by the time the NIH was able to file a patent application, information about the drug had entered the public domain. This negated the substance's status as "novel," a key requirement for patentability. The prize it had to offer to a CRADA partner was instead access to research findings developed before and during the agreement. In lieu of a patent, BMS received five years of marketing exclusivity after the FDA's approval of its Taxol application. This functioned as the equivalent of patent protection by preventing a competitor from gaining permission to sell the same product. As a result, generic paclitaxel did not reach the market until 2000.[138]

Because of the mismatch in bargaining strength, the NIH received a rather meager level of royalties for a life-saving drug that it was largely responsible for

developing. This is not unusual. The agency is often constrained in CRADA negotiations by limited competition for participation among qualified drug companies.
It is uncommon for more than one company to express interest in a particular
licensing arrangement. In about 30 percent of cases, the NIH receives no expres-
sions of interest at all. The result is that it frequently receives minimal royalties,
such as the 0.5 percent rate negotiated with BMS. However, the immediate financial return to the government is a secondary concern for policymakers. The central
goal is to harness the innovation and drive of private companies to bring promising new technologies to patients.

An Additional Life-Saving Use

The success of the CRADA between the NIH and BMS was only part of the story
of paclitaxel. Beyond its value in treating cancer, the drug also found an important
use in cardiac care.[139] After the oncology benefits had been established, researchers
discovered that it discourages the growth of scar tissue around the sites of metal
stents that are inserted into clogged arteries to prop them open.[140] Scarring can
lead to the redeposit of clog-inducing plaque.[141]

This second use of paclitaxel was again the offshoot of a government effort,
as two scientists working at the NIH conducted the initial research. Based on
the finding of value in protecting the sites of cardiac stents, the agency entered
into a CRADA with a company called Angiotech to commercialize this use of the
drug. Angiotech sublicensed its rights to Boston Scientific, which applied for FDA
approval to market paclitaxel for coating cardiac stents under the name Taxus. The
path to approval was eased by the drug's safety record in the previous clinical trials
involving cancer treatment. The product was approved for the new use, and it went
on to become a clinical and commercial success, with millions of paclitaxel-coated
stents sold worldwide and generating aggregate revenue of more than $3 billion in
the first year of commercialization.[142]

Paclitaxel and Public Policy

Paclitaxel is an example of a technology for which the CRADA system worked as
its congressional designers had intended.[143] The government created the conditions that let the private market carry the ball in bringing a clinically important
drug to patients. Through a series of laws that encouraged public–private collaboration and an initial government-funded research effort, a previously unknown
substance emerged from the woods of the Pacific Northwest to become a life-
saving product. The effort produced huge financial rewards for a drug company, a
device company, and a university that played an instrumental role in its development. Most importantly, it has extended the lives of millions of patients around
the world.

A VACCINE TO PROTECT TRAVELERS: HAVRIX FOR HEPATITIS A

Public–private partnerships have produced a variety of pharmaceutical products.
In addition to drugs, they have also served as the financial incubator for vaccines.

As preventive tools, vaccines often save more lives than medications targeting the same conditions.

Among the diseases that vaccines prevent are several to which many people give little thought until it is too late. These include disease threats for travelers that lurk in many foreign countries. Some of them are widely known, like malaria, but others are less apparent. When the local population develops immunity, the disease can hide insidiously, waiting for susceptible tourists to infect. Often, there are no obvious clues to warn visitors of the endemic nature of the disease in a region before they arrive.

The Nature of Hepatitis A

One such disease is hepatitis A. It is a viral infection that can cause acute liver damage and other debilitating effects, including respiratory problems, rashes, and joint pain.[144] Symptoms typically last for weeks or months.[145] In some cases, they can last as long as a year, and relapses are common. The disease can also be fatal. Estimates place the number of new infections each year in the United States at 25,000 and the number worldwide at 1.5 million.[146]

Hepatitis A is spread largely through contaminated food and water and generally results from poor sanitation. In areas where it is endemic, most of the population is exposed and acquires immunity at an early age. For instance, in Mexico, 95 percent of the population is infected by the age of 10. In some regions, the prevalence of antihepatitis A antibodies is 100 percent. Symptoms in children are usually mild, and those infected under the age of two may exhibit no symptoms at all. However, symptoms increase in severity with age. Mortality is more than four times higher in those over the age of 49 than in the overall population.[147]

There are no antiviral drugs to treat hepatitis A. A substance known as immune globulin can sometimes ward off symptoms, if it is given before they appear. However, it is expensive, must be given within a narrow timeframe, and is not always effective.

With local populations in endemic areas largely immune, the risk of acquiring hepatitis A mostly confronts visitors. Those most susceptible are typically from Western countries, where it is uncommon and so immunity is rare. Because manifestations of the disease appear infrequently in local residents, travelers are often oblivious to it. Less than one-quarter of Americans are aware of the disease, and a mere 2 percent realize that travel to endemic areas puts them at risk for acquiring it.

The Government Steps In

A serious disease that is invisible to those most susceptible to it and for which there is no effective treatment is a natural candidate for a vaccine. The government saw the need and stepped in. The National Institute of Allergy and Infectious Disease (NIAID), a component of the NIH, launched an effort to develop a vaccine in the early 1980s.[148]

The first step in the process was completed when one of NIAID's scientists, Dr. Richard Daemer, isolated a strain of the hepatitis A virus in cell culture.

This allowed other researchers to explore its genetic structure. Another NIAID scientist, Dr. Jeff Cohen, used the strain to derive a clone capable of causing infections. This could be studied to identify the components that made the virus virulent. In 1992, Dr. Suzanne Emerson, also of NIAID, found mutations in the clone that determined the virus's virulence and compared the genetic structure that she found with that of the wild strain. Other NIAID researchers then administered the inactivated virus to animals to see if it conferred immunity against infection by the virulent form.[149]

Collaboration with a Private Partner

Before this basic research into the nature of the hepatitis A virus had been concluded, NIAID looked for and found a private sector partner that could bring the fruits of the investigations to market: the pharmaceutical company SmithKline Beacham (now part of Glaxo SmithKline). In 1988, CRADAs were formed between SmithKline and both NIAIDA and the federal Centers for Disease Control and Prevention (CDC). Under those arrangements, SmithKline initiated an effort to develop a marketable vaccine under the auspices of one of its scientists, Dr. Erik D'Hondt, who worked in tandem with scientists at NIAID. The initiative determined that the safest kind of vaccine would be one using an inactivated virus, and a process was developed for growing one of commercial grade. The CRADA with NIH granted SmithKline nonexclusive rights to manufacture and sell it.[150]

Both NIAID and SmithKline conducted clinical trials of the vaccine's safety and efficacy in humans, a total of 43 separate trials in all. NIAID took responsibility for early-phase trials, which assess safety, as it had for preclinical studies in animals. Under a separate CRADA with the Walter Reed Army Institute of Research, SmithKline conducted large-scale efficacy trials in Thailand, including a test on 40,000 children. Those tests found the vaccine to be extremely effective, providing protection for 94 percent of the subjects.[151]

SmithKline named its vaccine Havrix and the FDA approved it for marketing in 1995.[152] In 1997, the CDC jump-started the market by awarding SmithKline a contract for a bulk purchase through the Vaccines for Children program, which provides free vaccines for low-income children.[153] That year, Havrix generated $370.6 million in sales.[154] In 2008, sales of Havrix along with a vaccine that SmithKline developed against another liver disease, hepatitis B, reached $1.12 billion.[155] Those revenues accounted for more than one-quarter of the company's total vaccine income that year.[156]

SmithKline went on to develop a vaccine that protects against both hepatitis A and hepatitis B, which it named Twinrix. That product received FDA approval in 2001.[157] A similar vaccine manufactured by Merck, Vaqta, had been approved in 1996. Subsequently, additional vaccines against hepatitis A were developed by Sanofi Pasteur, Avaxim, and Crucell.

Another Public–Private Success

Havrix and the other hepatitis A vaccines represent both commercial and public health successes. They have proven extremely effective clinically, and side effects from them are rare. They enable travelers from Western countries to avoid the risk of contracting one of the most common infectious diseases when they visit the rest of the world. This protection is especially valuable for members of the military. Before introduction of the vaccine, treatment of hepatitis A among American soldiers cost more than $200 million a year.[158]

It is unlikely that either the government or the private sector could have successfully developed Havrix or a similar vaccine against hepatitis A on its own. The basic research that NIAID began in the early 1980s held little promise of the kind of short-term payoff that could have attracted a private investor. However, a potential market was there, if a product could emerge from the development stage. In the end, an explicit public–private collaboration produced a substantial payoff, both for the companies that manufacture hepatitis A vaccines and for thousands of travelers who have been able to remain healthy after their wanderings.

THE NEXT ERA IN DRUG DEVELOPMENT AND THE PROMISE OF MORE SUCCESS STORIES

A new era in drug development dawned in the 1990s thanks to a new approach called *combinatorial chemistry*. It permits scientists to create libraries of thousands of compounds that can be tested as candidates to perform specific functions, like inhibiting HMG CoA reductase in the liver to block the synthesis of cholesterol. Within the time span of a few months, millions of such candidates can be tested for efficacy much more quickly and efficiently than they could have been previously.[159]

The new approach has begun to revolutionize private drug development. It is now the principle method for finding new medications of every kind, with dramatic speed. By way of comparison, the old technology had enabled Merck to synthesize, purify, and screen about 250,000 different chemicals in the 60 years between 1934 and 1994. In the four years between 1995 and 1999, using combinatorial chemistry techniques, it synthesized and tested 4.5 million of them.[160]

Like so many other technological advances that have bolstered the financial prospects of private pharmaceutical companies, combinatorial chemistry was devised by scientists who relied on the NIH for financial support. Beyond the pharmaceutical manufacturers that use it, a burgeoning new industry now supports its application. A raft of companies provides instrumentation, chemical reagents, and software. Through them, the government investment in advancing the process of drug development has sent ripples through yet another large swath of the private sector.

The "Free-Market" Pharmaceutical Industry and the Government

Let us turn to the fundamental question that underlies this chapter. How did the pharmaceutical industry, which has remained among the most profitable for decades, get that way? Certainly, entrepreneurship and innovation played a tremendously important part in maintaining the robustness of drug companies over the years. Market forces continuously prod private companies to devise new products and stay ahead of the competition. However, those companies must have raw materials to work with in their intellectual arsenal. For pharmaceutical firms, that is basic knowledge of human biology. Over the past three-quarters of a century, the greatest producer of that knowledge by far has been the US government.

The government's role in creating and maintaining the pharmaceutical industry can be highlighted by asking what the industry would look like in the absence of its government base. Without question, it would still exist. Pharmaceuticals date back almost as far as recorded history. Ancient Egyptian writings describe pharmaceutical preparations, as do the records of almost every early civilization.[161] Private companies, as well as individuals, have been manufacturing drug products since colonial times in America, long before there was an NIH to support research or an FDA to oversee quality.[162]

But what would that industry look like without the pillars of government support that emerged in the twentieth century? It would almost certainly be a shadow of its present self. Virtually every major drug that has supported private pharmaceutical profits over the past 50 years was developed with government support in one form or another. In no field of medicine would available treatments approach the range or effectiveness they do today. Cardiac care without statins, oncology care without paclitaxel, and AIDS care without AZT would fall far short of their present capabilities. In fact, it is impossible to name any medical specialty that does not today depend for its pharmacological tools, in some cases almost entirely, on the investment and innovation of the government.

COULD PRIVATE INDUSTRY HAVE THRIVED ON ITS OWN?

We know what the government has contributed, but it would also be fair to ask whether it is conceivable that the industry might have accomplished these or similar advances on its own. Without the NIH, might private entrepreneurs have mustered the resources to meet the basic science challenges that created modern medicine? Perhaps the same market forces that promote applied research in bringing products to market could have supported the advances in biology that underlie it.

To answer this question, we can look to the stories recounted in this chapter of some of the most important fruits of government intervention. Merck was ready to give up on statins before the NIH and the FDA stepped in with a helping hand. Government scientists combed the forests of the Pacific Northwest in search of anticarcinogens, eventually discovering paclitaxel, at a time when private companies showed little interest. The search for a vaccine against hepatitis A began when a government agency launched it.

As we look to the future of medicine, we can ask whether any private company could have devoted the resources to mapping the human genome, the essential first step in opening the door to genomic medicine. The investment required was huge, and the knowledge gained will require decades to commercialize. It is public information available to everyone, including competing companies, to take advantage of. What private investors concerned about a return on investment would have allowed their funds to be used in this way? Celera was able to join the effort only by piggybacking on findings generated by the NIH's initiative.[163]

It is inconceivable that private industry could have succeeded on its own in instances such as these. In none of them did pharmaceutical companies have the resources or the interest to act until the government led the way. The market imposes incentives for short-term financial gain that conflict with the nature of decades-long speculative research endeavors. The government, on the other hand, does have the resources and interest in promoting such enterprises. As history has shown, when the two sectors work in combination, with each focusing on what it does best, the rewards can be tremendous.

HAS THE GOVERNMENT ACTED WISELY?

Government support for the pharmaceutical industry has its share of critics. Many see the large amounts of money that are directed to it as an undeserved subsidy for an industry that could be amply profitable on its own. They point in particular to companies that patent discoveries based on NIH-funded research, thereby staking an ownership claim in a publicly funded resource. They ask why private ventures should be allowed to reap such rewards when taxpayers supported the underlying scientific advances.

CRADAs result in particularly disproportionate returns for private participants. In the case of Taxol, the NIH received $35 million on behalf of taxpayers under a licensing agreement with BMS after spending almost $500 million to test the drug. By the time the drug faced generic competition, BMS had earned over $11 billion. The company claimed that it invested $1 billion of its own money in applied research to bring Taxol to market, but, even with this expense, its rate of return dwarfed that of the NIH. Is it fair that a private entity should profit so handsomely from an invention that would not have been possible without substantial government investment?

Tax subsidies for research and development often garner especially harsh criticism. Do highly profitable companies really need a subsidy to invest in research when they would have to make the investment anyway to remain competitive? Perhaps the government already gives the industry enough research support through the NIH.

As described earlier, another common line of criticism concerns the rigor of FDA oversight. Several drugs with dangerous side effects have slipped through the vetting process, sometimes after receiving accelerated review.[164] The result has been recalls and additional warnings after reports of patient harm. An example is the drug rofecoxib (Vioxx), which was approved on an expedited basis as a treatment for arthritis pain, and its review failed to spot long-term cardiac hazards that a more careful process might have revealed.[165]

Critics place much of the blame for such lapses on the political clout of the pharmaceutical industry, which spends more than any other on lobbying. They also point to financial ties between the industry and many of the experts on whom the FDA relies for advice, which can create conflicts of interest. Critics on the other side see agency failings in the delay and expense it imposes on the drug development process. From either perspective, government oversight of drug safety leaves room for improvement.

Concerns are also raised about patents, which enable manufacturers to charge high prices for their products. Americans pay the highest amounts in the world for prescription medications, largely because the United States is the only developed country in which the government does not regulate prices. Moreover, pharmaceutical companies often enhance the volume of sales for their patented drugs with controversial strategies, such as advertising products directly to consumers who are ill-equipped to evaluate therapeutic claims, promoting drugs for uses that have not been approved by the FDA, and bestowing lavish gifts on high-prescribing physicians. Is this the reward we get as taxpayers for so generously building and reinforcing the industry's foundation?

To make matters worse, taxpayers unwittingly help the industry to perpetuate the arrangement. Government initiatives have enabled the pharmaceutical industry to become and remain one of the most profitable in the country, year after year. It then uses its financial resources to exert influence on politicians and regulators to expand these initiatives even further and even to launch new ones. The shape of the Medicare prescription drug benefit and of the ACA stand as testaments to the industry's considerable sway.

Perhaps taxpayers could be getting a better deal on their investment in the private pharmaceutical industry. The system of support could undoubtedly be improved in numerous ways. However, the point remains that, whatever the optimal level of support, government investment over the years has been, and remains today, crucial to the industry's well-being and to the development of many valuable new drugs. Regardless of the system's shortcomings, we have clearly gotten a robust and highly profitable set of companies and a cascade of important medications in return for the government's active involvement.

PUBLIC INVESTMENT AND PRIVATE INDUSTRY

Pharmaceuticals are developed, manufactured, sold, and distributed in the United States through the private sector. Private investment and competition among firms drive that sector's economics. Those dynamics characterize what is typically thought of as a "free market." However, the market does not exist because the government stepped aside and let private enterprise operate without constraint. Quite to the contrary, it functions precisely because the government has insinuated itself into almost every aspect of the business.

4

How the Government Created
the Hospital Industry

> Although it may be tempting to point at acute care hospitals as key
> shapers of health care, in reality they mostly function as pawns of
> Medicare.
>
> —ROBERT MARTENSEN, *AMERICAN MEDICAL ASSOCIATION JOURNAL OF ETHICS*[1]

American hospitals are big business. In 2008, the United States had 5,815 of them.[2] The private sector operated the vast majority, 4,710, and the government ran 1,105. All told, these institutions contained 951,045 beds, 820,514 of which were in private hands. The bill for the services they rendered totaled $718.4 billion, and it represented the largest single chunk of the country's health care costs.[3]

The pace at which this spending has grown over the past half century is striking. Hospital care in America cost $9.2 billion in 1960. The figure tripled to $27.6 billion in 1970, almost quadrupled to $101 billion in 1980, and is now approaching $1 trillion.[4]

Hospitals were not the only health care institutions to proliferate across America during the latter part of the twentieth century. Between 1985 and 2008, the number of skilled nursing facilities, the nursing homes that provide the most intensive level of care, tripled from 5,052 to 15,032. The number of end-stage renal disease facilities, which provide dialysis services, almost quintupled from 1,393 to 5,317. Outpatient physical therapy facilities increased in number from 854 to 2,781, hospices from 134 to 3,346, and ambulatory surgery centers from 336 to 5,174.[5]

What was driving this growth? Did more Americans find themselves in need of that much more care? Did the number of available treatments explode? The best way to answer the question is to look at the source of funding for the hospital industry's expansion.

Regardless of whether Americans actually needed the additional care they received, someone had to cover the cost. That someone was unlikely to be the patients individually, given the high price tag for the services involved. The largest source of funding was the only entity with the resources to meet such a daunting financial challenge—the government. And the principal source of public reimbursement for these proliferating health care institutions was the largest government health care program—Medicare.[6]

As the business of providing institutional health care grew, the nature of the businesses that make up the industry also began to change in important ways. None of these changes was more significant than the nature of their ownership. For-profit hospitals owned by private investors steadily increased in number in American health care as the industry was expanding overall.[7]

Traditionally, nonprofit institutions have dominated hospital care in the United States. Although this remains the case today, the proportion that these facilities represent has been declining since 1975, as has the number of beds they operate. However, for-profit hospitals have experienced the opposite trend. Their numbers have risen over the same timeframe, with particularly rapid increases since 2000. In 2012, they owned 20 percent of all hospitals.[8] The number of for-profit hospitals in the United States increased nearly by 14 percent, from 890 to 1,013, between 2006 and 2010.[9]

Why has the investor-owned sector of American hospital care grown in prominence? Once again, the question can be answered by understanding who pays the bills. For these hospitals, Medicare has served as an especially important source of reimbursement. As historian of medicine Rosemary Stevens has noted, the effect of Medicare may not have been intended or even foreseen by the program's architects, but it was nonetheless profound: "Through the reimbursement system the structure of the hospital system was also radically changed, despite the pious expectations of the Medicare legislation. The key here was hospital capital, and specifically, the mandated link between capital development and operating income."[10] When they created Medicare in 1965, government policymakers, wittingly or not, also created the hospital industry as we know it today.

Some would argue that government funding has been too generous and has forged an industry of excessive size with more hospitals than the country actually needs. An oversupply of hospital beds in some regions, including several major cities, has had the detrimental effect of exacerbating health care cost inflation. It engenders overhead expenses that are required to maintain the facilities, and it induces some facilities to fill their capacity by promoting unnecessary care. A hospital industry bloated by Medicare payments is also able to follow the pattern of other private health care sectors in devoting some of its government-bestowed financial resources to gaining political influence that it uses to maintain the spigot of funds. Nevertheless, regardless of whether the size and strength of the industry are too large or just right, they would be considerably different had the government not intervened.

The History of Hospitals

The history of the large sophisticated inpatient institutions that are the American hospitals of today tells the story of their government-supported growth. They have changed dramatically in size and structure from their early incarnations, prodded by waves of social, economic, and clinical forces. But no force has exerted more of an effect on them than a series of major public programs, most enacted during the latter half of the twentieth century.

THE FIRST INSTITUTIONS

The forebears of modern hospitals date back many centuries. The Romans established army hospitals to treat soldiers. During the Middle Ages, isolation houses for leprosy patients operated in Europe. Facilities that treated a broader range of patients and illnesses were established in greater numbers in Europe during the Renaissance, providing care that was enhanced by the spread of printed medical texts. Complex institutions that more closely resembled modern hospitals were commonplace in the Islamic world as far back as the twelfth century. They operated in many cities, including Cairo and Damascus and throughout much of Islamic Spain. At one point, there were sixty of them in Baghdad. Many trained medical students in addition to rendering care to patients, and many were subject to regular government inspections.[11]

American hospitals trace their origin to the middle of the eighteenth century. At that time, patients with financial means received most of their medical care at home from private physicians. Those unable to afford such personal service required a place of rest where their basic needs could be met. In the early part of the century, those who were poor and sick found shelter in almshouses that served the destitute. The first of these institutions to set aside a building specifically dedicated to housing the sick was the Philadelphia Almshouse, founded in 1729. In New York, the Publick Workhouse and House of Correction of the City of New York was founded in 1736. Over time, the New York facility increasingly focused on the needs of the sick and eventually became Bellevue Hospital. Funding for these institutions came primarily from taxes.[12]

In 1751, Benjamin Franklin, Dr. Thomas Bond, and several collaborators founded the first actual hospital in North America, Pennsylvania Hospital in Philadelphia, to provide comfort and care for the sick.[13] It was a successor to the almshouses that housed many of the poor.[14] In 1791, New York Hospital began operations along the same model, and, in 1821, Massachusetts General Hospital opened in Boston.[15] Many others followed over the course of the nineteenth century, including a large number founded by religious orders.

Hospital care at that time was fairly primitive, often tending more toward palliative care than toward attempts at actual cures. Available treatments were so limited that patients were as likely to acquire new infections during their stay as they were to overcome the illness that brought them in. A burst of hospital construction occurred during and immediately after the Civil War in response to the need to treat injured soldiers, but many closed soon thereafter. However, those that remained experienced a technological revolution in the years that followed. With it, they transformed themselves into centers of actual care. Among the key advances that led to this change were the development of anesthesia, which permitted complex surgery; antisepsis, which greatly reduced the chance of infection from any procedure; and x-ray imaging, which enabled physicians to visualize and treat internal injuries.[16] These technologies opened new possibilities for more complex surgical procedures that could no longer be performed in the homes of wealthy patients.[17]

A second development that contributed to a proliferation of hospitals at the time was a change in housing patterns. With increasing urbanization, houses tended to be smaller, and some families found accommodations in apartments. Tighter living spaces made it more difficult to care for ill family members at home.[18] Hospitals offered a ready alternative as a place to house them.

In response, the number of American hospitals grew substantially during the late nineteenth and early twentieth centuries. In 1873, hospitals numbered only 178, with a total of 40,000 beds. By 1909, there were 4,359 hospitals operating 421,065 beds. In 1945, there were 6,511 with 1,738,944 beds. The number of beds per population increased during this time from one for every 817 people to one for every 80.[19]

A third development that reinforced the trend was the rise in the status and influence of the medical profession. As their therapeutic powers increased, physicians were able to command more central positions in hospital operations. An organizational model emerged in which physicians formed independent medical staffs within institutions, with complete control over medical matters. At the same time, the medical profession was organizing itself more broadly to better standardize practices to improve quality. This effort received considerable assistance from the American Medical Association (AMA), which was founded in 1847 to promote and upgrade medical education. Its activities are discussed in more detail in Chapter 5.

The AMA took the seminal step in its effort to improve medical education almost 60 years later in 1910, when it requested a study by the Carnegie Commission to examine the quality of education in every medical school then in existence. A young education expert named Abraham Flexner conducted the study, and the account of his findings became widely known as the Flexner Report.[20] It led to a call for tighter standards and a greater emphasis on the clinical aspects of medical education. Medical curricula were transformed in response, with standards enforced by new accreditation rules for schools based on rigorous scientific and hands-on clinical training.[21]

By the early years of the twentieth century, every state had imposed licensure requirements for physicians, and medical education had been standardized and subjected to accreditation. Both of these steps helped to raise the quality of and public regard for the profession. To improve hands-on training, medical school curricula came to include instruction in hospitals, and postgraduate training through hospital internships and residencies was added during the early twentieth century as a requirement for entering actual practice.[22]

With these changes, by 1920, hospitals had established their place at the center of American health care. In 1922, their number had grown to 4,978. Most cities and large towns contained at least one community hospital, which served as a focal point for local medical care.[23]

The transformation of hospitals that had begun with developments in the late nineteenth century continued and accelerated over the course of the twentieth. In the years following World War II, they came to be seen as hubs for responding to all phases of life-threatening medical conditions.[24] During the latter part of the century, the industry experienced another dramatic growth spurt as hospitals were transformed into centers of advanced, high-technology treatment.[25] This most recent incarnation bears almost no resemblance to the institutional forebears of two hundred years ago. With it, the boundaries of hospital care have expanded tremendously as their capacity to render highly complex treatments and diagnostic services has exploded.[26]

During the latter part of the twentieth century, the growing capabilities and complexity of hospitals engendered a transformation in the corporate structure of many of them, as well. Institutional leaders saw the need for broader organizational arrangements that could add flexibility and tap into new resources. To accomplish this, starting in the 1980s, many larger hospitals began to expand into more comprehensive health systems that included physician practices, outpatient clinics, and ancillary providers, such as laboratories, radiology facilities, and nursing homes. Some health systems acquired several hospitals and merged them into single huge corporate entities.

Many such systems were formed throughout the country during the 1990s. A substantial number of them included major teaching institutions and were affiliated with medical schools. A few became especially prominent. Partners Health Care in Boston was formed by a merger between Massachusetts General Hospital and Brigham and Women's Hospital, both affiliated with Harvard Medical School.[27] New York Presbyterian Hospital in New York was formed through a combination of Columbia Presbyterian Hospital, the teaching facility for Columbia Medical School, and New York Hospital, which trained students at Cornell Medical School.[28] The University of Pennsylvania Health System in Philadelphia was created when the University of Pennsylvania acquired additional hospitals, physician practices, and ancillary care providers to form a region-wide system offering all levels of care.[29]

Major corporate changes such as these require financing. Costs had been rising for some time, but the evolution of hospitals into centers of high technology generated even greater financial demands.[30] They required new kinds of equipment, space to put it in, and professionals to operate it, including highly trained specialist physicians who command substantial salaries. Fortunately for the industry, the late twentieth century was also the time when the government implemented a series a large hospital funding programs. The trillions of dollars spent by these programs were key to enabling hospitals to meet these costs.

Direct Government Funding and the Hill-Burton Act

The federal role in building American hospitals dates to the nation's founding. In fact, in 1775, a year before the signing of the Declaration of Independence, the first government-funded hospital began operation in anticipation of the Revolutionary War. In 1798, the Marine Hospital Service was authorized by Congress to build and operate hospitals to care for ill sailors.[31] Other federal facilities were constructed over the years that followed, including a hospital in Washington, D.C. to care for the mentally ill, which was founded in 1855 and took the name St. Elizabeth's

Hospital in 1916. In 1871, Freedman's Hospital opened in Washington, D.C. to care for African Americans. In 1905, Congress authorized construction of a leprosy hospital in Hawaii. In the early twentieth century, several facilities were built throughout the South and Southwest to treat patients with trachoma, an eye disease that is a leading cause of blindness.[32]

Federal funding of private hospitals began in earnest during the early part of the twentieth century. It came in response to a growing need for external financial support to maintain increasingly complex operations. As expenses rose, hospitals found that donations were inadequate to cover their costs. Before 1900, patient fees covered about a third of hospital expenses. In 1939, the figure was two-thirds.[33] However, with many patients unable to pay the bills, supplementary sources of income were increasingly required. Much of the need was filled by the emergence of health insurance, as discussed in Chapter 6, but additional sources of income were also necessary to support the expanded role that hospitals had come to play.

In 1928, private donations still constituted the majority of funding for hospital capital construction. However, by 1935, government funding at the local, state, and federal levels had taken the lead. The federal share of the government contribution grew steadily, soon outstripping local and state expenditures. It received a substantial boost from several New Deal programs during the 1930s, which included initiatives to finance hospital care for particularly needy groups. The Social Security Act of 1935 authorized funding for state programs to provide medical care for crippled children, including their placement in hospitals when necessary.[34] The Act also created the Emergency Maternity and Infant Care program, which became effective in 1943. It allocated funds through state agencies for medical, nursing, and hospital obstetrical care for the wives and children of soldiers in the four lowest pay grades. Hospital services were arranged for beneficiaries on a contract basis. By one account, this program was largely responsible for banner years that hospitals experienced during World War II, when they enjoyed their highest levels of occupancy and income up to that time.[35]

The war years were also a time when direct federal support for hospitals accelerated substantially with the construction of new federal facilities for soldiers and veterans. Another boost came from the Lanham Housing Act, passed in 1941, which allocated funds for hospital construction in parts of the country that experienced rapid population growth because of the war and had inadequate community services to meet the increased need for inpatient care. States also expanded their aid for private hospitals during this time.[36] By 1947, two-thirds of the funds for hospital capital investments were coming from the government, compared with slightly less than a third from donations and other voluntary sources. Only 3 percent of funds came from private investors.[37]

Direct federal funding of hospitals grew dramatically in 1946 with passage of a major program to expand access known as the Hill-Burton Act.[38] That law financed the construction of new hospitals and the expansion of existing facilities on a scale that was unprecedented at the time.[39] It gave the federal government the central role in the financing of capital costs of American hospitals, a role that it never relinquished. The law's primary purpose was to improve access to hospital services in regions of the country where such access had been limited, particularly in rural areas.[40] Over the next 25 years, more than $3.7 billion was appropriated, representing grants to almost one-third of the hospitals in the country.[41] By 1968, the Hill-Burton Act had contributed to the financing of 416,000 hospital beds and 9,200 new medical facilities.[42] By 1975, it had assisted almost one-third of all hospital construction projects in the country and had funded close to 10 percent of the costs of all hospital construction since its inception.[43] By 1997, Hill-Burton had injected $4.6 billion in grants and $1.5 billion in loans to 6,800 health care facilities in 4,000 communities.[44]

Hill-Burton funding offered a lifeline to many rural hospitals and thereby to the regions they served, but it came with many regulatory strings attached.[45] Among them, the law required hospitals receiving funds to provide minimum amounts of indigent care, including emergency services, and to refrain from discriminating among patients based on race.[46] Participation in Medicare and Medicaid was added as a retroactive requirement in the 1970s.[47]

The law was distinctive not just for the amount of funding it authorized but also for the system of state-level planning that it created to allocate funding. This system laid the groundwork for a more comprehensive, state-based planning process that was implemented in the 1960s to determine which clinical services and facility improvements could be added at which hospitals.[48] In that regard, the law opened a new avenue for substantial federal involvement in the hospital industry.

The centerpiece of the planning process that grew from the Hill-Burton Act was a set of state-based programs known as "certificate-of-need." These programs divide states into planning regions, and each develops its own health care needs assessment. New facilities and services must obtain a certificate-of-need from the state in order to operate, and certificates are issued based on whether the proposed facility or service addresses an unmet need under the plan for its region. All states adopted these programs in response to a federal mandate in 1966, under the Comprehensive Health Planning and Services Act,[49] but the mandate was permitted to expire in 1986. Thirty-five states retain certificate-of-need programs today.[50]

Hill-Burton's combination of funding and regulation thereby created a blueprint for the distribution of American hospitals and for many aspects of their operations. It also fostered a tremendous expansion in the size and scope of the nation's overall hospital enterprise. Through the health planning process, it determined where new facilities would be located and new services would be offered, with a goal of extending care to broad segments of the population.

The government's role in shaping the distribution of hospital services may seem commonplace today. However, in 1946, when the Hill-Burton Act was passed, it was still a novel idea. It arose as a byproduct of President Harry Truman's desire for a national health insurance system that would guarantee coverage to all Americans. He did not succeed in persuading Congress to enact a universal coverage plan, but he was able to induce Congress to pass a mechanism to expand the availability of one category of health care services. In doing so, he set a precedent for direct government involvement in the hospital industry, which had major ramifications over the decades that followed.[51]

The Bedrock of Hospital Finance: Medicare

When President Truman realized that his hopes for a universal national health insurance program were almost certain to fail, he changed tack. In 1951, he decided to focus instead on a plan that would target the health care needs of a particularly needy and vulnerable group, the elderly. A plan to aid them would represent an incremental reform, but one that could be expanded by a future Congress to apply more widely. To diffuse concern among physicians that the plan would intrude on their autonomy, he limited it to hospital care. The initiative became known as the Ewing proposal, after Oscar R. Ewing, an adviser to Truman who led the effort to develop it.[52]

Even this stripped down plan failed to pass Congress, but it set the stage for a more sustained push about ten years later. President John Kennedy, in 1961, supported a similar plan to cover the costs of hospital care for the elderly, which was embodied in legislation known as the Anderson-King bill. Once again, the measure went down to defeat, but, with its introduction, the issue returned to the public's consciousness.[53]

In 1964, a year after Kennedy's assassination, Democrats won huge electoral victories. Lyndon Johnson won the presidential race in a landslide, and Democrats claimed 69 seats in the Senate and two-thirds of the House of Representatives. With these gains and public sympathy for Kennedy's legacy, Johnson saw the chance to reinvigorate much of Kennedy's social agenda. At the top of the list of unfinished business was passage of a health insurance plan for the elderly. It was given the name Medicare.[54]

The plan had a difficult gestation. Organized medicine in the form of the AMA fought it fiercely, fearing that government funding of health care would inevitably lead to government intrusion into medical practice. The story of Medicare's passage is filled with tales of backroom deals and compromises that Johnson successfully navigated as a skilled legislative tactician. At the end of June of that year, he emerged victorious, with a plan that covered both hospital and physician care for all Americans starting at the age of 65.[55]

One of the key deals that Johnson negotiated was for support from the hospital industry in return for a generous reimbursement formula.[56] Under the plan that he agreed to, hospital payments were based not on a predetermined fee schedule but on the actual amount that each facility spent providing care to Medicare patients. The more a hospital ran up its costs, therefore, the more it was reimbursed. Rather than rewarding efficiency, this payment scheme encouraged hospitals to deliver as much care as they could, regardless of medical necessity. As discussed later, Congress changed the system in the 1980s after the financial repercussions of this original plan had became apparent; however, for almost 20 years, Medicare reimbursement promoted explosive growth in the quantity of services rendered in hospitals across the country.

As part of the same legislative initiative, Johnson also gained passage of Medicaid, which covers care for the poor. This program is administered separately by each state, but it is funded jointly by the states and the federal government, which pays between 50 and 80 percent of the total cost, depending on the state's average income. States have some flexibility to set coverage parameters; however, they must do so within federal guidelines and are subject to federal oversight. Medicaid reimbursement rates are considerably lower than those of Medicare, so its direct impact on hospital finances has been less pronounced. Nevertheless, it has played an important role in shaping key aspects of the industry.[57]

Medicare has grown relentlessly since its inception, and it has, as the AMA had feared, led to substantial government involvement in many aspects of medical care. It affords the government a financial lever that has been used repeatedly to direct key aspects of hospital and physician behavior. However, it also has injected a large and growing source of funding into health care that transformed the size and scope of the hospital sector. This ultimately has worked to the benefit of all elements of the health care system, including hospitals and physicians, not to mention millions of elderly and disabled patients.

MEDICARE TODAY

Medicare today is divided into four components, two of which were part of program when it was first launched: Part A, which covers hospital and other inpatient services, and Part B, which covers physician and other professional and outpatient services. Their structure was modeled on the typical private plans offered at the time by the predominant insurers, Blue Cross and Blue Shield. In the 1990s, Part C was added to give beneficiaries the option to receive all coverage through a private managed care plan rather than through the traditional Parts A and B. This component of the program was originally known as Medicare + Choice but was substantially expanded and renamed Medicare Advantage in 2003.[58] In 2006, Part D was launched to cover outpatient prescription drugs.[59]

Medicare now covers the cost of care for almost 50 million beneficiaries.[60] Their ranks include not just the elderly, who comprise 38 million of the total. Eligibility also extends to 7.6 million who are totally disabled and about 19,000 who suffer from end-stage renal disease.[61] This last group gained Medicare eligibility in 1972. The program reached this size after growing inexorably since its enactment in 1965. Its total budget has risen at a pace of about 5 percent annually, and, in 2010, it exceeded $510 billion.[62] Of this total, $186 billion went for hospital inpatient care, and $140 billion was spent on outpatient services rendered by physicians and other health care professionals.[63] Federal and state contributions through its companion program, Medicaid, injected slightly more than $400 billion into the system.[64]

HOSPITALS TAKE OFF

As Medicare took off in size and scope, the fortunes of hospitals soared with it.[65] Medical historian Charles Rosenberg has described the situation this way: "The late twentieth-century hospital already existed in embryo, waiting only the nutrients of third-party payment, government involvement, technological change, and general economic growth to stimulate a rapid and in some ways hypertrophied development."[66] A new and reliable source of reimbursement in the form of Medicare meant that hospitals could provide many more services to many more patients, knowing the bills would be paid. In the words of another observer, "What cemented the centrality of hospitals was the passage of Medicare and Medicaid."[67]

The immediate effect of Medicare was to pour millions of dollars into hospital coffers in return for providing ever-greater amounts of expensive care. No longer bound by the fiscal constraint of devoting substantial resources to treating large proportions of nonpaying patients, hospitals were now limited only by their own ingenuity in finding services to provide and equipment to use in providing them. Medical sociologist Rosemary Stevens put it bluntly, "Medicare gave hospitals a license to spend."[68]

Hospital care in the United States cost a total of $9.2 billion in 1960.[69] In 1970, four years after Medicare went into effect, spending had risen threefold to $27.6 billion. In 2008, it reached $718.4 billion. The share paid by the government through the various programs that existed at the time stood at 42.2 percent in 1960. It rose to 55.2 percent in 1970, a figure that has remained fairly constant since. In other words, for almost half a century, more than half the revenue of American hospitals has consistently come from the government.

Of this massive government expenditure on hospital care, the share borne by the Medicare and Medicaid programs has grown strikingly. Medicare's portion of the nation's total hospital bill rose from 19.4 percent in 1970 to 29.4 percent in 2008, and Medicaid's from 9.6 percent to 17.1 percent over the same time period. In dollar terms, Medicare payments to hospitals and other health care facilities increased from $5.3 billion in 1970 to $236.6 billion in 2008, for a more than 40-fold increase.[70] Medicaid payments increased from $4.1 billion to $96.9 billion between 1972 and 2008, an increase of more than 23 times. This growth far outpaced the rate of inflation.[71]

From the perspective of the finances of hospitals, Medicare had two immediate effects. First, it increased the share of insurance reimbursement available to cover their budgets. At the time of Medicare's enactment, third-party payments accounted for 71 percent of all hospital revenues.[72] Just a few years later, that figure rose to 90 percent. Most of the increase in third-party payments was comprised of public funding, which represented just 8 percent of hospital revenue in 1961 but increased to 39 percent in 1971.[73] With the government and private insurers now paying most of the bill, hospitals had less need to rely on fundraising to cover their costs.

Heavier reliance on third-party reimbursement as the primary means of financing did more than just help hospitals make ends meet. It also allowed them to grow those ends markedly. More spending does not automatically bring in more donations, but it does bring in more third-party reimbursement under a system like Medicare's. With 90 percent of budgets covered by the government and other third-party payers, the sky could be the limit.

Once Medicare's generous cost-based reimbursement structure was in place, the effect on hospital spending was large and quick. As one observed noted, "It didn't take long for community hospitals, academic medical centers and doctors to realize that 'cost-plus' reimbursements and no overall budget caps meant they could realize their big dreams, especially those that required expensive facilities, staff, and trainees, and then dream new ones."[74] The average cost of an inpatient day in a semiprivate room increased at an annual rate of 5.6 percent between 1961 and 1966, the five years before Medicare's launch. The rate jumped to 13 percent between 1967 and 1971. Reimbursement for these higher costs bumped aggregate hospital revenue from $7,422 million in 1965 to $18,104 in 1971 and net income from $269 million to $547 million.[75]

The second major effect on hospital finances was to help facilities obtain funding in the bond market.[76] The sale of bonds is a major source of financing for non-profit hospitals, particularly for capital expansion projects such as new wings and new buildings. Under federal tax law, those who purchase the bonds of tax-exempt organizations like hospitals pay no taxes on the interest they earn. Bondholders are therefore willing to accept lower interest rates than they would if a for-profit corporation issued the bonds and the proceeds were fully subject to tax. As a result, hospitals can sell their debt at below-market rates, saving considerable sums.

However, even with this financial enhancement, the bonds are only as good as the underlying fiscal stability of the hospitals that issue them. Investors need assurance that the bonds they buy are backed by an organization with the wherewithal to pay them off. Medicare provides that assurance. Investors are reassured by the guaranteed stream of revenue from the federal government in the form of Medicare payments, which helps establish the creditworthiness of hospitals. The same dynamic also aids for-profit hospitals as they seek investments in equity markets. Easier access to credit for all institutions means more money with which to grow.

One feature of Medicare's design in particular helped support its value as a financial mainstay for hospitals—its structure as an entitlement.[77] This means it has no annual financial limit, and spending each year is determined by the needs of those who are entitled to receive benefits, not by a predetermined budget. The more health care Medicare beneficiaries receive, the larger the budget automatically grows, without any additional appropriation from Congress.

Medicare's entitlement structure funds American hospitals based on the overall amount of services that they, in their discretion, decide to provide. The result has been an accelerating burden on the federal budget, and one that may grow to an unsustainable size in future years. In the words of health economist Eli Ginzberg writing in 1996, "Medicare financing provisions loosened most of the financial constraints under which non-profit and for-profit acute-care hospitals had hitherto operated, a consequence that was not understood at the time and has largely escaped attention and analysis ever since."[78]

Capital expansion was only one consequence of Medicare's expandable source of funding. Another was an increase in hospital employment. Someone had to staff the larger and more technologically complex facilities. In the 15 years after Medicare's enactment, hospital employment grew from 1.4 million to 2.9 million, an increase of more than 200 percent.[79] During the same time period, total employment in the United States grew by only about 33 percent. The greater demand for hospital workers brought with it an increase in salaries. One study of hospitals in New York found that wages for the lowest paid workers rose from a level that was about one-third below the prevailing market rate to one that was about one-third above it during the first 15 years of Medicare's existence. The salaries of medical residents who train in hospitals rose by similarly impressive amounts, from a range of $3,500 to $6,000 at Medicare's inception to one of $15,000 to $20,000 15 years later. At the other end of income spectrum, Medicare brought about even larger gains in the income of physician specialists, as discussed in Chapter 5.

The dependence of American hospital finance on Medicare is strikingly demonstrated by what happens when some of it is taken away. In 1997, Congress slashed Medicare reimbursement for hospital services to ease the burden on the federal budget under a law known as the Balanced Budget Act.[80] In the two years that followed, spending under Part A of the program rose by a scant 0.1 percent.[81] Almost immediately, financial returns for hospitals fell precipitously and remained low for the next several years.[82]

ADDITIONAL GENEROSITY FOR HOSPITAL CONSTRUCTION

Beyond its role in reassuring investors, Medicare also enabled hospitals to expand and upgrade facilities in a more direct way through the mechanism that it used in its early years to reimburse for capital costs. As with operating expenses, Medicare paid hospitals for construction projects based on the actual costs incurred. All expenses for expanding and improving facilities were calculated and then multiplied by the percentage of the facility's patients covered by Medicare.[83] Since the elderly comprise a large proportion of the patients receiving care in many hospitals, this system covered a significant portion of their capital costs.[84]

Not surprisingly, the years immediately following Medicare's implementation corresponded with substantial growth in hospital construction.[85] As one observer noted, "From 1968 to 1971 the constant dollar value of medical facility construction increased at an average annual rate of 13.1%, a rate of increase not seen since the establishment of the Hill-Burton program twenty years before."[86]

Hospital building expenses in constant 1972 dollars grew from $3.1 billion in the four-year period between 1945 and 1949 to $16.6 billion in the period between 1975 and 1979.[87] The share of hospital construction in proportion to total non-residential construction during the same time period correspondingly rose from 10 percent in 1945 to 19 percent in 1975.[88] By infusing funds directly through reimbursement and indirectly through assurances to bond and equity investors, Medicare had turned hospitals into major players in the construction market.

The advent of Medicare did not coincide with an increase in the total number of hospitals or of hospital beds. These remained fairly constant from the late 1960s onward.[89] Instead, the funds provided by the program led to substantial improvements in existing hospital facilities and equipment and to the expansion of their technological capabilities.[90] One commentator observed, "Medicare payment policies generally have assured hospitals that they would be paid for the cost of new technologies. This assurance has had a direct effect on hospitals' decisions to adopt new technologies."[91]

It is possible that the hospital building boom would have extended even further had it not been for another government initiative that was designed to counteract it. As discussed earlier, "certificate-of-need" programs, a key part of the health planning process that began with the Hill-Burton Act, prohibited hospitals from constructing new facilities or adding new services unless they could demonstrate a community need.[92] This restriction thwarted many projects before they could begin. In 1986, Congress allowed the mandate to lapse, freeing states to decide for themselves whether to continue to limit hospital expansion. In those states that chose to drop certificate-of-need programs, about a third in all, large increases in hospital construction quickly ensued.[93] It is ironic that government policies designed to limit hospitals' growth were implemented in response to the effects of other government policies intended to encourage it. Nevertheless, the combined effect of the two sets of initiatives was a sizeable expansion of hospital facilities across the country.

Take a look at a nearby hospital. The odds are that its facility was replaced, expanded, or upgraded substantially within the past 40 years. It almost certainly has acquired expensive new equipment during that time. With few exceptions, the government provided much of the financing for those steps toward modernization, with Medicare taking the leading role. Now, try to imagine what the same institution would look like without this financial partner. It would be nothing like what it is today.

REIMBURSEMENT POLICY AND THE TRANSFORMATION OF HOSPITAL OPERATIONS

Medicare's influence on American hospitals stems from more than the magnitude of the funding it provided, as extensive as it has been. The manner of apportioning those funds was equally influential in shaping the overall nature of the enterprise. The initial approach of reimbursing hospitals for their costs strongly discouraged efficiency. As a result, expenditures for Part A of the program, particularly those for acute inpatient care, rose especially steeply during Medicare's early years. They jumped from $4.8 billion to $24.1 billion between 1970 and 1980, the largest percentage increase for any decade of the program's existence.[94]

Concerned about the unsustainability of this trend, policymakers searched for alternatives. Attention focused on a technique used in managed care. Known as "prospective payment," it determined reimbursement in advance of a patient's actual treatment. Under the first managed care plans, this approach took the form of "capitation" payments for primary care physicians, who received a set fee each month for each patient for whom they were assigned responsibility, without regard for the amount of care they actually rendered. Under this system, there is no reward for inefficiency. The challenge for policymakers was to apply the same concept to hospitals.

In 1983, Congress directed Medicare to implement a new reimbursement mechanism based on prospective payment. It determined payments not based on the actual costs incurred in providing care but on a set fee, calculated in advance, based on the patient's principal diagnosis. With limited exceptions, hospitals received the same reimbursement regardless of the amount they spent to treat each patient. This new payment structure created dramatically different financial incentives favoring hospital efficiency, which over time altered not only the nature of hospital care, but also the very structure of the hospital enterprise.[95]

The system that Medicare devised to implement prospective payment classifies every Medicare patient into a "diagnosis-related group" (DRG) according to his or her primary diagnosis. Each DRG is assigned a payment based on the cost to treat a patient of average complexity at a hospital of average efficiency. Payments are supplemented to cover three types of added costs. The first is the expense that teaching hospitals incur in training medical residents and fellows. These supplements are known as "graduate medical education" (GME) payments, and they mostly reflect the added burden of supervision.[96] The second is the expense that some hospitals bear of caring for a large proportion of indigent uninsured patients. These supplements are known as "disproportionate share hospital" (DSH) payments, and they are paid primarily to hospitals located in inner cities. The third is the added cost of treating those patients who require particularly complex care. That expense is recognized with supplements known as "outlier" payments, which are awarded on a case-by-case basis.[97]

WINNING AND LOSING SERVICES UNDER PROSPECTIVE PAYMENT

The DRG system created winners and losers among hospitals by making some conditions more profitable to treat than others. Profitable DRGs were those with high reimbursement rates that could be cared for efficiently. Among the most prominent of these was arterial blockages treated with cardiac bypass surgery.[98] Money losers required resources that were disproportionate to the economic reward. Pneumonia, for example, is a money loser because of wide variations in the time it takes patients to recover. This discrepancy in economic return presented hospitals with an incentive to concentrate their services on patients with the most profitable to treat conditions.

General acute care hospitals must provide a full range of medical services, so they cannot simply drop less remunerative treatments. However, they can encourage growth in profitable service lines and discourage it in others. Starting soon after the implementation of the DRG system, many hospitals expanded or created new lines of business in cardiac surgery. Some smaller hospitals that had never before offered procedures this complex decided to venture into the field. Larger hospitals with established programs sought larger patient volumes. Marketing campaigns to bring in more cardiac patients became more commonplace, with advertisements proliferating in many regions.[99]

Another lucrative line of business under DRG reimbursement is orthopedic surgery. Procedures to replace arthritic joints, such as hips and knees, were developed in the 1980s, and hospitals found they could provide them efficiently, which meant they could be quite profitable. As with cardiac surgery, new programs sprouted up and existing ones expanded, with many aggressive marketing campaigns to draw in patients.[100]

With this profit potential based on a restructured government reimbursement paradigm in place, the market took over. Hospitals in many regions that had been reluctant to tout their services began to behave like full-fledged market competitors, vying for patients who could be assigned the most lucrative DRGs. Today, it is difficult to avoid noticing advertisements in most regions of the country promoting the benefits of one hospital or another for treating lucrative conditions. Some institutions have dubbed themselves "heart hospitals," "spine centers," or "orthopedic institutes" to highlight their capabilities.[101] To all appearances, this looks like any other private market for a consumer good or service. But the driving economic force in this industry is not consumer spending, as it would be under the conventional "free-market" paradigm, but rather the structure of government reimbursement.

WINNING AND LOSING PHYSICIANS UNDER PROSPECTIVE PAYMENT

Commentators predicted soon after its implementation that the DRG payment system would exert a profound effect on hospital–physician relations.[102] They were right. The new reimbursement mechanism ushered in an entirely different approach by hospitals toward the composition and role of their medical staffs. Physicians now represented more than just a means to fill beds. They had become a competitive strategic asset.

The most important element in a medical service line is the physicians who render the care. With market pressures favoring those who treated the most profitable DRGs, many hospitals sought ways to restructure their medical staffs to encourage more of those practitioners to join.[103] To promote a financially optimal mix of physician specialties, in the 1980s, hospitals devised a system of basing medical staff membership on economic considerations through a process that became known as "economic credentialing."[104]

Traditionally, hospitals had welcomed any qualified practitioners who wished to practice within their walls. Under cost-based reimbursement, more physicians on a hospital staff meant the admission of more patients and therefore the generation of more revenue. By admitting patients, regardless of the kind of service, almost any physician could contribute to a hospital's bottom line.

This was not the case under the DRG system. With a reimbursement plan that rewarded efficiency, physicians in specialties that focus on profitable-to-treat diagnoses became money generators, whereas those who brought in patients with complex conditions that were difficult to treat represented monetary drains. Economic credentialing permitted hospitals to tilt the composition of their medical staffs toward those physicians most likely to generate the highest returns. Under this system, the hospital determines the maximum number of physicians permitted to perform each kind of service that the institution offers. The staff is closed to new members once the limit in their specialty has been reached. No new physicians, regardless of qualifications, are allowed to join. The number permitted to render services that are less profitable is set at the minimum needed, and the number allowed to provide more remunerative care is open-ended.

Some hospitals went one step further and changed their medical staffs from a structure composed of independent physicians to one in which medical professionals functioned as employees. Traditionally, physicians in American hospitals remained their own bosses. They rendered care for their own patients and billed either the patient or the patient's insurer directly. The hospital provided its clinicians with a place in which to practice, but did not pay them for their work.

Faced with an incentive to more tightly control the composition of their medical staffs, some hospitals chose to change this traditional relationship and employ some or all of the physicians who practiced within their walls.[105] Under this arrangement, physicians treat patients, and the hospital sends out the bills and collects the fees. It then pays the physicians a salary for their work. The advantage for the institution is that it can more closely supervise the care that is rendered and dismiss physicians who fail to meet standards.[106] Those standards include both clinical benchmarks and economic goals based on the revenues that the physicians generate.

In some markets, physicians took matters into their own hands. They formed their own for-profit hospitals that concentrated on treating patients with the most profitable DRGs. These facilities are known as *specialty hospitals*. Physician-investors used their power to make referrals to send only select patients to these facilities, often those with cardiac and orthopedic conditions.[107]

Although proponents of these institutions claim that they achieve better outcomes and efficiency by focusing on a narrow range of procedures, opponents claim that they siphon profitable patients away from general hospitals, which must still provide less remunerative services like emergency care and burn units. Specialty hospitals have another advantage in that they treat small numbers of uninsured patients, if they treat any at all. For this reason, some hospitals see specialty hospitals as a threat to their financial viability. Some have taken aggressive countermeasures, like trying to exclude participants in specialty hospital ventures from their medical staffs. Litigation has often ensued.[108]

Alarmed by the potential harm that specialty facilities pose to community hospitals, Medicare imposed a moratorium on payments to these institutions during the mid-2000s.[109] This significantly impeded their spread, as Medicare reimbursement was the primary instigator of their creation.[110] Nevertheless, they remain a serious competitive threat to hospitals in some regions, which adds another impetus for the adoption of economic credentialing and similar mechanisms to control the composition of their medical staffs.[111]

These changes in hospital–physician relationships transformed the character of the hospital industry in fundamental ways. Many individual institutions began to behave more aggressively, not just in competing for patients, but also in competing for physicians. Dealings with physicians became more businesslike, with written employment contracts often adding a layer of formality. Prominent physicians in specialties made lucrative by DRG reimbursement, such as cardiac care and orthopedic surgery, often found themselves the subject of bidding wars, sometimes resembling those for professional athletes. A world of gentlemen's agreements in nonprofit charitable institutions transitioned into a more conventional business environment, especially at larger facilities. Market forces came to dominate many aspects of hospital dealings with the medical profession, arising at their core from the guiding force of government policy.

PROSPECTIVE PAYMENT AND THE TRANSFORMATION OF ACUTE MEDICAL CARE

As dramatic as they were, the changes wrought by Medicare in the structure of American hospitals were only the start. The program came to alter the very nature of the care that hospitals rendered. For hundreds of years, hospitals were defined as facilities devoted to inpatient care. In the 1980s and 1990s, that model underwent a fundamental change.

The motivating force for this change was again the DRG payment system. Despite their efforts to game the system by crafting the shape of their medical staffs, many hospitals lost revenue under this new reimbursement paradigm. They were no longer able to generate income by adding tests, procedures, and inpatient days without external constraint. Admissions at community hospitals fell by almost one-quarter between the system's start in 1983 and 1995.[112] Average lengths of stay declined from seven days to fewer than six.[113] Financial margins declined along with them throughout the industry in both nonprofit and for-profit institutions.[114]

However, while hospitals were seeing their financial returns decline for rendering inpatient care, a different environment prevailed for outpatient services. Until 1992, the payment system for Part B of the program, which funds outpatient services, remained unchanged. That year, a new payment system was instituted; however, it did not change the underlying basis for reimbursement to prospective payment, as DRGs had done. Rather, it maintained separate fees for each service rendered and based them on a new schedule that was designed to reflect the actual work effort and expense required to provide each one.

The schedule is known as the Resource-Based Relative Value Scale (RBRVS). It sets reimbursement according to three factors—the level of training needed to perform a service, the resources needed to provide it, and the associated cost of malpractice insurance.[115] The goal in creating it was to base payments on the true cost of providing each service. The prior approach had been more haphazard because it based reimbursement on "usual and customary" charges in each market, which often bore little relation to the actual expense involved in rendering care.

Despite the change in methodology for calculating fees, RBRVS still paid physicians based on the quantity of services they performed. This maintained the incentive to provide as much care as possible. Although the new system changed the relative financial attractiveness of rendering various services, it did not change the underlying dynamic of earning more by doing more. DRGs, in contrast, placed an upper bound on the revenue potential of each patient admission, even for those conditions that are most profitable to treat.

Hospitals, like other private businesses, follow the money. They had learned over time to configure their services according to the incentives built into the structure of their reimbursement. Under the DRG system, revenues were capped for patients who were treated within their facilities, but the number of procedures rendered in outpatient settings under the RBRVS fee-for-service system had no upper limit. For outpatients, in other words, the more they did, the more money they could make.

The economic implications of this reimbursement dichotomy in the hospital setting were clear. Hospitals would do best by rendering whatever procedures they could on an outpatient basis. Outside of the hospital walls, the sky could remain the limit in producing revenue.

Hospitals were quick to respond to this new financial imperative. During the 1980s, outpatient facilities sprouted around the country, and numerous services were moved into them. The most common of these new centers of care were ambulatory surgery centers (ASCs) that performed many kinds of operations on an outpatient basis without an overnight stay. The stage had been set for their emergence with technological advances in surgical techniques that permitted many procedures to be performed in less invasive ways.[116] Among them were arthroscopic and endoscopic procedures that enable orthopedic surgeons to repair damaged joints, tendons, and other tissues and organs without the need for major incisions.[117] The technology behind these techniques was developed in the 1970s and 1980s and perfected on a wide scale on the large number of patients treated in newly opened ASCs.[118]

The move of many procedures to outpatient settings brought clinical benefits in addition to financial advantages. In particular, many of them can be performed with local, rather than general, anesthesia, which significantly reduces risks. Moreover, because they are less invasive, there is less room for error.[119] In addition to less invasive surgery, many outpatient centers offered a range of diagnostic services, especially in the field of radiology. These included x-rays, computed tomography (CT or CAT) scans, and magnetic resonance imaging (MRIs) that can be provided safely and effectively without an overnight hospital stay. A further advantage of outpatient settings is that they are often more convenient for patients.

The growth of outpatient care that began in the 1980s engendered direct improvements in some medical techniques as well. A prime example is the process of removing cataracts from the eyes. These are occlusions that cloud the cornea and can gradually block vision. Left untreated, they can lead to blindness. Before the outpatient revolution, removing them required major surgery with general anesthesia and long postoperative recovery times. The resulting discomfort for patients could be substantial. With the push to move care away from inpatient facilities, new techniques were developed that permit surgeons to perform the procedure on an outpatient basis using local anesthesia and to let patients return home the same day. Surgical risks are also substantially reduced. And, of course, the cost is also much less.[120]

Many physicians reacted to the relocation of care to outpatient settings with enthusiasm. In part, this was because, with Medicare offering fee-based reimbursement, it provided the opportunity to generate more income. Orthopedic surgery and diagnostic radiology, two specialties that are often practiced in out-patient settings, were among the biggest winners.[121] However, physicians stood to gain even more financially in another way—by acquiring ownership interests in the facilities. By investing in clinics in which they worked, physicians could share indirectly in a broader pool of revenue.[122] In addition to receiving payments for the services they rendered, they could receive part of the clinic's overall profits, which include additional reimbursement for use of the facility, itself.

Many hospitals aggressively courted physicians as partners in outpatient ventures.[123] They offered generous investment terms with the chance for sizeable returns. However, in some cases, they went too far, crossing the line that separates lawful economic partnerships from illicit kickback arrangements that improperly encouraged the referral of patients.[124] A flurry of federal enforcement activity ensued.[125] Nevertheless, the net effect of this activity was to bring large numbers of physicians into outpatient clinics, which enabled these facilities to grow in numbers and capabilities.

The movement of care to outpatient settings accelerated soon after Medicare implemented the DRG system for inpatients. Between 1983 and 1985, just after DRG-based reimbursement began, the portion of surgery performed in ASCs tripled from 1 percent to 3 percent, and total reimbursement for ASC procedures grew from $9 million to $71 million.[126] The number of physician and surgeon bills for services rendered at ASCs grew by 825.7 percent compared to only 111.1 percent for hospitals.[127] Ophthalmology is a specialty that saw particularly strong growth at ASCs. The percentage of Medicare ophthalmology bills for services rendered at ASCs increased from 7 percent to 12 percent during this time.[128] The effect of the outpatient revolution on medical specialties is considered in more detail in Chapter 5.

By the end of the 1990s, many large hospitals had developed substantial out-patient capabilities and used them for much of their operations. During the 1990s, average inpatient lengths of stay for Medicare patients shrank by 30 percent; however, overall hospital profitability rose.[129] By 1997, operating margins were higher than their levels had been when the DRG system began.[130] As hospitals adjusted to the new reimbursement environment, the paradigm of the industry was transformed from one of stand-alone institutions to amalgams of inpatient facilities and outpatient centers. The proportion of hospitals operating as part of larger systems more than doubled from about 30 percent in 1995 to 65 percent in 2001.[131] Many spread out through their regions with networks of facilities.[132] In regions with several of these medical conglomerates, competition among them intensified. Broad-based marketing campaigns were launched with billboards, newspaper, radio, and television advertisements to try to convince patients to seek out their services. Hospital advertisements became ubiquitous in some markets.

Outpatient care and specialty hospitals might well have expanded even without changes in Medicare's reimbursement paradigm. New technologies had begun to emerge independently in the 1980s that enabled physicians to perform many procedures less invasively away from inpatient settings. However, without

Medicare's redesigned payment approach, neither hospitals nor physicians would have encountered the same financial imperative to accelerate the transition. As a result, the transformation would, in all likelihood, have occurred more slowly and less pervasively. By altering the landscape of economic incentives, Medicare accelerated and directed a new approach to the very meaning of hospital care.

KEEPING TABS ON MEDICARE'S IMPACT

The impact of prospective payment on the behavior of providers is so pervasive that Congress established an oversight mechanism to monitor it. The 1983 law that implemented the DRG system created two new bodies to provide advice about the program's effects on provider behavior and clinical care.[133] These were the Prospective Payment Assessment Commission, which analyzed hospital care, and the Physician Payment Reimbursement Commission, which did the same for physician services. They were merged in 1997 into the Medicare Payment Advisory Commission, known as MedPAC.[134]

The mission of MedPAC is to consider broadly the effects of Medicare's payment structure on the health care industry. It considers the responses of providers to reimbursement incentives and of managed care companies under the program's Part C. Areas of particular concern include access to care and quality of care. To keep tabs on developments at the patient level, it conducts frequent surveys of beneficiaries to assess their experiences in obtaining care.[135] Based on the findings, it issues reports twice a year highlighting specific issues and presents testimony to Congress.[136] MedPAC's analyses often form the basis for adjustments to Medicare payment rates.

Clearly, Congress knew what it was doing when it directed Medicare to adopt the DRG system in 1983. The new payment structure was deliberately designed to encourage hospitals to abandon their inefficient ways, which required that they change their clinical behavior. The creation of MedPAC and its precursor bodies was an acknowledgment that the nature of those changes would be profound and unpredictable. The agency helps the government by generating information on the significant transformations it has wrought and by offering ongoing guidance accordingly.

MEDICAID'S CONTRIBUTION

Medicare provides the lion's share of government reimbursement for America's hospitals; however, its effects are substantially amplified by its companion program, Medicaid. By supporting care for more than 50 million low-income beneficiaries, as of 2013, who have no other means of payment for medical care, this funding source offers reimbursement for many services that would otherwise go uncompensated. It covers 14 percent of all hospital patients nationwide,[137] and this number will grow substantially under the Affordable Care Act (ACA). For hospitals that serve large indigent populations, especially those located in inner cities, this reimbursement is a lifeline.

The majority of Medicaid beneficiaries earn less than the federal poverty level, and 90 percent earn less than two times that amount.[138] With even the shortest of hospital stays often costing thousands of dollars, few of them could afford such care on their own, and few would have access to other sources of health insurance. Had the program not been created, virtually all of them would have joined the ranks of the uninsured. Many would avoid seeking care, dramatically shrinking the patient base for hospitals that now serve them. Others would receive care that would go unreimbursed, imposing significant costs on these providers. Although its payment rates are quite low, without Medicaid, the number and size of hospitals serving inner cities and rural areas would be a fraction of what they are today.

Medicaid offers particularly important financial support for some hospitals in its supplementary payments for treating a disproportionate share of indigent patients. As under Medicare, hospitals that treat a high proportion of patients who have no insurance at all receive additional reimbursement in recognition of the financial burden of doing so. These payments can mean the difference between financial life and death for these institutions.

Between payments for services rendered to beneficiaries and the supplements for indigent care, Medicaid directs a substantial amount of spending to institutional care. The portion of its budget devoted to inpatient hospitals was only 12.5 percent in 2008, but this translated into $7,070 per beneficiary, up from $4,919 in 2000.[139] Nursing homes received 16.1 percent, which amounted to $123,501 per beneficiary, a sizeable jump from the $79,330 the program spent in 2000.

As with Medicare, Medicaid has grown dramatically since its inception, and it continues to do so. Enrollment increased from 42.8 million to 58.2 million just between 2000 and 2008.[140] Spending rose from $168.3 billion to $294.2 billion during this time. Many of these beneficiaries are above the age of 65, making them eligible for both programs and thereby able to receive particularly generous coverage. The number of Medicaid beneficiaries below age 65, whose care is paid for solely by Medicaid, grew fourfold between 1984 and 2009 from 14 million to 42.4 million.[141] Another 15 million beneficiaries may be added by the ACA.[142]

Without Medicaid, the mix of services in many hospitals would also look quite different. Medicaid is the single largest source of payment for childbirth in the United States, providing reimbursement for 40 percent of all births.[143] Few inner-city hospitals could afford to offer this service with almost half the patients uninsured.

Medicaid also serves as the financial lynchpin for the hospital care of children. Pediatric hospitals represent only 5 percent of those in the country, but they provide almost all of the hospital care for children with complex conditions.[144] Half of their patients are covered by Medicaid, which insures one-third of all children in the country.[145] Beyond their role in caring for America's sickest children, pediatric hospitals train more than 40 percent of all general pediatricians in the country, 43 percent of all pediatric specialists, and over half of all pediatric researchers.[146] Medicaid provides key funding for this educational role through Children's Hospital Graduate Medical Education payments, which supplement reimbursement for medical care in a similar manner to Medicare's GME payments for training in general acute care hospitals.[147]

Medicaid's support for children's hospital care is reinforced by another program that extends health care coverage to children in families with limited incomes. The Children's Health Insurance Program (CHIP) covers more than 6 million children who do not qualify for Medicaid and have no access to private insurance. It is authorized and funded at the federal level and administered by each state.[148]

Medicaid and CHIP together provide a financial foundation for the care of a large proportion of America's children in much the same way that Medicare supports care for the elderly and disabled. Pediatric hospital care would look quite different without these programs, and the country would almost certainly have fewer children's hospitals. Those that still existed would operate on a smaller scale. What is more, obstetrical services in general hospitals would be more limited. Hospitals would, of course, still provide care for America's youngest patients. However, they would do so on a more limited basis, and major segments of the industry that provide this care would be significantly smaller.

THE OTHER SIDE OF THE BARGAIN: EMERGENCY CARE AND OTHER MANDATES

The huge sums of money that the government pours into the hospital industry to maintain its financial base come with substantial strings attached. Federal funding is rarely a free lunch. Many of the strings are contained in rules that determine eligibility to receive reimbursement from Medicare. With them, the program not only sustains American hospitals but also shapes various important aspects of their operations. For the most part, they impose quality standards to ensure that beneficiaries receive adequate care.[149] The most significant is a rule mandating that hospitals maintain accreditation with the Joint Commission, which surveys facilities regularly for compliance with standards governing virtually every aspect of their operations. However, most hospitals would comply with Joint Commission standards even without Medicare's requirements because they are also obliged to do so by most private insurers.

Beyond the quality standards, Medicare imposes other important operational requirements. The most substantial of them requires that hospitals provide basic emergency services to all who seek such care, without regard to insurance status. This obligation is embodied in the Emergency Medical Treatment and Active Labor Act, commonly known as EMTALA, which Congress enacted in 1986.[150] Under that law, hospitals that participate in Medicare must assess and stabilize all patients who present themselves in the emergency department before inquiring about their ability to pay.[151] This has ensured that acute care hospitals serve as crucial public health safety valves, standing ready to respond to patients in the most dire need, regardless of whether they can afford the bill.

However, aware that they must be seen regardless of their financial situation, many indigent patients have also turned to emergency rooms as sources of routine care. As a result, many hospitals, particularly those in inner-city areas, have come to serve some of the same functions as community health centers. In such neighborhoods, alternatives for receiving care tend to be scarce, so these de facto clinics largely define health care in their communities. With emergency room care often costing thousands of dollars for even routine procedures, this role can place a substantial burden on the finances of the hospitals involved.[152]

However, inner-city hospitals that serve largely indigent communities still have a means of financial recourse. They can recoup much of the lost revenue by charging higher rates to private insurers. This added expense is then incorporated into the premiums that the companies charge their customers. In paying these inflated rates, those with private insurance effectively subsidize, although unwittingly, the free emergency care that hospitals are mandated to provide for the indigent.

Whether they operate on a nonprofit or for-profit basis, virtually all American hospitals participate in Medicare. The program's emergency room rules, therefore, guide important elements of community and payer relations across the industry. The care available to everyone in America is thereby shaped, at least in part, by the rules imposed by this massive government program.

The Medicare program also insinuates itself into hospital operations in other, less intrusive ways. Numerous operational dictates have been added over the years, with the threat of removal from the program or adjustments to reimbursement as the means of enforcement. For example, under the Patient Self-Determination Act passed in 1990, hospitals must ask all patients on admission whether they have an advance directive, a document describing their wishes should they lose the capacity to make their own medical decisions, and to assist patients who do not have one in obtaining it.[153] Under the Health Information Technology for Economic and Clinical Health Act (HITECH) passed in 2009, hospitals face financial penalties for failing to adopt computerized records systems.[154] Under the ACA, they must publicly report data on patient outcomes. That law also offers financial incentives for forming "accountable care organizations," which are alliances with physicians and other providers to improve outcomes and efficiency.[155] In addition, the ACA prods hospitals to improve clinical effectiveness by, among other means, penalizing the readmission of too many patients within 30 days of their discharge. The strings attached to Medicare reimbursement to guide hospital operations seem perpetually to multiply.

Indirect Funding Through a Tax Subsidy

Many forms of government support are direct, like Medicare and Medicaid. They explicitly allocate funds for specific purposes. Others operate more subtly. They incentivize activities without an overt allocation. This kind of support commonly takes the form of tax breaks.

For hospitals in the United States that operate on a nonprofit basis, financial support through the tax code is an essential economic resource. By qualifying for tax-exempt status under section 501(c)(3) of the federal Internal Revenue Code, they gain several important financial advantages.[156] They can avoid federal and state taxes on any income that they earn; local taxes on their real estate holdings, which are often substantial; and state and local taxes on the sale of goods and services.[157] As noted earlier, tax-exempt status also permits investors who purchase hospital bonds to earn interest tax-free, allowing hospitals to pay lower interest rates when they issue debt.[158] And, of particular importance to some institutions, it grants donors a tax deduction for money they contribute.

In return for receiving a tax exemption, nonprofit hospitals must abide by an additional set of rigorous regulatory requirements. The tax code prohibits them from letting any part of their earnings benefit private individuals, from engaging in substantial lobbying for or against legislation, and from participating in political campaigns.[159] To avoid benefiting private parties, any financial dealings between hospitals and their physicians must comply with various restrictions so that favored staff members are not overcompensated.[160] Hospitals must also demonstrate on a continuing basis that they provide substantial benefits to their communities, for example by maintaining open emergency rooms that treat indigent patients without charge (an obligation that is reinforced by EMTALA), by participating in Medicare and Medicaid, and by including community representatives on their boards.[161]

The aggregate value of the tax subsidy that nonprofit hospitals receive in return is considerable. In 2002, they avoided about $6 billion in federal taxes and an equivalent amount in state and local taxes for a total annual benefit of over $12 billion.[162] By forgoing this revenue, the government effectively injected this amount as additional funding into the industry. It also uses the leverage that comes with this largess to shape the business practices of the recipients through the various regulations circumscribing their behavior.

Of course, a substantial number of hospitals operate on a for-profit basis. They receive none of these financial favors and therefore avoid the restrictions that come with them. However, this segment of the industry still faces regulatory accountability for its financial dealings, although it answers to different authorities. By selling stock to raise funds, the companies that own for-profit hospitals fall under the jurisdiction of the federal Securities and Exchange Commission (SEC), the Federal Trade Commission (FTC), and other agencies that regulate corporate finances. They are also beholden to the investment banks and other financial institutions that underwrite their efforts to raise capital.

Observers disagree on whether nonprofit status and tax exemption affect the behavior of health care institutions. Some believe that by maintaining public missions and governance by community boards, nonprofit hospitals remain sensitive to local needs. Others counter that for-profit hospitals provide as much uncompensated care and that they respond to the same health care regulatory agencies that enforce quality standards.[163]

Whatever the actual effects of tax-exempt status may be, by favoring nonprofit hospitals with special treatment, government policy encourages many institutions to maintain this type of structure. Along with the financial benefits they receive comes another layer of regulatory oversight through which the government further shapes their behavior. The tax exemption also confers additional billions of dollars in subsidies on the hospital industry, further reinforcing its economic base.

How Medicare Built Two Key Industry Sectors

The history of two segments of the American hospital industry tells the story of the government's foundational role especially vividly. These are the for-profit chains that have come to dominate care in many regions and the academic medical centers that mint new generations of physicians and conduct much of the research that advances medical science. Both grew during the second half of the twentieth century from relative obscurity into huge enterprises that serve as mainstays of American health care. They have reached a level of such prominence that their influence now extends throughout the entire economy. And both emerged from a crucible of government policy.

THE FOR-PROFIT GIANTS

Perhaps nothing demonstrates the transformative effect of Medicare more poignantly than its role in fostering the most market-driven segment of the hospital industry, investor-owned chains. For-profit hospitals are a relatively recent phenomenon in the industry's history. Nonprofit institutions trace their origins in America to the mid-eighteenth century, but for-profit facilities first appeared in the 1920s.[164] The early ones were small, mostly taking the form of physician-owned cooperatives. Many were little more than large clinics. For the most part, they were established in rural areas of the South and West that lacked easy access to larger nonprofit institutions. Although they were investor-owned, the investors tended to be small groups of physicians in search of a place to provide inpatient care. Ownership stakes rarely spread to the broader public, and they held little interest for the world of professional investors.[165]

The size and scope of for-profit hospital care changed dramatically beginning in the 1960s. Investor-owned institutions spread throughout the country and came to include many major facilities. In some cases, even large academic medical centers adopted a for-profit model.[166] Most of these new profit-making enterprises were part of national chains that owned large numbers of facilities.[167]

First Among Giants: Hospital Corporation of America

The first national chain to form is still the most prominent today: Hospital Corporation of America (HCA). This giant enterprise began as a single hospital, Park View Hospital, in Nashville, Tennessee, founded in the early 1960s by Dr. Thomas Frist, Sr.[168] By the mid-1960s, it had grown to the point where Dr. Frist needed outside help to run it. He found assistance in 1968, in a new physician-owned management firm that called itself Hospital Corporation of America. The hospital and its manager merged to form a new enterprise under that name.[169]

With this partnership in place, HCA immediately launched a major expansion in size and scope. It acquired additional existing hospitals, built new ones, and entered into contracts to operate others. HCA had a number of powerful advantages, with its combination of physician ownership, management expertise, and access to private capital. By the beginning of 1969, its network included 11 hospitals, and it filed an initial public offering to sell shares to the public. With this step, Wall Street and the hospital industry joined together for the first of what would be many successful joint endeavors.

With significant investment capital behind it, HCA's growth took on an even faster trajectory. By the end of 1969, it owned 26 hospitals containing a total of 3,000 beds. Expansion continued through the 1970s, and, in the 1980s, it acquired four other chains, General Care Corporation, General Health Services, Hospital Affiliates, and Health Care Corporation. By the end of 1981, it owned or operated 349 hospitals containing more than 49,000 beds, which together generated operating revenues of $2.4 billion. In 1987, the number of facilities stood at 463.[170]

The company continued its growth through deal making into the 1990s. In 1994, HCA merged with Columbia, one of its largest rivals. That company had gained prominence with the acquisition the previous year of Galen Health Care, formerly known as Humana. The combined enterprise then acquired Medical Care America, along with several other companies that operated various kinds of health care facilities. With its new size and resources, HCA put in place a comprehensive nationwide provider network that grew to include more than 350 hospitals, 145 outpatient surgery centers, 550 home care agencies, and several other ancillary providers. Together, they employed 285,000 workers and produced $20 billion in annual revenues.[171]

Starting in the late 1990s, the company changed direction. Rather than expanding in whatever way it could, it began to pare itself down to focus on its core businesses. It divested several facilities and nonhospital businesses, and spun off two smaller chains, LifePoint and Triad Hospital Groups. In 2006, it took itself private, the third time it had done so, in a deal led by an investor group that included affiliates of Bain Capital, Kohlberg Kravis Roberts, Merrill Lynch Global Private Equity, and Dr. Frist. With a value of $33 billion, the transaction was the largest leverage buyout in history up to that time.[172]

In 2008, the company achieved a milestone. Its services represented 20 percent of all hospital care in the country. It returned to public status in 2011, with an initial public offering valued at $4 billion that was, once again, the largest to date. In 2012, after four decades of dealings with Wall Street, the company's chain had come to include 163 hospitals and 105 freestanding surgery centers located in 20 states and in England. It boasts that it invests $1.5 billion each year in maintaining and upgrading its facilities.[173]

HCA tends to locate its hospitals in smaller cities and in rural areas. It has a particularly strong presence in the South, with a large number of hospitals in Florida and Texas.[174] Its strategy is to focus in areas where a lack of significant competition permits it to play a leading role.[175] It thereby tends to dominate hospital care in the regions where its facilities operate.

Other National Chains: Community Health Systems and Tenet

HCA leads the industry, but other large for-profit hospital chains also dot the country with their facilities. Among them is Community Health Systems, which began its corporate existence in 1985 and has grown through numerous corporate transactions over the years since.[176] In 1996, it was acquired in a leveraged buyout by an affiliate of Forstmann Little & Co., but it went public again in 2000. In 2007, it acquired Triad Hospitals, which had been spun off by HCA, thus adding more than 50 facilities to its system. Revenue in 2010 reached $13 billion.[177] Today, it has 133 hospitals in 29 states that include a total of 19,800 licensed beds.[178] These facilities employ more than 90,000 people. The company also provides management services to more than 150 independent facilities.

Like HCA, Community Health Systems locates its facilities in regions with hospital markets that it can dominate. More than 60 percent of its hospitals are the sole ones in their market. As a result, in these areas, the health care system is defined by investor-owned hospital care.

A third giant chain, Tenet Healthcare Corporation, grew from the first for-profit hospital management company in the country, American Medical International, which was founded in 1960. Tenet was created when that company merged with National Medical Enterprises in 1985. It grew dramatically in the 1990s and early 2000s, through a series of acquisitions of both for-profit and nonprofit hospitals around the country. Tenet experienced a rocky stretch when a series of criminal investigations and revelations of ethics violations shook it in the early 2000s and led it to replace its leadership in 2003. It spun off a number of facilities at that time. Today, the chain includes 50 hospitals and 90 outpatient centers in 13 states with more than 57,000 employees.[179] It boasts of being the second-largest investor-owned hospital chain in the United States. Revenues in 2010 exceeded $9.2 billion.[180]

Medicare and the For-Profit Hospital Industry

These three chains together produce annual revenues of more than $40 billion. They employ more than 430,000 people. Their prominence has certainly captured the attention of Wall Street, considering the series of buyouts and large public offerings in which they have been involved in recent years. As these numbers reflect, they have become a major presence in the American economy.

Many factors account for the rise of these industry titans. For one, hospital care has grown more complex and expensive over the past several decades, requiring investments that private equity markets are particularly well suited to provide. For another, economies of scale in a more sophisticated industry, particularly in purchasing and in clinical services, have strengthened the position of larger health care organizations relative to stand-alone institutions. During the 1980s and 1990s, another boost came from changes to laws in many states that made the legal environment more favorable to for-hospital ownership and removed some barriers to their expansion.[181]

Nevertheless, despite all of these favorable developments, for-profit hospital chains could not have grown and spread without a large and steady source of funding. To truly understand how these organizations arose and how they are sustained today, it is necessary to look to the foundation of the financing for the $40 billion in income they generate each year. The largest single source of that funding over the past half-century has been Medicare. The rise of the for-profit hospital sector is directly attributable to the program's generosity.[182] In the words of Rosemary Stevens, "[T]he importance of federal policy in stimulating a capitalistic hospital system cannot be overstated."[183]

It is not surprising that two of the largest hospital chains established themselves and started on paths to substantial growth in the 1960s. HCA and Community Health Systems began modestly in the early 1960s, and both embarked on major expansions toward the end of that decade. In the interim, Medicare was launched and, with it, a significant infusion of reimbursement became available. With this financial footing, the for-profit sector was poised for further expansion when Medicare changed its reimbursement method to the DRG-based system in the 1980s. For-profit hospitals were quick to devise ways to game the system by leading the movement of care to outpatient settings and partnering with physicians in the process. In the words of two veteran health policy analysts, "Medicare's different reimbursement systems made it a target to aggressive entrepreneurs whose tactics had become attractive to a growing number of hospital executives worried about the effects of managed care on their institutions. With corporate forces gaining influence, for-profit hospital chains found a niche and became a growth industry."[184]

As the for-profit chains grew, an increasing number of nonprofit hospitals converted to for-profit status, often to facilitate their acquisition by national corporations. The pace at which these conversions took place tells an interesting story. The rate held steady at about 10 a year during the first two decades of the chains' existence. The number spiked in the early 1980s, reaching a peak of 29 in 1986, but soon returned to the prior level.[185]

What forces lay behind this pattern? The answer, once again, was the market-structuring role of Medicare. When the program revised its method of reimbursing hospitals to the DRG system in 1983, many executives of nonprofit institutions became concerned that the new approach would substantially shrink their revenues. One response was to seek access to the considerable financial resources of the private equity market, which was available with a for-profit corporate structure. To that end, conversion to for-profit status and acquisition by a national chain seemed an attractive option. By the end of the decade, when experience with the new reimbursement scheme proved less damaging than feared, the pace of conversions slowed. Medicare had acted, and the private market responded.[186]

Without Medicare, there would undoubtedly still be a place for profit-making hospital chains. They have existed in one form or another since the 1920s. But they could not have reached anything close to their present size without a major source of capital. By creating Medicare, the government supplied the needed funds. Today, these facilities dominate institutional health care in many parts of the country, inspire some of the largest transactions on Wall Street, and employ almost half a million people. They exert a powerful influence throughout American health care and indeed throughout the entire economy.

THE TEMPLES OF LEARNING: ACADEMIC MEDICAL CENTERS

As important as for-profit hospitals have become to many regions of the country, their influence in American health care is dwarfed by another segment of the industry. The largest, most expensive, and most influential institutions of all are the facilities that train future generations of physicians and conduct the research that continually extends medicine's scientific horizons. These are academic medical centers (AMCs), the 800-pound gorillas of the industry. Within their corporate structures lie collections of individual institutions, medical schools, ancillary health care providers, and the practices of thousands of physicians. And no segment of the hospital industry owes its size and robustness more to Medicare than these sophisticated centers of teaching and research.

The United States has 136 medical schools, which provide students with hands-on training in hospitals as part of their education.[187] To fill the need for training sites, more than 1,000 hospitals serve as teaching facilities for these schools.[188] Of these institutions, 125 qualify as full-fledged AMCs.[189] They rank among the largest of hospitals, containing an average of almost 600 beds.[190] Between them, they train over three-quarters of all physicians in the United States.[191]

AMCs are big business. They employ more than 6,000 full-time workers on average, and one-fifth of them employ more than 10,000.[192] Nationwide, AMCs and their medical school partners employ almost 1.9 million people.[193] In addition to their direct employees, AMCs also retain the services of independent physicians who have medical school faculty appointments and supervise trainees. The average AMC has a complement of 1,410 faculty members, and one in eight has more than 2,000.[194] That adds up to more than 100,000 medical school faculty members working at these institutions nationwide.[195] Each year they train about 100,000 medical residents.[196]

Beyond their importance in training new generations of physicians, AMCs play an outsized role in providing clinical care. They represent just 6 percent of all acute care hospitals in the country but provide 20 percent of all inpatient care and 40 percent of all charity care.[197] These are the institutions that Americans usually turn to when highly specialized treatment is needed.[198] AMCs operate 75 percent of all burn care units, 80 percent of level I trauma centers, 50 percent of surgical transplant services, and 62 percent of pediatric intensive care units.[199] With their range of specialized capabilities, they provide 22 percent of all cardiac surgery, usually for those cardiology patients who are most seriously ill.[200]

AMCs are also powerful economic engines in their communities. Their payrolls, which include many highly paid physicians and executives, contribute considerable purchasing power to local economies. By one estimate, every dollar of government support for AMCs brings $3.84 in economic activity to the states in which they are located.[201]

This economic influence, coupled with the clinical capacities of the AMC enterprise, has left a major mark on American health care. In the words of one observer:

> In the course of the years, the teaching hospital has developed into one of society's most important institutions and as such has consequently assumed

a dominant role of leadership in the health field, fusing its dual purpose of education and caring for the sick into the single objective of improving the health of all the people.[202]

The Origin of the AMC Enterprise

The origin of AMCs can be traced to the birth of the first formal medical education in the United States. That dates to 1765, with the opening of the medical school of the College of Philadelphia, later to become the University of Pennsylvania.[203] Three years later, in 1768, King's College of New York, which later became Columbia University, added a medical department. Over the following decades, medical schools were added at Harvard in 1783, Dartmouth in 1798, and Yale in 1810. Over the course of the nineteenth century, they continued to proliferate, with the opening of over 400 more. However, most were of extremely low quality, and many did not stay in business for long. In 1900, there were 155, and the number fell to 75 over the course of the next 60 years, a result in many cases of the influence of the Flexner Report, which identified quality lapses in many of them.[204]

The better schools relied on hospitals as training sites. To ensure reliable access, some opened their own facilities, and others entered into formal affiliation arrangements with independent institutions. Professors from King's College's new medical department founded New York Hospital in 1776, although it was not able to open until 1791 because of the disruption of the Revolutionary War.[205] Harvard Medical School moved from Cambridge to Boston in 1807 to gain easier access to hospitals where students could be trained. Massachusetts General Hospital, which opened in 1821, met much of that need.[206]

The trend of combining hospitals and medical schools took an important turn in 1867, with the $7 million bequest of Johns Hopkins, a wealthy Baltimore businessman, to found a hospital and university. His vision was that the two institutions be intertwined so that the hospital would function as an integral part of the university's medical program and medical training would take place in a working hospital. He directed that the boards of trustees of the two institutions be interlocking to guarantee that the two components would remain joined.[207]

Johns Hopkins' vision became the model for American medical education. In the early twentieth century, changes in curricula spurred by the Flexner Report relied on the model of rigorous scientific and clinical training pioneered at his namesake university.[208] In particular, it led the way in hands-on hospital training.

In response, over the decades that followed, every medical school in America forged formal ties with a teaching hospital and sometimes with several. Today, it is taken for granted that medical schools are situated in university settings and include hospital training as part of the educational process.[209] These facilities also serve as centers for university-based biomedical research. They contribute facilities and equipment both for investigations into basic science and for clinical studies of the patients whose illnesses they are treating. Many are located in inner cities, where they also provide essential health care services to indigent populations that have few alternative sources of care.

The AMC Powerhouses of Today

With these expansive missions, teaching hospitals have grown into large and complex enterprises. In combination with their affiliated medical schools, they have evolved into entities that bear little resemblance to the stand-alone facilities from which they emerged. The combination of teaching and research missions give AMCs the capability to offer cutting-edge care, to set national standards of care, to test the latest technologies, and to serve as providers of last resort for the most seriously ill patients. These institutions are also the proving grounds for most new drugs, devices, procedures, and other technologies that are used throughout the country and the world. And they are the crucibles that forge new generations of medical practitioners.

AMCs now dot the country, often dominating the market for hospital care in their regions. In New York City, New York-Presbyterian Hospital, the training site for the medical schools at Columbia and Cornell Universities, operates 2,389 beds, employs more than 18,000 people, and generates $3.2 billion in annual revenue.[210] Montefiore Hospital, an affiliate of the Albert Einstein College of Medicine of Yeshiva University, operates 1,491 beds with more than 17,000 employees and $2.87 billion in annual revenue.[211] And these are just two out of several AMCs in the City.

Partners Health Care in Boston, a health system that includes Massachusetts General Hospital and Brigham and Women's Hospital, the two main teaching facilities for Harvard Medical School, operates a total of 2,564 beds. It is the largest employer in Massachusetts, with 54,000 people on its payroll.[212] It generates $8 billion a year in revenue, 40 percent of which comes from government programs.[213]

The University of Pennsylvania Health System owns three hospitals in downtown Philadelphia. Together, they contain 1,714 beds, employ 21,000 people, and generate $4.3 billion in annual revenue.[214] At the other end of the state, the University of Pittsburgh operates a health system that includes 20 hospitals, including the flagship University of Pittsburgh Medical Center. They contain 4,500 beds and, with 55,000 employees, represent the second largest employer in Pennsylvania.[215] The system brought in $9 billion in revenue in 2011.[216] More than 40 percent of that sum came from government programs.[217]

These institutions, and others like them, dwarf the others in their regions in size, financial impact, and technological sophistication. They act as major foundations not only of local employment but of overall economic vitality, as well. They not only help to support entire regional economies, but some of them have been instrumental in reshaping economies, such as those of Boston and San Francisco, into high-technology engines.[218]

AMCs and Medicare

Operating institutions on this scale is tremendously expensive. AMCs must maintain state-of-the-art facilities with cutting-edge equipment that embodies the latest technologies. They must attract and retain the most highly trained and skilled physicians. And they tend to treat the sickest patients who require the most intensive care. To do so, they generate costs well above those for other kinds of hospitals. A 1998 analysis pegged the average cost to treat a patient at $8,548 in an AMC, $6,047 in a stand-alone teaching hospital, and $5,238 in a nonteaching community hospital.[219]

To maintain their high cost structure, these mainstays of the American hospital industry rely on government programs to a greater extent than smaller institutions. Almost a third of their revenue comes from Medicare.[220] When that reimbursement is combined with payments from Medicaid, the total represents close to half of all revenue for most of them.[221] Almost a third of their Medicare payments reflect the costs of training medical students, residents, and fellows, and another 12 percent represents the added expense of treating an unusually large share of indigent patients.

Medicare's GME payments not only recognize the cost of actual training but are also designed to reflect the higher concentration of complex conditions, seriously ill patient populations and more sophisticated equipment and technology that characterize academic institutions.[222] They include two components. One is a pass-though for the direct costs of salaries for medical residents. The other is a supplement to the DRG reimbursement for each patient to compensate for indirect costs, in particular the reduced productivity of physicians who must supervise trainees.

The net result is a substantial financial boost for AMCs that reached $9.5 billion in 2010.[223] The value of indirect GME payments alone reached $6.5 billion in 2012.[224] In addition, some states pay GME supplements to AMCs through their Medicaid programs. In 2009, these totaled over $3 billion.[225]

This generosity has been instrumental in keeping many AMCs financially afloat.[226] Of all hospital types, these institutions tend to have the lowest overall operating margins. However, their margins for treating Medicare patients are the highest. This means that without Medicare to boost their financial returns, many would have no alternative financial source with which to counteract a perennially shaky bottom line.

By reimbursing the cost of patient care and the additional expense of training new physicians, Medicare and Medicaid have been the driving financial force that enabled the teaching hospitals of the mid-twentieth century to become the AMCs of today. Before the creation of these programs, teaching hospitals had spent much of their resources providing free care to indigent patients.[227] Their faculty members supervised this care without compensation and earned most of their income from private practice. Medicare and Medicaid offered a source of reimbursement for many of the indigent, thus freeing faculty physicians to perform more nonclinical duties, such as teaching and research, and permitting the institutions to devote more of their resources to upgrading their facilities. By alleviating the burden of uncompensated care, therefore, these programs allowed AMCs to assume their present mission of education and research. As a study of AMCs in several major markets concluded, "This system of training and faculty development became practical only when governments began supporting the care of indigent and elderly patients."[228]

Had Medicare and Medicaid never been enacted, teaching hospitals would still exist, as they had for more than half a century before these programs came into being. But the teaching hospitals of the early and mid-twentieth century bore little resemblance to the academic powerhouses of today. They were considerably smaller, conducted much less research, and contributed a fraction of the financial stimulus to their local economies. Without Medicare and Medicaid, we would not have AMCs in their present size and form, and the entire academic medical enterprise, not to mention the financial fortunes of many parts of the country, would be considerably reduced in size.

The Government and the Hospital Industry of Today

The government initially intervened in the hospital industry to help patients. The first major federal program, the Hill-Burton Act, responded to the lack of accessible facilities for those in rural areas. Medicare responded to the limited availability of insurance for the elderly and totally disabled, and Medicaid was designed to serve the same purpose for the poor. Private companies would find it difficult to bear the risk of insuring such needy populations with little prospect of generating profits in return.

But it is impossible to support the demand side of a market without affecting the supply side, as well. The government programs that opened the door for millions of customers who needed hospital care could not help but transform the institutions that rendered that care. These effects are largely invisible to the beneficiaries who are at the core of the government's mission, but those in the industry and outsiders who invest in it see them every working day.[229]

Medicare and Medicaid survive today as hypertrophied versions of their initial forms. They inject a total of more than a trillion dollars a year into the health care system and account for close to half of the industry's revenue. It is impossible to provide support like that without profoundly affecting the recipients. Medicare now explicitly accounts for the role it has assumed as the guiding force for its hospital participants when it sets reimbursement rates for them.[230] It also has a mechanism to regularly gauge its effects on hospital operations and patient satisfaction in the advice of the Medicare Payment Advisory Commission.

Medicare's role in underpinning the financial viability of the hospital system is now so firmly established that it has been recognized by the Supreme Court.[231] In the case of *Fisher v. United States*, a 2000 opinion involving criminal health care fraud, the Court considered whether Medicare payments should do more than merely provide compensation for services rendered.[232] It concluded that Medicare's function is much broader and now includes responsibility for insuring the general availability of health care. The Court declared, "The payments are made not simply to reimburse for treatment of qualifying patients but to assist the hospital in making available and maintaining a certain level and quality of medical care, all in the interest of both the hospital and the greater community."[233]

As the largest single payer for hospital services, Medicare could use its market position to impose draconian reductions on payment rates. Indeed, federal budget pressures may force it to do so at some point in the future. However, for the time being, Medicare is not administered with an eye to obtaining care as cheaply as possible. To the contrary, it is operated as a partner that strives to sustain the industry it funds.[234] In the words of two veteran health policy analysts, "Medicare has an interest in assuring access to needed services for the beneficiaries it serves; correspondingly, it has no interest in abusing its position of market power to the detriment of its beneficiaries and the delivery system."[235]

Government support for hospitals took another giant step with passage of the ACA in 2010. That law seeks to cut by at least half the number of Americans without health insurance, which means fewer patients with no means of payment. This is a significant financial boost, especially for struggling inner-city hospitals that see large numbers of indigent patients in their emergency rooms. In return, the ACA reduced some elements of Medicare reimbursement that were intended to compensate for the indigent care burden; however, the net effect is to provide yet further reinforcement of the industry's economic base.[236]

With this relatively secure financial footing, hospital care today comprises a commercial enterprise that behaves in many ways like a typical private industry. The business of operating hospitals is marked by intense competition and aggressive corporate behavior. The government has partnered with a major private sector economic force, yet the independence of that force is more apparent than real, leading one observer to note, "Although it may be tempting to point at acute care hospitals as key shapers of health care, in reality they mostly function as pawns of Medicare."[237]

HOSPITALS WITHOUT THE GOVERNMENT

With the government explicitly committed to the vitality of the hospital industry and implicitly dedicated to directing its behavior, the same question can be asked concerning hospitals that was asked of other key components of America's health care system. What would it look like without the massive public support that sustains and structures its revenue base? Clearly, hospitals would still exist. They have operated in one form or another for thousands of years and have been part of American health care for more than 250 years. However, they would look quite different in many ways.

For one, far fewer of them would serve as mainstays for health care in indigent communities. Without the mandate to serve all who seek emergency care, many would turn uninsured patients away from their emergency departments. Without the Hill-Burton Act's indigent care requirements and the rules for maintaining tax-exempt status, less care of any sort would be provided to those with no means of payment. And without Medicare and Medicaid funding, few could afford to render charity care, even if they wished to. Poorer citizens would find it difficult to obtain services in many institutions, and inpatient care would resemble more of a luxury than an entitlement.

With a smaller revenue base and less commitment to serving all of their neighbors, hospitals would also play less central roles in the economic life of their communities. They would be less likely to function as financial mainstays of many cities and towns and as primary sources of employment. With hospitals leaving a smaller financial footprint, the economies of their regions would be quite different and, for the most part, much smaller.

Perhaps more significantly, the country would have fewer hospitals, and many of those that survived would be smaller. They would also face considerably greater financial constraints in building and maintaining facilities and equipment. The high-technology marvels that we take for granted today as part of the health care environment would be much harder to find, and the quality of care in those that existed would be lower. Through the incentive structure that prospective payment created for greater efficiency and increased emphasis on outpatient care, Medicare has engendered significant improvements in quality that are seen throughout the entire health care system.[238]

In recent decades, the hospital industry has consolidated considerably. Many facilities have merged into larger systems, and some smaller ones have closed. Reimbursement pressures and an increasingly competitive environment have made it difficult for all but a few institutions to survive on their own without access to the resources of strategic and financial partners. This has produced more concentrated markets in many regions dominated by a few major players. Had the government not encouraged a wave of hospital expansion in the mid-twentieth century, these industry changes might have occurred much sooner.

The most dramatic difference would be in the number of major medical centers. More than any other component of the industry, the behemoth health systems of today owe their size and shape to a foundation of government programs. The Hill-Burton Act provided the financing for a first round of construction and expansion in the decades following World War II. Medicare financed a second round during the latter part of the twentieth century. Medicaid added another boost by sustaining the financial viability of centers located in inner cities, where many AMCs are situated. It is difficult to imagine that Temple University Hospital in Philadelphia, New York-Presbyterian/Columbia University Medical Center in New York, Johns Hopkins in Baltimore, UCLA in Los Angeles, or numerous others could have reached their present size and depth of capabilities on their own while serving the poor inner-city communities that surround them.

AMCs are also the base for much of the country's biomedical research. Their scale permits sophisticated investigations in a range of fields that would be impossible in smaller institutions. Without support from another government agency, the National Institutes of Health (NIH), they could not have built the laboratories, hired the staff, or maintained the research infrastructure that sustains advances in biomedical science.

Nor could the for-profit sector of the hospital industry have grown to a substantial size. For-profit hospitals rely on Medicare to supply payment for many of their services and to reassure investors of their financial stability. Without government reimbursement, the number of profit-making facilities would have remained small, and the large chains that today own the majority of them would not have formed.

COULD THE INDUSTRY HAVE THRIVED WITHOUT THE GOVERNMENT?

Despite its position as the largest single source of funding for health care, the government is, of course, not the only one. Private insurers still provide about half the reimbursement that the industry receives. Might the private market have played a similar supporting role had the government not stepped in? The national chains that own many of today's for-profit hospitals and the large national insurers have access to considerable resources. Might they have used their financial wherewithal to support the same level of industry growth?

Private funding might well have made up some of the shortfall had the government not created the industry's economic base. However, it is difficult to imagine that this support would have reached the same level of generosity as the government's. Private firms rarely have the excess capital to invest in promoting the country's basic needs. The pressures of market competition preclude them from diverting significant funds from immediate business concerns to support long-term societal goals like medical education, biomedical research, and indigent care.

Moreover, most hospitals serve a clientele that is largely old and often poor. What private institution could earn a profit caring for those populations without a reliable source of third-party funding, and what private insurer could stay in business selling them coverage? Medicare and Medicaid were created because the private market was unable to meet this need. Without these programs, there would have been no source of reimbursement for millions of the most frequent customers for hospital services. In the absence of payment for much of their market, it is difficult to imagine that hospitals could have attracted the private capital through either the equity or bond markets that they need to function as they do today.

Hospitals and American Health Care

A smaller and less robust hospital industry would have engendered a very different kind of health care system at all levels. One significant difference is that hospitals would have offered far fewer opportunities for physicians. A smaller number of facilities providing a more restricted scope of services could not have supported the range of highly trained specialists who render advanced care to severely ill and injured patients today. Nor could they have supported the level of income that attracts many physicians into specialized fields of practice. The medical profession and all of the other kinds of professionals who rely on hospitals to maintain their practices would function in a very different manner had the government not inserted itself so aggressively into health care.

Government policies may well have created a larger hospital industry than the country really needs. Experts often bemoan an oversupply of inpatient capacity in many regions, which adds costs and inefficiency to the overall health care system. Public initiatives have certainly lacked precision in pursuing their goal of fostering a large national complement of technologically capable and financially stable institutions. Nevertheless, regardless of whether those policies overshot the mark, Americans still have them to thank for the level of access to advanced institutional medical care they enjoy and for the economic stimulus this access engenders.

5

How the Government Created
the Medical Profession

[Medicare] made us rich, as simple as that.

—CHARLES FISCH, FORMER PRESIDENT, AMERICAN COLLEGE OF CARDIOLOGY[1]

No profession enjoys more prestige than medicine, and few enjoy higher incomes. The average cardiologist earned more than $300,000 in 2010, and the average orthopedic surgeon more than $350,000.[2] Even in the lowest earning specialty, pediatrics, the average practitioner took in over $150,000. Almost one-third of all physicians earn more than $250,000 a year.[3]

The income advantage of American physicians is largest for specialists. The median incomes of two of the top-earning specialties, orthopedic surgery and radiology, were more than double those of the principal primary care fields of internal medicine, family practice, and pediatrics.[4] But even the lowest-earning physicians took home well more than the average American worker. The median household income in the United States in 2010 was $51,914, about a third that of pediatricians.[5]

Physician incomes in America are also well above those in most other countries.[6] American primary care physicians earn more than their colleagues anywhere else in the world, more than double the median for similar practitioners in Europe. American specialists rank third behind the Netherlands and Australia but still earn almost three times the median for other developed countries. These differences hold both in absolute terms and in relation to each country's gross domestic product.[7]

Beyond its outsize earnings, the medical profession in the United States also holds a special importance in other ways. Physicians play the dominant role in determining the size and direction of almost every dollar spent on American health care. Their clinical decisions guide 90 percent of the funds that flow through the system.[8] With this power to shape expenditures, the profession serves as the financial gateway for the entire health care industry, which generates a total of more than $2.5 trillion a year in economic activity.

The medical profession did not always enjoy this vaunted status. Before the start of the twentieth century, it was a largely disorganized, an occasionally disreputable, and an often low-paid vocation.[9] Formal training was inconsistent and often seriously deficient. More practitioners gained their skills as apprentices rather than as students in universities, and those who attended formal medical schools often obtained only a rudimentary education, unless they went to one of the top institutions.[10] Once in practice, many physicians earned more of their incomes selling patent medicines than rendering actual clinical care.[11] Until the middle of the nineteenth century, medical practice was largely nonstandardized, with practitioners in different regions rendering widely differing treatments for the same maladies.[12] With formal training the exception, few physicians worked in, or even maintained regular contact with, hospitals.[13] Respect for the profession was low, and the incomes of many practitioners were meager.

How did the medical profession evolve from one of low status and limited earnings into the paragon of American professionalism that it is today? The shift was largely instigated by the profession itself, with the American Medical Association (AMA), founded in 1847, serving as the driving force. Over the next hundred years, the Association used various strategies to improve the lot of physicians so that, by the middle of the twentieth century, the medical profession's standing had been transformed.

But the story of American medicine's advance did not end there. Starting in the 1960s, another wave of change brought even greater influence and riches. It is what created the modern medical profession as we know it today. While the AMA and other professional groups offered support, another player added the essential ingredients of authority and funding: the government.

Medicare, Medicaid, and other government payment programs today account for 31 percent of all physician income.[14] The program with the greatest effect is Medicare, which alone is estimated to fund almost 23 percent of all physician earnings nationally. In some specialties, the proportion is even larger. American cardiologists, for example, earn almost 40 percent of their income from Medicare, and nephrologists, who treat kidney disease, earn almost two-thirds. The government did not create the medical profession, but it did provide the key ingredients for the field's remarkable ascent.

Some would argue that government initiatives have been too favorable to physicians and that they enable practitioners to earn incomes that are excessive. High physician salaries are often singled out as a major driver of America's substantial health care cost burden. As with other industry sectors, physicians have learned to use the financial rewards that public programs have bestowed on them to maintain and enhance the monetary flow. Specialty societies routinely lobby Congress to sustain ample levels of Medicare reimbursement. Moreover, as described later, representatives of medical specialties have insinuated themselves into the Medicare rate-setting process to ensure that payments remain at levels they consider acceptable.

To be sure, for their part, many physicians complain about inadequate Medicare payments, particularly for primary care. However, they continue to enjoy incomes above those of colleagues in most other developed countries thanks in large part to Medicare's support. Perhaps it has not succeeded all the time, but, to a large extent, the medical profession has been able to capture much of the regulatory process that oversees it. And regardless of whether that process confers financial rewards that one considers reasonable or excessive, without it, the profession would enjoy a fraction of its present wealth and standing.

The Medical Profession Through History

The story of the medical profession in the United States shows the remarkable nature of its rise. A combination of self-help and government intervention produced a professional juggernaut. Much of its success can be attributed to the ways in which these two forces have often functioned as one and the same.

THE FIRST ATTEMPTS AT STANDARDIZED OVERSIGHT

When the AMA was established in the middle of the nineteenth century, few viewed physicians as the adherents of a rigorous scientific calling. Their power to actually effect cures was limited at best. Many of them still used leeches and blood-letting as standard therapies.[15] Moreover, clinical standards varied widely for the treatments that did exist, and vigorous rivalries raged between different schools of practice. Some alternatives to traditional allopathic medicine, such as homeopathy and osteopathy, held considerable sway.[16] Medical practice itself was not even recognized as a single profession, with physicians, surgeons, and pharmacists vying to treat patients with similar conditions.[17]

The Association's founders sought to change that state of affairs and the public perception of the medical profession that went with it. Their goal was to place the profession on a scientific footing through formal education and systematic oversight of quality.[18] This was a formidable task in 1847, given the profession's uneven state. In seeking to reverse the medical profession's standing, the Association pursued two complementary strategies. One was to upgrade and standardize medical education with rigorous scientific training and clinical experience. This was the primary element in the organization's founding mission.[19] The other was to introduce a system of formal licensure through which entry into practice would be restricted to qualified individuals. The two goals worked in tandem, as completion of a more demanding course of study served as a prerequisite for obtaining a license.

Government-imposed standards for medical practice were hardly a novel idea. They are described as far back as far as the first century A.D. in India and China and in 1140 in Italy.[20] England adopted a medical licensure system in 1518 under King Henry VIII with the chartering of the Royal College of Physicians, which had a mission to "grant licenses to those qualified to practice and punish unqualified practitioners and those engaging in malpractice."[21]

Despite this long history, licensure was not required for medical practice in mid-nineteenth-century America. A few state programs had been enacted in the early part of the century, but all were later abandoned. The AMA set about not only to promote licensure but to do so on a uniform national basis. The focus was on a system based at the state rather than federal level. Local bureaucracies, the

AMA believed, would be more responsive to physician concerns than a central-ized apparatus that served the entire country.[22]

The first state to respond to the AMA's call and adopt a modern regulatory scheme for physician licensure was Texas, which implemented its system in 1873. Over the course of the next 40 years, every other state followed suit, with legisla-tures across the country adopting more than 400 statutes regulating medical prac-tice.[23] Each created its own medical board to supervise the grant of licenses. A key aspect of the process was the administration of an examination testing knowledge of the field, which was standardized across all of the states. To add a further ele-ment of consistency to their standards and operations, all of the boards joined together in 1912 to form a coordinating body, the Federation of State Medical Boards (FSMB).[24]

The boards brought many disparate schools of medical practice, including allopathic medicine, homeopathy, osteopathy, and hydropathy, together under one oversight mechanism. In creating a single regulatory process, licensure laws encouraged standardization of the various forms of practice as a means to enhance quality.[25] The notion of doing so was considered somewhat novel at the time. One contemporary account felt it necessary to justify a new law in Pennsylvania as "a perfectly satisfactory basis for the settlement of disputes and contentions among the several schools of medical practice by placing them all on an equality before the law."[26]

ADDING RIGOR TO MEDICAL TRAINING

The cornerstone of the licensure programs was the requirement that applicants receive a diploma from an accredited medical school that offered an approved curriculum. Accreditation of schools is granted by an organization known as the Liaison Committee on Medical Education (LCME), which operates under the AMA's auspices.[27] This prong of the Association's campaign was in some ways more of an accomplishment than the adoption of licensure laws by all of the states. It imposed rigorous standards through a process over which it, rather than the government, retained direct control.

The AMA's campaign to oversee medical education began in earnest in 1904, when it established an expert panel, the Council on Medical Education, to devise a plan for reform.[28] The Council's first order of business was to recommend uniform requirements for training. Among these were mandates that prospective physi-cians complete four years of high school, four years of medical training, a fifth year of education in basic sciences, and a one-year hospital internship. The Council also recommended the basic elements of knowledge and skills that physicians should learn and the resources, such as libraries and laboratories, that medical schools should possess to teach them.[29]

With these standards in mind, the next step was to measure whether each of the medical schools then in existence met them. A preliminary review based on the pass rates of graduates on licensure examinations found acceptable results for only about half the schools. However, rather than publicly releasing the findings, which could have generated a political backlash, the AMA asked a reputable outside organization to conduct a separate investigation of its own.[30]

The group that the AMA turned to for an independent assessment of America's medical schools was the Carnegie Foundation for the Advancement of Teaching, which, as discussed in Chapter 4, hired a young educator named Abraham Flexner to visit and evaluate every one of them. He described his findings in a report published in 1910, and it led a revolution in the structure of American medical education.[31] The Flexner Report concluded that more than half the schools in the country failed to meet AMA standards, and it recommended that they be closed. The findings led some marginal schools to disband on their own, realizing that they could not afford the improvements needed to meet the minimum standards. Other schools disappeared through mergers. Overall, the number of medical schools shrank dramatically in the wake of the Report, but, among those that remained, standards rose markedly. With the pool of schools winnowed down to the most rigorous and financially stable, many states sought to improve quality further by adding an extra entry requirement of at least one year, and later two, of college.[32]

Having established the criteria for medical education, the AMA took on the responsibility of supervising their implementation going forward. It created a set of nonprofit organizations, including the LCME, with which it remained affiliated to accredit various parts of the educational enterprise. The LCME is a partnership between the AMA and the Association of American Medical Colleges (AAMC). It provides basic accreditation for medical schools in the United States and Canada.[33] The Accreditation Council for Graduate Medical Education (ACGME) accredits postgraduate residency and training programs. The Educational Commission for Foreign Medical Graduates (ECFMG) certifies graduates of foreign medical schools to enter ACGME-approved programs in the United States. These latter two groups also operate in conjunction with the FSMB.[34]

Under this new bureaucratic oversight structure, medicine began to take on the attributes of a standardized and rigorous profession. Practice was increasingly based on scientific principles and knowledge, which brought the profession new clinical effectiveness. What had been largely a cottage industry grew into a major business enterprise that adopted increasingly sophisticated modes of operation and an expanding array of technological tools.

THE MOVE TO SPECIALIZATION

The next significant step in medicine's advance was the formal recognition of specialization as a distinct form of practice. It may have seemed a minor development at the time, but, over the course of the mid-twentieth century, it came to define the underlying character of medicine as a profession in the United States. A license confers legal authority to provide any medical service; however, many kinds of care require special expertise that only a limited number of physicians possess. In the decades following the winnowing of the profession in the wake of the Flexner Report, much of medical practice had fallen into that category. These aspects of care could only be rendered competently with a refined set of skills and specialized knowledge. Those who hold them are known as specialists.

The AMA created a formal structure to certify competence in medical specialties in the 1930s.[35] It based the regime on a series of boards that set standards and measured abilities in various fields. The first was the American Board of Internal Medicine (ABIM) founded in 1936.[36] Today, there are 24 such boards in fields ranging from long-established disciplines such as radiology and surgery to newer arrivals such as medical genetics and preventive medicine.[37]

Since the inception of the ABIM, specialization has come to define much of the medical profession. The transformation gained particular momentum in the 1950s, when the proportion of medical students planning to enter general practice fell from 60 percent to 16 percent, and the proportion looking to specialize rose from 35 percent to 74 percent.[38] Over the decades since, this pattern has remained fairly constant. Today, primary care physicians, the modern-day equivalent of generalists, comprise less than 40 percent of the profession. The rest practice in medical specialties or in surgery, treating the most complex and serious conditions and rendering the most technologically sophisticated care.[39] These physicians, as noted, also command the highest incomes, earning on average more than twice the salaries of their primary care colleagues.[40]

PHYSICIANS AND HOSPITALS

By enforcing practice standards, the regulatory apparatus composed of government agencies and professional organizations underlies much of the medical profession's prestige and status. However, it is only one of several mechanisms that do so. Among the most significant of the others is the oversight process of the hospitals in which most of them practice.

The educational reforms of the early twentieth century placed hospitals at the center of physician training. At the same time, physicians were able to cement a dominant role in running these institutions. Until the early twentieth century, hospital boards of trustees held most of the power and influence.[41] Their members tended to represent the social and economic elites of their regions. As medicine advanced in the late nineteenth century and the care rendered to inpatients became more complex and effective, the physicians who provided it gained greater importance.

For example, by 1890, surgery had moved almost entirely to hospital settings from private homes, where much of it previously had been performed.[42] By that time, the standard of care had come to include the use of technological tools that only an institution could provide such as general anesthesia, aseptic operating procedures, refined handling of tissues, and surgical pathology.[43] By the end of the century, the role of physicians who rendered such advanced procedure-oriented care had been formalized as the most powerful component in the structure of most institutions.[44]

Physicians exert their dominance in hospital operations as members of autonomous medical staffs that oversee all medical care. These function as separate divisions over which the administration has no direct control. American hospitals are required to maintain this structure under criteria imposed by their accrediting body, the Joint Commission (formerly the Joint Commission on the Accreditation of Health Care Organizations [JCAHO]).

Accreditation guidelines of the Joint Commission not only mandate that hospitals maintain medical staffs, they also grant physicians substantial latitude in directing the functioning of these bodies. Most importantly, medical staffs control their own membership, deciding who is qualified to join and what privileges to render particular clinical services they may exercise. Control over membership includes the authority to police physician behavior and to decide when infractions by members merit discipline or expulsion. Of particular importance to member physicians are the procedural safeguards available before an adverse action may be taken against them. The Joint Commission requires that physicians facing discipline be afforded "due process," a fair proceeding that permits them to present their side of the story, a protection that few other professionals enjoy. More generally, medical staffs also oversee all clinical functions carried out in hospitals, from the handling of tissue samples, to the maintenance of medical records, to the assessment of patient outcomes.[45]

Recent trends have chipped away at some aspects of this structure, and hospital administrations play an increasingly powerful role in overseeing their medical staffs. As described later, many hospitals now directly employ some or all of the members of their medical staffs, which confers greater power to guide their behavior. However, physicians continue to hold key elements of authority in most institutions and thereby to exert considerable influence over the provision of inpatient care.

PHYSICIANS' ECONOMIC AUTONOMY

Medicine during the first half of the twentieth century was defined not only by the nature of clinical practice but also by a distinctive economic structure. Physicians practiced predominantly in solo settings or with a single partner, and larger groups were the exception. The business model for those entering the profession was either to "hang out a shingle" to attract patients on their own or to practice with an established colleague. Although the profession was gaining substantial sophistication on the scientific and technological side, it remained essentially a cottage industry in its economic aspects. Many practitioners cherished such an environment in which they could maintain their professional autonomy and function as their own boss.

Over the course of the second half of the twentieth century, that pattern began to change. By 2008, solo and two-physician practices comprised less than one-third of the profession.[46] Almost a fifth of physicians practiced in groups containing more than five members, and 6 percent practiced in groups of more than 50. Another third worked for larger organizations that were either hospitals, medical schools, health centers, or health maintenance organizations (HMOs), and a majority functioned as employees rather than as outright owners of their practices. With these shifts, the work environment for physicians has increasingly come to resemble the businesslike environment of most other professions. However, even under this new professional paradigm, they still enjoy a special place in society, with respected status and high earnings.

MEDICAL PRACTICE AFTER ITS FORMATIVE YEARS

Through the creation and maintenance of licensure, standardized education, and hospital medical staff authority, the medical profession was able to define its own structure and determine the nature of its regulatory oversight. It exercised unique power to shape its own working environment in hospitals and in independent practice settings. By the mid-twentieth century, it had come to enjoy remarkable social and economic status, in stark contrast to its standing of just half a century earlier. But an even greater leap lay ahead. This one came at the instigation not of the profession itself, but of an unlikely partner—the federal government.

The public sector gave medicine a level of financial reward and technological sophistication that the profession's leaders of a century earlier could hardly have imagined. Its role in transforming the lot of physicians began in earnest in the 1960s, with a series of programs that addressed perceived deficiencies in the profession's reach and scope. Of these, the most influential by far was Medicare, which expanded the reimbursement landscape for physicians and showered them with hundreds of billions of dollars in revenue. With this dramatic infusion of funding, it also transformed the underlying nature of medical practice. However, Medicare, important as it was, served as merely one of several initiatives that worked in combination to advance the economic standing of medical practice.

The Federal Government and the Medical Profession: First Steps

The federal government's first intervention in the structure of the medical profession focused on the distribution of its services. With its quality and value clearly established, the ability of patients to access physician care became increasingly important. By the 1950s, government policymakers foresaw a major threat to American health care in a looming national shortage. Increasing demand for medical care combined with a growing population and the greater availability of insurance to cover the cost led to predictions that the supply of practitioners would soon become inadequate. All Americans, it was feared, could find physician services difficult to obtain, and prices could consequently rise precipitously.[47]

Coupled with this threat was a maldistribution of physicians who were already in practice. They tended to cluster in suburbs and affluent urban areas, where they could serve a higher-income clientele that was more likely to have the financial resources to pay for their services, either on their own or through insurance. This pattern of concentration left shortages in poorer regions, both in inner cities and in rural areas, with consequent deficiencies in access to care.[48]

An answer to both problems was seen in an expansion of medical school enrollment to enhance the pipeline of new practitioners. To this end, Congress in 1963 acted to increase the supply of physicians by allocating funds for medical school construction and loans for students through the Health Professions Educational Assistance Act.[49] Amendments enacted two years later continued the programs and expanded their scope to provide funds to increase enrollment at existing schools.[50]

The Act succeeded in dramatically increasing the size of the medical education enterprise. Eighty-seven medical schools operated in the United States in 1972, nine years after the funding programs began. By 1982, there were 127, an increase of almost 50 percent. Along with larger enrollments at many established schools, the number of graduates doubled, from 7,409 a year to 15,135. With a larger national complement of physicians, the ratio of physicians to population increased markedly from 140 per 100,000 in 1960 to 202 per 100,000 in 1980.[51] By 2010, the country had 850,000 physicians in active practice.[52] The number had risen from 781,000 just 10 years earlier in 2000.[53]

In the end, this effort to manage the physician workforce successfully increased the supply, but it did not eliminate either of the underlying problems it was intended to solve—growing cost pressures and a maldistribution of practitioners. Fees charged for services continued to rise, and access remained limited in many poorer regions. Nevertheless, the profession emerged much larger, and with bigger numbers came greater influence.[54]

The academic medical enterprise also solidified its standing at this time and with it came a new line of opportunities for physicians. As academic medicine grew in size with higher enrollments, it also expanded its role as the foundation of research-based innovation. In large part, this resulted from another funding source that grew during the latter half of the twentieth century, this one supporting biomedical research. The primary vehicle for allocating this support was the National Institutes of Health (NIH), which, as described in Chapter 3, began operation in the 1930s to advance basic biomedical science. The agency's budget grew from about $30 million in 1950 to $14 billion in 1998, with about 80 percent of it supporting research by private investigators at universities and institutes across the country.[55] The NIH's budget continued to grow at a rapid pace in the early 2000s, and it exceeded $30 billion in 2012.[56] In constant 1938 dollars, it today would be close to $1 trillion.[57] Particularly dramatic increases occurred in the periods between 1956 and 1968 and between 1998 and 2004.[58]

Most NIH-funded projects are housed in medical schools. With higher student enrollments and larger numbers of faculty members working in them, these institutions were well positioned to take advantage of this new form of governmental generosity. The growing federal interest in supporting biomedical investigation led them to expand their missions from one focused primarily on education to one in which research received equal status. With this dual focus, the institutions that trained physicians were able both to reinforce the standing of their graduates with new capabilities for practice and to create new opportunities for them to generate revenue.

NIH funding transformed the entire health care system. It would be difficult to find any corner of American medicine that does not avail itself of new equipment, drugs, or devices that were made possible in whole or in part by this form of government support. As the gatekeepers who prescribe these products and the practitioners who use them, physicians are in as good a position to reap the benefits as anyone.

Federal funding for medical school construction and expansion expired in the 1980s, but its cessation did not mark the end of federal efforts to influence the size and shape of the physician workforce. Programs that administered grants and loans to medical students continued under the auspices of the federal Health Resources and Services Administration (HRSA), a component of the Department of Health and Human Services.[59] These initiatives offer aid to those future practitioners who plan to enter primary care and to practice in underserved regions.

Were it not for government funding of medical school expansion, America would likely have about half as many physicians as it does today. They would be harder to find, and practitioners in many specialties would be a rarity in many regions. Without federal funding of research, the capabilities of the physicians who practice would be considerably more limited, and medical schools would play a more minor role. America undoubtedly would still have a robust and profitable medical profession. That was the state of physician practice in the mid-twentieth century before concerted federal involvement began. But its reach and scope would be a fraction of what we are familiar with today.

CONTROL OF ENTRY INTO THE PROFESSION FROM ABROAD: FOREIGN MEDICAL GRADUATES

The federal government also controls the size and shape of the physician workforce indirectly by overseeing the entry of foreign medical school graduates into the American market. The states set standards for their licensure, and the federal government determines the number of visas granted to non-American physicians. Those seeking admission to medical residency programs must pass the ECFMG's tests of basic science skills and of proficiency in English.[60]

Each year, about 25,000 graduates of schools outside of the United States enter residency programs in American hospitals, including many Americans who attended medical schools abroad.[61] They account for one-quarter of all American hospital residents. Of those who train in American hospitals, about three-quarters remain in the country to practice when their training ends.

Foreign medical graduates significantly enlarge the overall physician workforce. In 2000, America had 155,629 of them, up from 83,571 in 1980.[62] Over that time, their proportion in the population rose from 42 per 100,000 people to 63, corresponding with an increase in the overall physician supply from 202 per 100,000 people to 276.[63] Many foreign medical graduates take residency slots in primary care that are left unfilled by those trained in American schools. By admitting them to practice in the United States, the government helps to fill part of the country's need for generalist practitioners, while many of their American-educated colleagues enter higher-paying specialties.

The Government and the Medical Profession: The Transformation Wrought by Medicare

The nation's large complement of physicians could only thrive if it had a source of payment for its services. This is true for all practitioners but especially so for specialists, who perform the most complex and expensive procedures. Their services can cost many thousands of dollars.

Those most likely to need specialty care are the elderly, as the incidence of most serious ailments, from heart disease to cancer to neurological disorders, rises with age. However, health insurance can be difficult to obtain in the private market after retirement. There is no employer to offer coverage as a workplace benefit, and insurers are reluctant to issue individual policies to older applicants who have a greater chance of becoming ill. Because of this, half of the elderly in America lacked health insurance before the mid-1960s.[64]

That situation changed in 1965, with the enactment of Medicare. Through it, the government granted coverage for most medical needs to every American age 65 and older. Physicians could provide whatever services they felt a patient required, and the government would cover the cost. Over the ensuing decades, this funding source dramatically changed the nature of the medical profession. It gave physicians a boost similar to the one described in Chapter 4 for hospitals.

The scope of Medicare's coverage extends beyond the elderly who were its original intended beneficiaries. It also covers those below the age of 65 who are totally disabled and eligible for Supplemental Security Income under the Social Security program. In 1972, the scope was extended further to include patients below the age of 65 who suffer from end-stage renal disease (ESRD), the irreversible failure of the kidneys to function properly.[65] About a quarter of those whom Medicare covers fall into these categories of nonelderly beneficiaries. By adding them to the program, Congress not only provided a lifeline to millions of people with nowhere else to turn for pressing health care needs, it also greatly expanded practice opportunities for physicians who specialize in treating them and for facilities that provide them with institutional services. In particular, today, thanks to Medicare, renal dialysis centers represent a significant industry.[66] Nevertheless, the elderly represent the bulk of Medicare beneficiaries, and it is the financing of health care for this population that has given the medical profession its most significant support.

As described in Chapter 4, Medicare's structure consists of four parts that provide different kinds of coverage. Initially, it was composed of two complementary funding programs—Part A to reimburse the cost of hospital and other inpatient care and Part B to reimburse the cost of physician and other outpatient professional services. Two other components were added to the program over the years. Part C, which was created in 1997, permits beneficiaries to opt out of Parts A and B and receive coverage for all care through a subsidized private insurance plan. Part D, which was added in 2003, provides coverage for outpatient prescription drugs.[67] Part B is the component of Medicare that is primarily responsible for boosting the medical profession.

MEDICARE AND STRUCTURE OF THE MEDICAL PROFESSION

For many physicians in clinical practice, particularly those who treat a large share of older patients, Medicare serves as an indispensible source of reimbursement for the services they provide. In paying for physician care for the nation's elderly, Medicare has turned the treatment of this population into an extremely profitable business opportunity. No other country spends anywhere near as much on the care of its elderly citizens. In 2007, the United States spent about $34,000 for the average Medicare beneficiary.[68] Second-place Norway spent about $18,000, slightly more than half that amount. Most Western countries spend less than $11,000. Beyond its overall support for physician incomes, Medicare shapes the structure of medicine by determining the relative attractiveness of various specialties with differential reimbursement rates.

PHYSICIAN TRAINING

After completing medical school, new doctors generally spend an additional three to five years receiving hands-on training as residents and fellows in hospitals. This is when they hone their skills as apprentices in their chosen specialty. These physicians-in-training also play an important role in the clinical care that their hospitals provide. However, as discussed in Chapter 4, they require considerable supervision, which detracts from the institution's overall productivity. The additional demands on physicians who supervise them can add as much as 83 percent to the cost of care in hospitals with large training programs.[69] Without a means to recoup this expense, hospitals would find it difficult to participate in the training process.

To ensure the flow of new physicians into practice, Medicare covers the cost, providing the only dedicated source of funding for postgraduate medical training.[70] Before the program's inception, hospitals had been forced to bear the expense themselves.[71] Medicare's support takes the form of supplements to the reimbursement of teaching hospitals to recognize their added financial burden. These supplements are what make the minting of new generations of physicians economically possible for many institutions.

The supplements are incorporated into the prospective payment system that Medicare has used since 1983 to reimburse hospitals. As discussed in Chapter 4, that system bases payments on the diagnosis of each patient. Diagnoses are grouped into one of 745 categories known as "diagnosis-related groups" (DRGs). Each DRG is assigned a value based on the resources needed to treat it. That value is translated into a reimbursement amount according to the cost to treat a patient whose condition is of average severity at a hospital of average efficiency.[72] Since the added expense of supervising residents and fellows substantially reduces the efficiency of teaching hospitals, they must operate with less than average efficiency, so the DRG payments fall short of covering their costs. To compensate for this, Medicare adds two kinds of supplements to the amount it pays for each DRG, which are known as "graduate medical education" (GME) payments.[73]

Direct GME payments cover the direct costs of training, such as the salaries and benefits of residents and fellows and of physicians for the time spent supervising them. These supplements essentially pass these costs through to the government. Indirect GME payments account for the reduced efficiency of patient care when trainees are involved. They are based on the ratio of full-time equivalent trainee positions to hospital beds and paid as an add-on to the reimbursement amount for each DRG. Together, these additional sources of revenue turn the training function of academic hospitals into a financially viable proposition.[74]

GME supplements are expensive. In 2010, they cost the Medicare program $9.5 billion, of which $6.5 billion went for indirect payments and $3 billion for direct costs. In addition, 40 states spent a combined total of $3.78 billion to support graduate medical training through their Medicaid programs. These amounts funded training for 115,000 new physicians, which adds up to about $100,000 per year per trainee.[75]

Through GME supplements, Medicare controls the purse strings for postgraduate medical training.[76] This gives it a lever with which to shape important aspects of the country's physician complement. By deciding how many training slots it will pay for, it sets the number of new physicians who will enter the workforce. Since there are generally enough slots for graduates of American medical schools, the number is particularly important in determining how many foreign-educated practitioners can train in the United States.[77] Medicare, therefore, has substantial power to create or alleviate a physician shortage and to set the balance between American and foreign-educated practitioners.

In 1997, Congress capped the number of residency slots that Medicare can fund at the 1996 level, and warnings were sounded of a physician shortage as a long-term consequence.[78] A frequently discussed remedy would add more slots but allocate them to primary care to correct the specialist tilt in the composition of the physician workforce.[79] This idea remains part of public debates today. Whatever Congress decides, it is clear that the funding of medical training will continue to mold the size and shape of America's physician workforce in a very direct way.

MEDICAL SPECIALIZATION

The concept of specialization within medicine dates back at least as far as the Romans. It began to take on special importance in clinical practice in the eighteenth century, when many physicians found they could earn extra income by focusing their work on certain procedures that were in high demand. Among these were tooth extractions and assistance with childbirth. Specialization as a practice style first emerged in Paris in the 1830s. Over the next decade, it spread to other major European cities and then to North America in the 1850s and 1860s. The enticement of greater earning potential caused the proportion of specialists among American physicians to begin growing in the early twentieth century, and it continued to do so over the decades that followed.[80]

Although postgraduate internships had become a standard part of professional training for all physicians by the 1920s, the process of obtaining additional preparation to enter a specialty was still quite variable at the time.[81] Some physicians became specialists by completing residencies in Europe, and some took postgraduate coursework, which could last as little as a few weeks. One provider of specialty education, the University of Pennsylvania School of Medicine, offered 15 kinds of courses varying in length from 4 to 12 months.[82]

The AMA took the lead in efforts to standardize specialty training, as it had in standardizing all of medical education, by devising and implementing a self-regulatory scheme. In 1927, it applied its specialization standards to hospital residency programs and published a list of 270 that it approved for training in 14 medical areas.[83] The number of positions in specialty training programs grew over the years that followed from 808 in 1940, to 4,000 in 1950, to 22,000 in 1960, and to 45,000 in 1970.[84] Today, there are 7,700 residency programs in 103 fields based at more than 1,700 institutions throughout the country.[85] At any one time, a total of 115,000 physicians participate in them.[86]

Once the AMA had established a formal educational process, the next step was to create a procedure to certify those who received the training as competent to practice in their specialty. This was accomplished with the creation of the ABIM and other specialty boards starting in the 1930s. By the end of that decade, 12 boards were in place.[87]

The attractiveness of specialization for physicians received a large boost from a set of government policies in the years following World War II. The military had favored board-certified specialist physicians over their primary care colleagues during the war by granting them higher ranks and higher pay.[88] This differential remained in place after the war, making the extra training worthwhile for the many physicians who entered military service. The government added further encouragement for medical specialization through the GI Bill, which funded tuition and living expenses for physician veterans who wanted to add specialty training to generalist credentials.[89] The Hill-Burton Act also assisted in the growth of medical specialization by expanding the capacity of hospitals across the country.[90] Its effect on the overall hospital industry is discussed in Chapter 4. By pumping funds into inpatient facilities and enabling them to grow in size and clinical capabilities, that law also helped hospitals to expand their offerings of specialty services along with the residency programs that trained new physicians to provide them.

On a more fundamental level, the federal government promoted specialization by supporting the creation of tools that physicians needed to render technologically complex care. The NIH has funded most of the research that underlies the advances in basic biomedical science of the past 70 years, as discussed in Chapter 3. These discoveries have generated much of the scientific knowledge behind the implements of specialized care, including many innovative drugs, devices, and new forms of equipment.[91]

In the wake of these programs, the profession had gained a pronounced tilt toward specialization by the mid-twentieth century. In 1940, fewer than 25 percent of physicians considered themselves specialists.[92] Nine years later, the proportion had grown to 37 percent. By 1955, the figure had reached 44 percent. By 1966, it stood at 69 percent, and that percentage has remained relatively steady since.

MEDICARE'S SPECIALIST-FRIENDLY RATE-SETTING PROCESS

Having laid the groundwork for the medical profession's specialty focus by the mid-twentieth century, the government then served as the primary force in maintaining it through Medicare. The program that provides the largest single source of payment for physician services uses a complex reimbursement process that is skewed to favor specialists. By consistently keeping specialty practice more remunerative, Medicare has ensured that successive generations of physicians see it as the most financially attractive career path.

The story of Medicare's specialty bias started in its early years. When the program began, it reimbursed physicians based on the prevailing payment rates in their region. These were known as "usual and customary" charges. The system mirrored the one used by Blue Shield plans at the time for privately insured patients. These rates reflected the profession's general understanding of the relative worth of different services and of the various specialties that rendered them. In 1965, the profession's attitudes already assigned technologically complex care the highest value.[93]

By the late 1970s, it had become evident that the monetary values assigned to physician services through this system encouraged the overuse of procedures, thereby engendering considerable excess costs. Policymakers increasingly came to realize that the market that generated these charges undervalued services involving patient interaction and counseling, which are the stock in trade of primary care. This differential was exacerbated by improved techniques for rendering many complex procedures that had initially been expensive to perform.[94] Payments stayed the same as the procedures improved in efficiency, which substantially enhanced their profitability. Similar efficiencies were not possible for cognitively oriented primary care.

In an attempt to address this imbalance, Congress amended the Medicare law to change the physician payment scheme to a fee schedule designed to rationalize payment rates. It took effect in 1992, nine years after hospital reimbursement had been shifted to the DRG system to accomplish a similar goal. The new system continued to base reimbursement on a payment for each service rendered, but it did so in a manner that was intended to more accurately reflect the true cost to perform these services.

The system is known as the Resource-Based Relative Value Scale (RBRVS), and it compares the financial burden of rendering each kind of service that a physician can provide. The concept behind it originated in efforts in the early 1950s to devise a reimbursement mechanism that based physician payments on the actual cost of care.[95] The initiative was the work of the California Medical Association (CMA). Its plan was to calculate the cost and effort required to provide each of the hundreds of procedures a physician can render. The results for each one were recalculated as multiples of an index service, which was assigned a value of one. These relative values were then multiplied by a "conversion factor" representing the payment amount assigned to the index service. If, for example, a procedure was determined to require five times the expense and effort to deliver as the index, the fee schedule would set reimbursement for it at five times the conversion factor.

A system that bases physician compensation on a ranking of relative costs to provide care may seem objective on its face, but the CMA scheme titled heavily toward specialists from the start. The original relative values were set to reflect the payment rates already in effect, based on the reasoning that prevailing market rates must already have incorporated actual practice expenses. However, these rates also reflected the dynamics of the reimbursement system in use at the time. That system routinely paid for expensive medical procedures, such as surgery and radiological imaging, but rarely covered office visits, which represent most of the work of primary care.[96] The difference in coverage was reflected in differences in fees for the two kinds of services, since it is easier to charge a higher price when a third party is paying the bill. The CMA thereby perpetuated an inherent bias in payment rates, while purporting to promote objectivity. Its plan gradually came to influence insurance reimbursement throughout the country, and it formed the starting point for setting "usual and customary" Medicare payments when the program began operation in the mid-1960s.

RBRVS was intended to recalibrate payments based on a more rational application of the original CMA methodology. To accomplish this, the cost of each physician service was divided into three components for analysis—the work effort; the practice expense for personnel, equipment, and supplies; and the cost of malpractice insurance.[97] The physician work component, which accounts for 52 percent of the total, reflects the time needed to perform each service, the technical skill and physical effort involved, the mental effort and judgment required, and the stress engendered by any potential risks to the patient. The practice expense, which accounts for 44 percent, reflects the proportion of each specialty's revenues needed to cover the cost of maintaining a practice. The malpractice insurance cost accounts for 4 percent and directly reflects the expense of coverage.[98]

As with the CMA scheme, RBRVS used the results of these calculations to compare services, about 7,000 in all, to produce a value for each in relation to the others. These amounts were then multiplied by a conversion factor representing the monetary value of an index service, which in 2010 was about $36.[99] This process was intended to produce results that were independent of the values that prevailed in the market at the time.

Policymakers anticipated that by rationalizing pricing to more accurately reflect actual practice costs, RBRVS would reimburse complex medical procedures at much lower multiples of primary care visits than the old system and that the more cognitively oriented services of primary care doctors would accordingly rise in value in relation to them. However, preexisting biases concerning the nature of specialty care crept in over time nevertheless. Although the relative values set by RBRVS initially tilted the payment system more toward primary care, it did not take long for the pendulum to swing back the other way.

PERPETUATING THE SPECIALIST BIAS

How is it that a payment system designed to right the reimbursement imbalance toward specialty care came to have the opposite effect? Few predicted when

RBRVS was launched in 1992 that the ultimate winners would be the very physicians it was designed to disfavor. Yet, as it turned out, between that time and 2011, rather than shrinking, the income gap between specialists and primary care physicians grew from 61 percent to 89 percent.[100] Was this the result of the underlying workings of the free market readjusting priorities that the government sought to artificially impose? In fact, it was anything but.

The perennial dominance of specialty care under RBRVS results in large part from the difficulty of lowering prices once they have been set. Economists call prices that persist at historical levels "downward-sticky."[101] Just as the system of usual and customary charges had not been able to adjust prices downward for complex medical procedures as they became easier and more efficient to perform, RBRVS was not able to reduce them when they exceeded the actual cost of rendering care. It is easy to give people more money but quite another matter to take it away.

The stickiness of prices for procedure-oriented specialty care is maintained by a mechanism that is built into the regulatory process but largely hidden from public view. Each year, CMS reevaluates the rankings of medical services within the system. Based on its findings, it makes adjustments, mostly to account for changes in the physician work component for each procedure. The cost of maintaining a practice and the price of malpractice insurance in each specialty can be measured fairly straightforwardly, but assessing the effort and stress involved in rendering care requires assessments that are inherently subjective. The most efficient way to make them is to rely on input from the physicians involved.[102]

CMS receives this input in the reevaluation and adjustment process from a committee that is organized and managed by the AMA. It is known as the Specialty Society Relative Value Scale Update Committee, or RUC for short.[103] It meets three times a year, sometimes for as long as four days at a stretch, in the AMA's hometown of Chicago. The committee's charge is to consider whether the time, skill, and mental effort required to render any of the services on the payment scale has changed.[104] Every five years, it conducts a more complete review that considers every service on the scale.[105]

The RUC officially functions in an advisory capacity only. CMS retains the final word on whether the scale should be adjusted each year and, if so, by how much. However, the RUC's recommendations might as well be considered binding, as the agency has accepted them 94 percent of the time. This is, in part, a consequence of the close relationship between advisor and advisee. CMS medical officers and staff attend all RUC meetings and routinely contribute to the discussions.

The RUC is comprised of 29 voting members.[106] The AMA selects one of them directly and appoints the chair. Medical specialty societies appoint 21 of the other members, subject to the AMA's approval. Those slots are awarded to fields that account for the highest percentages of Medicare expenditures. In addition, two seats are designated for internal medicine, one for general primary care, and one for another specialty. The internal medicine seat is sometimes occupied by a subspecialist within the field; for example, one of its recent occupants was an oncologist.[107] Unlike the 21 dedicated specialty seats, these spots rotate, so that none of the four additional members serves for more than two years. As might seem evident from this structure, specialists perennially dominate the RUC. In 2011, 23 of its members were physicians representing specialty societies, and only five represented primary care.[108]

Another advisory committee, this one composed of representatives of 109 specialties, gives the RUC further advice in its deliberations. That committee is extremely influential in the rate-adjustment process because it initiates the mechanics of calculating each procedure's work effort. It does this by reviewing the results of a survey that each specialty society sends to its members asking them to rank the procedures they perform according to the time, difficulty, and skills required. Members of the advisory committee use the findings of the survey to propose changes to relative values for consideration by the RUC. In addition to weighing these general recommendations, the RUC usually hears directly from advisory committee members who practice in the specialties involved.

Needless to say, physicians who advise the RUC about services they perform have a strong interest in the group's ultimate decisions. Defenders of the RUC contend that the group corrects for such conflicts in its deliberations.[109] However, the influence of self-interest is difficult to avoid. In the view of a former RUC member from the field of family practice, battles between specialties are common, with alliances and deal making characterizing much of the process.[110] Representatives of a field will often support an increase in a value calculation in another field in return for a vote in favor of their own demands.

The end result of this process is that the vast majority of RUC recommendations to CMS call for the values of procedures to increase. During the group's first 15 years, it recommended changes in 2,739 procedure codes, only 400 of which involved cuts in the practice expense component.[111] Most of the increases it recommended were for procedures performed by specialists. In the annual review that the RUC conducted in 2000, of the 870 procedures assessed, increases in relative values were recommended for 469 of them, no change for 311, and reductions for only 27.[112] Action was deferred on the remaining 63.

Another important reason that the RUC's recommendations for upward adjustments persistently favor specialty procedures is that in this competitive, deal-making environment, primary care has the least leverage. Specialists introduce a steady stream of new procedures into their clinical arsenal that require evaluation. Primary care, in contrast, adds new ones infrequently because it relies to a greater extent on patient counseling. Those procedures that it does provide tend to be less complex and to place fewer demands on physicians in terms of time and stress. This leaves their representatives on the RUC with fewer bargaining chips to use in negotiating trade-offs with other fields.

Primary care is further disadvantaged by a provision in the Medicare law that requires the aggregate of all adjustments to relative values for physician services each year to be budget neutral. This means the trade-offs among specialties amount to a zero-sum game in which increases for one procedure must be offset by decreases for another.[113] Therefore, when a specialty society succeeds in convincing the RUC that its work deserves higher reimbursement, a corresponding cut must be found somewhere else. With fewer expensive new procedures to bring to the bargaining table and less negotiating clout, primary care is often the place where a fee reduction is found. In 2008, for example, the practice expense component for a routine primary care visit was adjusted down to 0.8806 of the index value from 0.92, which is where it would have been had CMS's standard methodology been used without consideration of the RUC's advice.[114] Although the RUC's recommendations have occasionally called for primary care reimbursement to rise at the expense of payments to specialists, these instances are extremely rare.[115]

For these reasons, primary care physicians complain often about the structure and composition of the RUC, and conflicts regularly arise in its deliberations.[116] In 2005, negotiations over a proposed increase for primary care became bitter when agreement on a small increase was blunted by Medicare's budget neutrality requirement.[117] In 2007, a push to add an additional primary seat to the RUC was defeated. Advocates for primary care argue that the RUC's tilt toward specialty care contributes to a national shortage of primary care capacity.[118] Studies of medical student attitudes certainly reflect this. Between 1990, two years before implementation of RBRVS, and 2007, two national surveys found the percentage of medical students planning to enter general internal medicine dropping from 9 percent to 2 percent.[119]

The RUC's methodology is not the only one that could be used to measure the work required to render physician services. Advocates for primary care, such as the American Academy of Family Practice Physicians, point to other approaches that they feel are more objective.[120] For example, surgery logs could be used instead of personal recollections to measure the time needed to perform surgical procedures. Nevertheless, the RUC retains its influence, and through it, that of the medical profession's specialty wing. Because many private insurers follow Medicare's lead in setting reimbursement rates, the RUC's impact extends to the larger health care system beyond Medicare. The consequences shape more than just the nature of a government spending program. They guide the career choices of new physicians and thereby the composition and structure of America's physician workforce.

MEDICARE'S OVERALL EFFECT ON THE SPECIALTY TILT

Medicare did not create the medical profession's specialist glut. More than two-thirds of physicians were already choosing specialty practice at the time of its inception. However, Medicare has done much to enshrine the pattern by reinforcing the income gap between specialists and primary care physicians, despite the efforts of policymakers to accomplish just the opposite. In 2004, a decade after RBRVS was implemented to shrink the earnings differential, the four lowest-earning fields were all in primary care—internal medicine, general pediatrics, family practice, and geriatrics.[121] Every form of specialty practice ranked above them.

The most lucrative specialties rely heavily on Medicare to maintain their high earnings. The program supplies almost 40 percent of the revenue for the highest earning specialty, hematology-oncology. When Medicaid and other government programs are included, the figure is 50 percent. Medicare funds more than

60 percent of the revenue collected by nephrologists, in large part because it covers the treatment of ESRD for patients of any age. For cardiology, Medicare's contribution is more than 30 percent, and all government insurance combined accounts for almost 45 percent.[122]

Among primary care fields, the story is different, with Medicare contributing less to practice revenue. Internal medicine receives less than 30 percent of its revenue from Medicare, even though its practitioners treat a large proportion of elderly patients. The total contribution from all government programs to that field of practice is less than 40 percent. Family practice, which focuses on treating non-elderly patients, receives only about 15 percent of its revenue from Medicare and less than 30 percent from all government programs combined. General pediatrics receives almost nothing from Medicare and just over 20 percent from the government in any form.[123]

The exception to this trend is the primary care field of geriatrics, which receives almost three-quarters of its revenue from Medicare and almost 80 percent from all government programs combined. However, the services rendered by these physicians fall near the bottom of Medicare's payment scale. Much of their work involves counseling, which receives low rankings in the RBRVS system. Moreover, because counseling elderly patients can be extremely time-consuming, the volume of patients that practitioners can see is more limited than it is in other branches of primary care. Nevertheless, although Medicare is stingy in its reimbursement, the field of geriatrics would not exist at all were it not for the program, which provides the lion's share of its reimbursement.[124]

Medicare's payment structure also leads hospitals to favor certain specialists in the composition of their medical staffs. As discussed in Chapter 4, since the advent of DRGs, hospitals have actively sought ways to tilt the composition of their medical staffs in favor of specialists who treat patients with the most lucrative DRGs. They do this both by capping the number of other physicians to whom they grant clinical privileges and by recruiting specialists with offers of lavish salaries.

Through this indirect effect of the DRG system, Medicare has turned hospitals into unwitting accomplices in reinforcing the bias toward specialty care in American medicine.[125] As with the other incentives that it bestows on specialty practice, the effects were unintentional. In fact, Medicare's official position is ostensibly one of neutrality as to the shape of the medical profession and the relationships between physicians and hospitals. However, its influence is undeniable. In the words of one observer, "Medicare takes no official position, but its passivity should not be taken for inaction, as its policies and practices shape almost every aspect of the hospital and physician relationship."[126]

Although unintentional, Medicare's stamp on the structure of the medical profession has nonetheless been dramatic. During the 30-year period beginning in 1975, 10 years after Medicare's enactment, the number of physicians in general and family practice increased by about 60 percent, from 46,347 to 74,999. The number of office-based specialists, on the other hand, increased at almost three times that rate, from 126,112 to 329,344. The number of specialists who treat large proportions of elderly patients increased particularly rapidly. The number of cardiologists more than tripled from 5,046 to 17,519, the number of neurologists grew almost fivefold from 1,862 to 10,400, and the number treating pulmonary disease jumped by almost sevenfold from 1,166 to 7,321.[127]

Medicare's support for specialization can also be seen in a proliferation of specialties that began soon after the program's inception. The number of different specialty certificates that were available to physicians through the American Board of Medical Specialties held fairly steady in the range of 21 to 36 between 1940 and 1970.[128] That number jumped in 1970, five years after Medicare's enactment, to 55, and it continued on a steadily accelerating trajectory to reach 124 in 2000. The total number of distinct specialties with accredited training programs grew during that time from 31 to 103.

MEDICARE AND PHYSICIAN ENTREPRENEURSHIP

The Medicare reimbursement changes that promoted physician specialization also gave some physicians tremendous opportunities to gain even greater riches as entrepreneurs.[129] As described in Chapter 4, the switch to DRG payments led many hospitals to shift services to outpatient settings because that system caps the amount of reimbursement that can be generated for inpatient care to a sum determined by each patient's diagnosis. Outpatient care, on the other hand, generates a separate fee for each service rendered under both the original Medicare formula and under the RBRVS system, so the revenue to be gained from each patient is limited only by the provider's ability to find services that they can offer. Hospitals therefore stood to enhance their Medicare revenues by performing as many procedures as possible outside of their core facilities.

The setting for these procedures was commonly new outpatient centers that offered tremendous earning potential for the physicians who practiced in them. As described in Chapter 4, many hospitals also offered participating physicians opportunities to invest in these centers to earn additional returns. Many physicians also established outpatient facilities on their own, which often grew into extremely lucrative ventures. When physicians own the facilities in which they practice, the earnings potential is multiplied. This is because, in addition to gaining reimbursement for the services they provide, they can share in payments that Medicare also makes for use of the facility.

Physicians who invest in facilities where they practice enjoy a unique advantage over other kinds of entrepreneurs. They hold the power to determine when a customer needs to use their services. When a patient requires medical care, it is his or her physician who guides the decision making on which procedures to obtain and where to obtain them. Physicians with ownership interests in an outpatient center can use this power to direct patients to their own businesses, and Medicare gives them the incentive to do so as much as possible.[130]

In some instances, physicians abuse this power.[131] They refer patients for services that are not truly needed or refer them to their own facilities when others might do a better job. Two laws address this potential for abuse. The anti-kickback provisions of the Medicare statute prohibit the payment or receipt of financial inducements for referring patients under the Medicare program, and a set of provisions known as the Stark Amendments prohibit the referral of patients to facilities with which the physician has certain kinds of financial relationships. The role of these laws in altering the structure of physician practice is discussed later in this chapter. However, even under these laws, physicians still hold wide discretion to determine the amount and location of each patient's care. This confers the ability to maintain the flow of business to their ventures to an extent shared by entrepreneurs in few other businesses. It also makes them especially attractive partners to hospitals and outside investors seeking ways to profit from the health care system.

Some physicians have taken this power to generate business one step further and established their own hospitals that focus on providing particularly remunerative procedures. As described in Chapter 4, these are known as "specialty hospitals" because they offer services limited to certain specialties. By focusing on procedures that are particularly well reimbursed under the DRG system, such as orthopedics and cardiac care, they can avoid the money losing services that general hospitals must provide. In effect, they skim the most profitable business from general hospitals, which must continue to provide necessary but financially draining services such as emergency rooms and intensive care units.[132]

Outpatient care centers and specialty hospitals represent considerable business opportunities for entrepreneurial physicians. By partnering with hospitals or with outside investors, they stand to gain substantially higher earnings than even the most lucrative specialty practice would yield on its own. These medical care ventures have paved the way for a new breed of physician who combines clinical skill with business acumen.

The economic environment in which these physician-entrepreneurs function is anything but a free market. It was created by Medicare and is sustained by Medicare's reimbursement mechanisms.[133] The program is instrumental to them, first by providing the pot of money that funds the care they provide. Beyond this, it also structures the process for making that money available in a way that encourages outpatient care in certain favored specialties. The DRG system rewards hospitals for partnering with physicians in these specialties on generous financial terms, and the RBRVS system amply compensates practitioners who render services in centers that they own. One overview of Medicare's prospective payment system observed that "distortions in Medicare DRG payments for inpatient services were a catalyst not only for stimulating a major expansion in specialty hospitals but also for orienting community general hospitals toward overprovision of surgical services in general and cardiac surgical services in particular."[134] The entrée of physicians into the world of business did not begin with Medicare, but the program built this branch of the profession into a major economic force.

A Case Study: The Specialty of Cardiology

The story of Medicare's transformative effect on the medical profession is especially vivid in the history of one specialty in particular—cardiology. Of all fields of medicine, none has benefitted more from the program's influence. With a large proportion of elderly patients, it was well positioned to reap the rewards of a generous reimbursement system oriented toward a geriatric population. Thanks to Medicare, cardiology practitioners are today among the most well-equipped technologically and perennially among the highest paid. But it was not always this way.

The origins of cardiology date back as far as medicine itself. Physicians have understood the importance of the heart and circulatory system for thousands of years. Papyrus scrolls from ancient Egypt describe the heart as the center of a system of blood vessels, although they contain few other details.[135] Hippocrates, in ancient Greece, offered a description that was only slightly more detailed.[136] Early explanations of the heart and its role can also be found in the Old Testament and in the Talmud.[137]

A more complete understanding came in the seventeenth century, with the invention of the microscope and more sophisticated techniques of dissection. Using these tools, William Harvey, an English physician, described the basic elements of the circulatory system and the role of the heart in 1628.[138] His work paved the way for further investigations that, over the next 200 years, revealed basic elements of their physiology and function. By the early twentieth century, the core knowledge that lies behind cardiology practice had been established.

Practitioners of cardiology began the process of organizing it into a formal specialty in the United States in the years immediately following World War I.[139] The first steps were taken in New York, Boston, and other large cities with major hospitals. Leaders in the profession brought together physicians who worked in cardiac care from different professional perspectives to mold them into a unified field based on their common focus on heart and circulatory ailments. Their constituents included physiologists who studied the causes of disease, private practitioners who treated patients, academicians who focused on teaching and research, and public health–oriented physicians who emphasized prevention.

Cardiology had begun to coalesce as a coherent specialty a decade earlier, with the invention of a powerful new technological tool that expanded the diagnostic capabilities of practitioners in all of these settings—the electrocardiograph (EKG). This device, which permits physicians to analyze electrical activity in the heart and to spot abnormalities, was first used in 1902. It opened previously unimagined clinical possibilities, and its uptake was rapid. By the mid-1920s, it had become a mainstay of practice, with almost 500 in use in the United States by 1926.

Skill at using the new technology helped to define practitioners of cardiology as distinct from other physicians.[140] At the same time as its widespread adoption, another medical advance, the chest x-ray, was entering into common use as a means to visualize structural abnormalities in the heart and other organs. Together, these two technologies led to a revolution in cardiac care in which a range of maladies could be accurately diagnosed for the first time. "We are living in an era of diagnosis," boasted a prominent Philadelphia practitioner in 1926.[141]

Soon thereafter, cardiologists, along with members of other nascent specialties, began to enjoy higher earnings than their primary care colleagues. A surgeon writing in 1935 noted the striking difference in average incomes, with specialists earning in the range of $10,000 a year and general practitioners only about $3,900.[142] Technologically centered care was quickly bringing financial benefits along with it.

CARDIOLOGY'S PROFESSIONAL ORGANIZATION

As cardiology coalesced as a field, many of its practitioners saw the need for a national organization to promote its further development. Such a body began to take shape in 1924, in the form of the American Heart Association (AHA). The following year, its journal, the *American Heart Journal*, began publication to spread news of developments in the field. In 1940, the AHA established an examination to certify specialists in cooperation with the ABIM. In 1949, the American College of Cardiology (ACC) was founded to advance the education of practitioners and to advocate for their interests.[143]

Once it had been established as a recognized specialty with a formal process of board certification, the ranks of cardiologists grew steadily and continued to do so over the next 50 years. In 1941, only six physicians trained for board certification in the field, none in formal programs. In 1949, 15 physicians received training in seven programs. By 1960, 72 programs were in operation, training 142 new cardiologists. In 1994, the high point, the country had 214 programs that turned out 2,791 cardiac specialists.[144]

THE STIMULUS OF MEDICARE

Much of the expansion of cardiology during the latter part of the twentieth century was concentrated in a particularly rapid growth spurt in the 1960s. During that time, the number of training programs grew almost fourfold, from 72 to 280, and the number of cardiologists in training increased almost ninefold, from 142 to 1,260.[145] This growth in numbers marked the specialty's first response to its greatest stimulus since the invention of the EKG—the creation of Medicare. The program gave those patients most likely to need cardiac care, the elderly, full health care coverage, and, in response, the demand for services soared. In the words of one observer, "By insuring the elderly against acute illness, Congress created a system that favored cardiology, which, by the mid-1960s, was focused on diagnosing and treating acute flare-ups of chronic disorders such as coronary artery disease."[146] In more concrete terms, when asked how Medicare affected the field, former ACC president Charles Fisch declared, "It made us rich, as simple as that."[147]

The specialty of cardiology also benefitted from the growth of private health insurance during the middle of the twentieth century. As discussed in Chapter 6, the first private plans were created in the 1930s, and their uptake increased dramatically during and just after World War II. Before private coverage had become widespread, many physicians who treated heart ailments did so without the assurance of payment. In 1936, a past president of the American Association for Thoracic Surgery issued this warning to new physicians of the financial risks of focusing their practice on heart surgery: "It is fair at this time to warn the young man who hopes to make thoracic surgery his one and only field of professional endeavor that 75 to 90 percent of all thoracic surgery must be done without hope or expectation of financial remuneration."[148]

The combination of Medicare and private insurance changed that. Together, they transformed what had been charity work into one of the most lucrative professional endeavors in the country.

MEDICARE AND THE TRANSFORMATION OF CARDIOLOGY PRACTICE

Third-party reimbursement created the financial foundation for cardiology's growth. At the same time, changes in the underlying nature of practice expanded the range of services for which practitioners could bill and the kinds of patients to whom they could render care. Advances in technology, such as cardiac pacemakers, stents to prop open clogged arteries, and drugs to treat a range of disorders, brought the field well beyond the era of the electrocardiogram and permitted medical cardiologists to shift the focus of their work in the years following World War II from treating congenital and rheumatic heart disease to caring for coronary artery disease and its complications.[149] On the surgical side, thoracic surgeons who had focused on the care of tuberculosis patients in the 1930s gained the ability during that time to treat malfunctions of the heart and blood vessels.

These advances in clinical practice had significant economic effects beyond simple increases in the volume of work that cardiologists could perform. Congenital and rheumatic heart conditions are relatively uncommon, so they provide physicians with a limited pool of patients. Coronary artery disease, which results from a narrowing of arteries caused by fat deposits, is widespread, which means greater practice opportunities for medical cardiologists.[150] Tuberculosis occurs more frequently among the poor, who are less able to afford the bills for care on their own and less likely to have private insurance. Heart ailments, in contrast, strike people of all socioeconomic levels, providing a more lucrative patient base for surgeons. With these changes in the population of patients who could be treated, the new technological capabilities helped the field's financial horizons to expand exponentially.

The government stood behind this growing technological sophistication through the funding of biomedical research by the NIH. As discussed in Chapter 3, the NIH has been the driving force behind the proliferation of new products that brought growth and profitability to the pharmaceutical industry during the latter half of the twentieth century. As the single largest source of biomedical research support in the world, it has also transformed the technological tools available to practitioners in several fields of medicine, few of them more so than cardiology.

With new clinical capabilities and a larger pool of patients that it could serve, cardiology was well positioned to reap the benefits from the new sources of payment that became available in the 1950s and 1960s. Coming as they did on the heels of a technological revolution, Medicare and private coverage arrived at a particularly opportune time. In the words of one observer, "Medicare and private health insurance reimbursement policies helped transform cardiology from a technology-oriented into a technology-dominated specialty."[151]

As technological advances opened new therapeutic horizons, NIH research funding and Medicare reimbursement worked in tandem to spur cardiology's growth. In the 1960s, the NIH concentrated much of its support for research on the study of diseases whose treatments were most likely to receive Medicare reimbursement. Of almost $80 million devoted by the agency to heart-related research in 1966, almost two-thirds was allocated to understanding conditions that primary affect the elderly—atherosclerosis, heart failure and shock, hypertension, and myocardial infarction.[152] Only about one-eighth of NIH's cardiology-related funding was directed to congenital and rheumatic heart disease, which had been the specialty's focus in the early part of the century. More research funding led to more sophisticated and expensive treatments for which Medicare provided a ready source of reimbursement. These two government programs thereby worked hand in hand to transform cardiology from a clinical niche into a preeminent player in medical care.

One technology in particular, cardiac pacemakers, clearly demonstrates the synergistic effect of government research support and generous reimbursement for care. These devices correct defects in the electrical impulses that generate heartbeats to ensure that the heart maintains a steady rhythm. They came into common use in the early 1960s. However, they are expensive to implant and require regular monitoring by a physician. Most of the patients who receive them are elderly, and few of them could afford the cost before the advent of Medicare. Lacking other sources of funding, some patients in the days before Medicare resorted to holding fundraisers. This situation changed once the program was in place and payment was assured. Almost immediately afterward, sales of pacemakers rose dramatically, and they became a new staple of cardiac practice, as well as lifesavers for the patients who needed them.[153]

The growing importance of government funding to their professional future was not lost on members of the specialty. In 1965, the ACC decided to move its headquarters from New York to the Washington, D.C. area to be closer to the government policymakers whose decisions were increasingly determining their fortunes. The College chose a location just outside the capital, in Bethesda, Maryland, near the campus of the NIH. The new headquarters was also convenient to the National Library of Medicine and the Surgeon General's Office. Former College president Samuel Fox remarked that the move gave the organization "opportunities to engage in things with the federal government."[154] There were many "things" for them to engage in, indeed.

The ACC took advantage of those opportunities many times during the next several decades. It directed much of its attention to lobbying Congress to grant steady budget increases to the NIH. In 1972, it hired a legislative assistant to enhance the group's visibility before Congress and various administrative agencies.[155] In 1981, amid talk of steep federal budget cuts that could imperil research funding and Medicare reimbursement, it established a full-time government relations department.[156] In 2009, it ventured into the policy arena through litigation, suing the Department of Health and Human Services to block proposed cuts to Medicare reimbursement.[157]

RECENT FURTHER EXPLOSIONS OF TECHNOLOGY

Over the decades since Medicare's enactment, the therapeutic horizons of cardiac care have continued to expand. Many tools that are commonly used today for diagnosis and treatment—medical, surgical, and pharmacologic—were barely imaginable as part of routine care in the 1960s. Implantable defibrillators, catheterization, stents, cardiac bypass surgery, valve repair and replacement, statins, and beta-blockers, to name just a few, have extended the capabilities of cardiologists and saved countless lives. All of them owe at least part of their development to research funded by the NIH.[158]

New facilities for rendering cardiac care became available during this time, as well. With more powerful tools for saving lives, practitioners needed better-equipped settings in which to use them. In the 1960s, the notion emerged of creating special units in hospitals where intensive treatment could be provided to extremely ill heart patients. These became known as "coronary care units." The first ones were established in the early 1960s, and by 1965 when Medicare was enacted, the United States had 50 of them. Two years later, in 1967, the number had grown sevenfold to 350, and five years after that in 1972, to 2,300.[159]

Of all the tools that cardiologists gained in the middle of the twentieth century, none did more to expand the capabilities of the field than therapeutic catheterization. The technique allows a physician to insert a probe known as a catheter through a patient's veins and navigate it to the heart to diagnose and treat disorders, most notably arteries clogged with plaque formed by the buildup of fat. It was developed in the early 1940s, and, in 1945, the first cardiac catheterization laboratory was established at Johns Hopkins Hospital.[160]

Initially, cardiac catheterization was used only to visualize the heart and arteries to diagnose conditions. However, subsequent enhancements turned it into a powerful therapeutic tool, as well. In 1960, balloon catheters were invented, which permitted cardiologists to perform several kinds of procedures through a catheter without surgery. In 1969, a version was patented that could actually remove plaque that caused arterial obstructions.[161] Its first use in the United States came in 1978, to treat angina pectoris, and it soon spread rapidly.[162] The procedure, known as percutaneous transluminal coronary angioplasty (PTCA), is now performed more than 300,000 times a year.[163] It is a safer and less costly alternative to cardiac artery bypass grafts (CABG), the surgical technique that had been the prevailing form of treatment.

PTCA revolutionized cardiology.[164] In addition to its clinical benefits, it effected an important change in the structure of practice. For the first time, medical specialists rather than surgeons could perform a therapeutic procedure to treat angina, a condition that afflicted as many as 5 million Americans in 1978.

At about the same time, catheterization found yet another powerful application. The technique of invasive clinical electrophysiology enabled practitioners to diagnose disorders in electrical impulses in the heart by attaching electrodes to catheters.[165] It also enabled them to use catheters to insert pacemakers to correct these disorders. Both of these uses were major advances over surgical incisions, which previously had been necessary.

With PTCA, electrophysiology, and other invasive techniques at their disposal, a subfield within the specialty, interventional cardiology, was born. It applied powerful tools to diagnosing and treating once intractable heart and blood vessel conditions. Since the preponderance of patients on whom these tools are used are above the age of 65, Medicare serves as the financial foundation for these forms of care. Moreover, Medicare's RBRVS reimbursement system, which provides a payment for each service rendered, has strongly encouraged cardiologists to use their growing clinical armamentarium to the maximum extent possible, while the system's specialist-friendly payment calculations have inflated the prices they receive each time they do. This generous source of payment for a growing array of intricate and expensive procedures has led interventional cardiologists to enjoy even higher incomes than those of their colleagues in the rest of the field.[166]

THE SPECIALTY'S FINANCIAL REWARDS

The effect of these technological advances on the financial fortunes of cardiologists was profound. During the period between 1973 and 1979, as the pace of development of new clinical tools began to accelerate, median incomes of cardiologists grew faster than those of any other medical specialty.[167] The increase was 55 percent in those six years, whereas for the profession overall it was about half that, at 28 percent. Cardiologists today are among the top earning specialists, with an average income in 2011 of over $300,000.[168] Some segments of the field earned much more. Invasive cardiologists averaged over $472,000 and cardiovascular-pediatric surgeons over $725,000.[169]

As America's population ages over the coming decades, cardiac care is likely to grow even more prominent. And, if present trends in the prevalence of obesity continue to hold, cardiology's role stands to be reinforced even further, since the condition leads to a surfeit of heart disease. The field has contributed powerfully to increases in life expectancy over the past several decades, and it promises to bring even more advances in America's health going forward. At the same time, it has rewarded its practitioners generously. None of this would have been possible without the foundational support provided in various forms by the government.

Consolidation of the Physician Workforce

Federal programs like Medicare and NIH funding have shaped the composition and remuneration of medical practice directly for half a century. In recent decades, other government initiatives have done so indirectly. These include laws that promote an ongoing shift in the structure of practice toward larger arrangements.

A declining number of physicians ply their trade in solo or two-person settings. Practices have been growing in size for several decades, and many of them no longer function autonomously.[170] Larger health systems increasingly serve as the organizational structures in which physician practices are housed.

Driving this trend to a large extent is a series of federal initiatives that have different primary objectives but exert powerful secondary effects on the business of providing medical care. Through the 1990s and early 2000s, the decline in the proportion of physicians in one- and two-person practices was especially dramatic. Between 1997 and 2005, the percentage of practitioners working in these arrangements fell from 40.7 percent of the country's physician workforce to 32.5 percent. The trend was most pronounced for surgeons and medical specialists and least for primary care.[171]

Beyond the consolidation of the profession into larger practice groups, the proportion of physicians who have an ownership interest in their own practice also declined. Between 1997 and 2005, the percentage dropped from 61.6 percent to 54.6 percent. Once again, the greatest change was for surgeons and medical specialists and the smallest for primary care. The proportion of practices owned by their member physicians stood at 70 percent in 2002 and at about 67 percent in 2005. By 2008, it had fallen to less than half.[172]

Where did the physicians leaving small practices go? Most went to larger practices with between six and 50 members. Their proportion increased from 17.6 percent to 31.1 percent between 1997 and 2005. Many others went to practices that operate as part of medical schools, which increased their share of the total from 7.3 percent to 9.3 percent. Hospitals own a growing portion of these practices, and, since 2008, more physicians have worked in them than for themselves.[173]

What lies behind the shift? Some point to a larger number of women in the profession who seek the security of an employed position in balancing work and family demands.[174] Others point to the growing complexity of medicine itself, which requires increasingly sophisticated equipment and other resources to effectively render care. These are beyond the means of most smaller physician groups.[175] Another explanation is the exploding cost of medical education. Higher tuition leaves graduates with larger loan repayment burdens. The average level of debt for graduates of private medical schools grew from $120,000 in 2001 to $160,000 in 2006. Debt-ridden physicians are more likely to seek more stable practice settings that cover the cost of staff, equipment, and other needs.[176]

However, the shift in medical practice structure has also coincided with the growth of several disparate government initiatives that have had the effect of making practice in larger groups more attractive. Three in particular exert this effect most powerfully. None of the three is specifically directed toward that end, but each of them lessens the appeal of remaining in a traditional autonomous practice arrangement.

CONSOLIDATION AND THE ANTITRUST LAWS

The first initiative is antitrust enforcement. The laws that proscribe anticompetitive behavior affect practice structure by setting the parameters for negotiations between physicians and one of their primary sources of revenue—managed care insurers. As these companies grew in size during the final decades of the twentieth century, they gained substantial bargaining clout. Physicians have sought to counter it by banding together to bargain in groups.[177] Solo practitioners and smaller practices have little leverage in such matters because any one of them is easily expendable from the insurer's point of view.

However, in 1982, the Supreme Court placed an important limitation on this strategy. In the case of *Arizona v. Maricopa County Medical Society*,[178] it ruled that collective activity by independent physicians to set the prices they charge insurers constitutes illicit collusion under the antitrust laws. The Court found that since each practice is a separate business, it must bargain over payment rates on its own.

Nevertheless, the decision did leave physicians with an alternative. If they combined their practices into a single economically integrated entity, they would cease to function as competing businesses. Therefore, they could no longer be viewed as colluding. However, this approach came with an important condition. The practices that comprised the entity had to abandon their individual business autonomy.

The implication for the structure of physician practice arrangements was clear. The main hope of gaining the upper hand with managed care companies lay in sacrificing the independence they enjoyed in separate groups for the strength offered by a larger organization. As managed care proliferated in the years after the *Maricopa County* case was decided, insurers have shown increasing assertiveness in bargaining over rates. In response, growing numbers of physicians have sought safety in numbers in the only way they legally can—by joining larger practices, many of which are owned by hospitals and other large organizations. For practitioners caught between the aggressiveness of insurance companies and the threat of antitrust enforcement, group practices offer an increasingly attractive route to financial security.

CONSOLIDATION AND THE LAWS RESTRICTING REFERRALS

Statutes that penalize practitioners for offering or accepting monetary rewards in return for referring patients have also made consolidated physician practice more appealing. Since the late 1970s, the government has been increasingly aggressive in enforcing these prohibitions. An effective way to insulate a practice from legal jeopardy is to incorporate it into a larger entity.

Laws limiting payments for referrals stem from abuses that have been prevalent under the Medicare program since its inception. With the government picking up the tab for care, many providers, including physicians, have sought ways to increase their volume of Medicare-eligible patients, knowing that payment for the services was guaranteed. The most reliable source of new patients for many providers is referrals from their colleagues, and the best way to encourage them is often to offer financial rewards in return.

Payments for referrals are considered unethical by the AMA because they can warp physician judgments.[179] To the extent that they result in recommendations for unnecessary care, they also add costs to insurance arrangements, especially to Medicare, which is the biggest arrangement of all. To safeguard the integrity of Medicare, along with Medicaid and other government health care programs, Congress made them illegal.

As described earlier in this chapter, there are two federal laws that prohibit the payment or acceptance of a monetary inducement for referring patients covered by Medicare or Medicaid. The first is the anti-kickback provision of the statute under which Medicare operates, which makes it a felony to pay, offer to pay, receive, or solicit anything of value in return for referring a patient whose care may be reimbursed by a government program.[180] In 1985, in one of the first federal court decisions to apply the law, *United States v. Greber*, a federal appellate court enunciated the rule that a violation may be found if any intent of the parties to a financial transaction is to influence referrals.[181]

This broad prohibition encompasses many kinds of health care business relationships in its sweep, some of which can serve legitimate purposes. For example, hospitals commonly rent office space to staff physicians. Surgeons sometimes invest in ASCs where they perform outpatient procedures. Hospital emergency departments employ physicians who admit patients who are seriously ill. To differentiate legitimate from illegitimate transactions, the Department of Health and Human Services has issued guidelines describing the elements of these and other permissible arrangements. They are known as "safe harbors" because they render the arrangements safe from prosecution.[182]

The second law is the Ethics in Patient Referrals Act, commonly known as the Stark Amendments.[183] It denies reimbursement under Medicare and Medicaid for nine designated health care services when the patient was referred by a physician who has a financial relationship with the provider who rendered the care. There are exceptions for legitimate arrangements that are similar to the safe harbors under the anti-kickback provisions of the Medicare statute.

For physicians, hospitals, and other providers wishing to enter into financial relationships, these laws can present significant obstacles. The penalties for entering into an improperly structured transaction range from disqualification from receiving Medicare reimbursement to heavy fines to up to five years in prison. The rules that define legitimate transactions under the safe harbors and related regulations are complex and often difficult to interpret.

However, there is one clear way to avoid the dilemma—to combine several providers into a single entity. If all providers who render care in the entity do so as part of an integrated organization, there is no actual referral of patients from one to another. If, for example, a primary care physician refers patients to a specialist colleague and both practice within a single large group, they can, under most circumstances, insulate themselves from liability.[184] By creating this zone of safety from prosecution for physicians who join their practices together, federal laws have again encouraged consolidation into larger groups.

CONSOLIDATION AND HEALTH REFORM

Two recent federal initiatives lend a more deliberate impetus to the transition of medical practice into large integrated entities. The first is a provision in the health reform law passed in 2010, the Affordable Care Act, that authorized experiments with a new form of health care integration known as an accountable care organization (ACOs).[185] This is a collection of providers that work in collaboration to meet targets for efficiency and clinical outcomes set by the Medicare program. Commonly, it includes a hospital and a number of affiliated physicians, who are typically paid for meeting quality benchmarks or with other alternatives to a fee for each service rendered.[186] If an ACO is successful in meeting its goals, the Medicare program supplements the reimbursement it receives.

The goal behind the creation of ACOs was to promote coordination between providers at different levels of care. To that end, policymakers sought to nudge the prevailing payment paradigm for physicians away from traditional fee-for-service arrangements that characterize much independent practice to a compensation system tied more closely to actual patient outcomes. From the perspective of physicians, they represent yet another reason to move beyond private small-group practice into consolidated organizations.

The second initiative was a law passed in 2009 to promote the widespread adoption of computerized medical records, the Health Information Technology for Economic and Clinical Health Act, commonly known as the HITECH Act.[187] It allocated $20 billion in incentives to physicians for adopting and using electronic medical records (EMRs) in a meaningful way to replace paper charts.[188] It also imposed reductions in Medicare reimbursement for those who fail to use them. A primary goal of the legislation was to facilitate better coordination of care among providers through easier exchange of information. Better coordination and improved recordkeeping can also reduce the chance for errors.[189]

However, even with government assistance, EMRs are extremely expensive and can strain the budgets of small physician practices.[190] Moreover, the learning curve for physicians who are unfamiliar with them can be long and steep. For many independent practices, the economic and logistical challenges of adopting EMRs can be close to insurmountable.

Implementation of EMR systems is a different story in larger health organizations, which enjoy a number of advantages. Most notably, in applying one computer system to the needs of an entire network of physicians, they benefit from substantial economies of scale. Large provider organizations are also able to maintain staffs of technology experts to put systems in place and to train physicians in their use. The pressures to adopt EMRs thereby add another incentive for physicians to abandon independent practice in favor of work in larger integrated settings.

GOVERNMENT POLICIES AND PHYSICIAN PRACTICE STRUCTURE IN THE AGGREGATE

These government programs have not transformed the structure of physician practice arrangements on their own. Advances in the technological sophistication of medicine and social trends that have altered the nature of America's professional workforce have also played important roles. However, federal laws have unquestionably accelerated the move to larger physician groups. In the absence of the legal pressures they create, the allure of joint practice arrangements would be far less compelling. The result would be a medical profession more closely resembling the cottage industry of years gone by.

The Medical Profession and the Government

It is ironic that the medical profession fought the creation of Medicare so bitterly during the political battles over its enactment in the 1960s. The AMA launched a particularly aggressive campaign in opposition, including a passionate appeal by then-actor Ronald Reagan warning that the program could turn the entire economy into a Soviet-style system.[191] Just before the program's passage, only 38 percent of physicians in one poll supported any kind of national insurance program for the elderly, even one that covered only hospital services.[192] Some physicians even talked of boycotting Medicare once it began operation.

Those attitudes changed soon after the program was enacted. Just 10 months later, and before it had even gone into effect, support among physicians had grown to 70 percent.[193] Six months after implementation, the proportion had risen to 81 percent. Today, many physicians would be unable to maintain financially viable practices without it.

The change in attitudes should not be surprising. This government initiative now underpins much of the profession. It supports the high income levels that prevail and makes it economically possible for physicians to render technologically complex care. It also shapes the composition of the profession by maintaining its strong bias toward specialty practice with particular generosity to those who engage in it.

In light of the high economic and social standing that the medical profession enjoys today, the same question can be asked about it that was asked about other major segments of the health care industry. What would it look like had the government not launched the programs that sustain it? Where would it be without Medicare reimbursement, the physician workforce programs of the 1960s, NIH support for technological advances, or numerous other programs that have promoted and facilitated its growth?

Clearly, the profession would still exist. Physicians have served as the backbone of medical care for thousands of years. They practiced long before third-party reimbursement had been invented and long before government regulations circumscribed their professional conduct. Medical practice even predates the creation of formal educational programs to train those who engage in it.[194]

However, it is only within the past hundred years that medicine has achieved the status and income that characterize its position in American society today. Until the late nineteenth century, the profession's therapeutic powers were limited, and the reputation of its practitioners was uneven at best.[195] It gained stature with the advent of state regulation that imposed requirements for entry. That brought the weight of government authority to bear in the enforcement of standards that were developed and maintained by the profession itself. The combination of government sanction and self-regulation by private practitioners formed one of American health care's first public–private partnerships, albeit an implicit one. Through it, medicine underwent a transformation into a respected and lucrative occupation by the 1920s, and, by the middle of the twentieth century, it stood atop the country's hierarchy of professions.

With its standing established, medicine was ready to move to yet higher levels of esteem and income in the latter part of the twentieth century, this time based on a foundation built by the federal government. The NIH invested tens of billions of dollars in the advancement of biomedical science, which yielded a parade of new tools that physicians could use to diagnose and treat illnesses. Workforce management programs added thousands of new slots to medical schools and effectuated a doubling of the number of practicing physicians. And, most importantly, the Medicare program spent billions of dollars each year on reimbursement for the services that physicians provide and on training to turn medical school graduates into the practicing physicians of the future. Beyond these funding programs, the federal government shaped the nature of physician practice by reinforcing the heavy tilt toward specialty care and encouraging the migration of physicians from independent practices into larger provider organizations.

Perhaps, the health care system could benefit from a smaller medical profession. Many medical services could be delivered at lower cost by other kinds of clinicians, such as nurse practitioners and physician assistants, who command lower salaries. An array of government policies has impeded such cost-saving arrangements by reinforcing the grip of the medical profession over the provision of a large swath of medical care. Moreover, programs to increase the size of the physician workforce may have gone too far and created an oversupply of practitioners in some specialties and in some regions.

The public policies that put the medical profession in its present position have certainly engendered their share of unintended consequences. The policymakers who crafted them failed to foresee many of the implications of their decisions. Nevertheless, the questionable nature of some policy outcomes does not mean that the programs were any less effective in nurturing the profession in numerous ways. Whatever their effects on the overall health care system, they have been instrumental in building medicine into a paragon among professions.

American physicians today enjoy a level of influence, prestige, and financial reward greater than their colleagues in any other developed country.[196] The rise of medicine in the United States represents a model of success that other professions seek to emulate. Yet, behind it lies more than just the hard work and dedication of the practitioners involved. The medical profession owes much of its success to the hand of its indispensible ally, the government. Without significant public intervention, the profession today would be smaller, less remunerative, and less clinically effective. Physicians would have fewer services to offer and would earn less for rendering them. And with a smaller and less capable medical profession, the entire health care system would stand on shakier ground.

6

How the Government Created
Private Health Insurance

> By subsidizing the cost of health insurance and out-of-pocket medical
> spending, the tax provisions encourage both the use of health-care
> resources and the development of more elaborate forms of medical care.
>
> —CONGRESSIONAL BUDGET OFFICE[1]

> We have become so accustomed to employer-provided medical care that
> we regard it as part of the natural order. Yet it is thoroughly illogical.
>
> —MILTON FRIEDMAN, *THE PUBLIC INTEREST*[2]

Private health insurance is a multibillion dollar industry in the United States.
In 2012, the top 10 firms generated more than $300 billion in revenue.[3] Their com-
bined profits were more than $10 billion. The largest firm, UnitedHealth Group,
was the 22nd largest corporation in the country.[4] In 2009, the health insurance
industry as a whole was 28th in return on assets, ranking higher than all other
lines of insurance.[5]

America is unique in the size of its overall health care sector. In 2009, it
accounted for more than 17 percent of the country's gross domestic product, the
largest proportion by far of any country in the world.[6] The Netherlands was second
at 12 percent. Many developed countries were much lower. Japan devoted only
about 8.5 percent of its economy to health care. In dollar terms, the United States
spent almost $8,000 per person. Second-place Norway came in at only $5,300.[7] All
told, America's health care bill totaled $2.7 trillion in 2011.[8]

Of the country's huge investment in health care, about 33 percent was financed
through private health insurance in 2010.[9] That is the highest proportion of private
health care finance in the developed world.[10] Although private coverage is available in many other countries, its scope is generally more limited, and it funds a
much lower percentage of overall national expenditures. In no other country does
it cover more than about 15 percent of the total health care bill.[11]

At the same time, the United States maintains an extraordinarily expensive
set of public health care finance programs. Medicare spends about $554 billion
a year on coverage for the elderly and totally disabled. Medicaid spends almost
$408 billion on coverage for the poor.[12] Other government programs, includ-
ing the Children's Health Insurance Program (CHIP), the Veterans Health

Administration, and Department of Defense coverage for active military personnel and their dependents, spend another $90 billion.[13]

In other words, as large as it is, the government's role in health care finance clearly has not crowded out the private sector. In fact, the amount spent on private health insurance has risen relentlessly over recent decades, in step with public programs. It totaled just $4.8 billion in 1960 and just $14 billion in 1970.[14] By 1990, it had risen to $204.8 billion, by 2000 to $405.8 billion, and by 2009 to $712.2 billion. At the current rate of growth, it will be a trillion-dollar industry before too long.

What accounts for the size, robustness, and steady growth of America's private health insurance industry in a system that leaves so much room for public programs? Did clever entrepreneurs spot an untapped market niche? Did unconstrained consumer demand create a private juggernaut to meet it? As with the rest of American health care, the reality is quite to the contrary. Private entrepreneurs did respond to commercial opportunities, but the vibrant private sector they built was only possible with the help of a silent partner. That partner, once again, was the government.

The history of private health insurance in the United States is marked by a series of seminal government policies that underlie its very existence. Unlike many other health care sectors, health insurance had not existed for thousands of years before taking its modern form. Rather, it is an invention of the twentieth century that arose in response to a combination of private initiatives and government programs that created the conditions for its emergence.

Some would argue that these programs have led the industry to become too large and powerful. Its mechanisms for administering policies and paying claims add overhead costs to the health care system while contributing nothing to the actual provision of care. The profits that it generates for investors represent sizeable sums that leak out of the system without adding more or better health care.

The political power that the health insurance industry has acquired with its size is reflected in numerous lobbying successes. Supporters of a single-payer approach to health care finance point to its opposition as an important impediment to the achievement of their goal. The industry's influence was notably displayed in the process of crafting President Barack Obama's health reform initiative, the Affordable Care Act (ACA), which relies primarily on private insurers to extend coverage to the uninsured. The Act not only increased the size of the market for individual policies substantially, it did so without the inclusion of a public insurance option, as some had advocated. Ironically, it is the nurturance of the government that has given the industry the wherewithal to shape public policies such as these, thereby enabling it to sustain its continual growth.

The Development of Private Health Insurance in America

Before the early part of the twentieth century, there was little need for health insurance. Medical care was provided either on a charity basis or paid for directly by patients out of their own pockets. Hospitals were compensated sporadically for the care they provided because their patients tended to be very ill and poor, with few financial resources. Physicians charged fees that most of their patients could afford, and they could write off the bills of those who could not. There were few prescription drugs, and those that were available were relatively cheap.[15]

THE FIRST FOCUS OF HEALTH CARE COVERAGE: THE WORKPLACE

Early efforts to establish insurance arrangements to defray the cost of health care focused on injuries in the workplace in the late nineteenth century. In a country that was rapidly industrializing, hazardous jobs in factories, mines, and construction sites often led to serious injuries. Several unions, railroad brotherhoods, and industrial corporations created funds to protect workers in individual industries. In some cases, benefits extended to general health care. For example, the Northern Pacific Railway Company created the Northern Pacific Beneficial Association to provide medical and hospital care to employees and their families.[16] It administered benefits through a network of affiliated physicians and hospitals. However, unlike some European countries, in which public health insurance programs were gaining a foothold at the time, insurance for health care expenses outside the workplace was uncommon on either a public or private basis in the United States.[17]

The first attempts in America at broader health care coverage remained focused on the workplace. In the early twentieth century, each state established a workers' compensation program to provide comprehensive protection against the costs of work-related injuries and illnesses in all industries. They followed the model of similar arrangements that were gaining popularity in Europe. These programs required employers to purchase private insurance coverage for their workers against both medical expenses and lost wages caused by work-related mishaps. These arrangements remain in place in every state today.[18]

This limited form of coverage followed a pattern that eventually came to characterize much of American health care. The government, in this case at the state level, implemented a regulatory scheme that defined the products to be offered and set the parameters in which the private sector could sell them. The mandate for employers to purchase workers' compensation insurance created demand for policies, and regulatory requirements defined their contours. The ACA contains a mandate that all individuals maintain coverage, and regulations define the elements that the coverage must contain.[19] Although the architects of workers compensation may not have realized it at the time, they had designed a public–private partnership whose structure would eventually permeate the American health care system.

THE FIRST GENERAL HEALTH INSURANCE:
PROVIDER-SPONSORED COVERAGE

The crucible for general health care coverage beyond the confines of the workplace was the Great Depression of the 1930s. By the time it arrived, hospitals had reached a level of technological sophistication that required a source of payment for the services they rendered. However, with unemployment rampant, many of them found their patient base lacking financial means. Baylor University Hospital in Dallas, Texas devised a solution in 1929, in the form of prepaid care. The hospital offered to provide a group of 1,500 schoolteachers with up to 21 days a year of hospital care for the fixed sum of $6 a month, paid in advance. With this modest beginning, American health insurance was born.[20]

The concept of prepaying hospitals for the cost of care succeeded at Baylor, and it soon spread to other hospitals. In the early 1930s, it was broadened further to include multiple institutions under a single coverage plan, with the first such arrangements launched in California and New Jersey. They were known formally as "hospital service plans" but took the popular name "Blue Cross."[21] They operated under the supervision of the American Hospital Association, which promulgated principles for their conduct in 1933.[22] The Association granted formal approval to plans that met its standards along with permission to use the Blue Cross designation. Most coverage was sold through employers because of the ease of administering policies for groups of beneficiaries, although in some regions the plans sold policies directly to individuals.

These first health coverage plans contained distinctive features that distinguished them from traditional insurance arrangements that covered other kinds of risks. As an initial matter, since they were designed to bolster the financial support of hospitals rather than as profit centers in their own right, they were structured on a nonprofit basis. This lifted the burden of having to generate sufficient revenue to pay dividends to shareholders. However, Blue Cross plans also faced another more significant economic hurdle. Laws in every state require licensed insurance companies to maintain large financial reserves as safety valves in the event of major unexpected claims. Nonprofit plans established by health care providers lacked access to the funds that were needed to comply.[23]

To enable Blue Cross plans to surmount this obstacle, many states granted them special exemptions from reserve requirements. New York was the first to do so, in 1934. Under the special rules it adopted, as long as the plans retained their nonprofit status and remained under the control of member nonprofit hospitals, they could maintain lower levels of reserves than traditional insurance companies. The states reasoned that the plans did not need substantial backup funds to protect against large claims because they could guarantee coverage by directly providing services through their member hospitals. Over the next five years, 25 other states enacted similar measures.[24]

A model similar to Blue Cross was first applied to physician services 10 years after Baylor launched its experiment. The first such plan was introduced in 1939, in Sacramento, California. It operated on a nonprofit basis with physicians controlling the board of directors, and it took the popular name "Blue Shield." Additional plans were launched in a number of other states over the next several years, and they received regulatory flexibility concerning reserve requirements similar to that granted to Blue Cross plans. However, the concept spread more slowly than had Blue Cross because physician charges presented less of a financial challenge to patients than those of hospitals.[25]

With the special regulatory status granted to Blue Cross and Blue Shield plans, state governments had helped to give health insurance an initial foothold as a new kind of financial product. It was health care providers who had devised the idea for the product, but their success depended on help from lawmakers and regulators who developed new legal mechanisms to accommodate it. The public gradually took to the notion, and it grew in popularity through the 1930s and into the early 1940s.[26]

THE FEDERAL ROLE IN ENCOURAGING PRIVATE COVERAGE

Although it had become quite popular, health insurance was not yet established as a staple of America's financial infrastructure at the start of World War II. That changed during the War. The seminal step in the transformation was a policy decision by the government, this time at the federal level. It seemed a relatively minor action at the time. Those who made it had no intention of igniting a revolution in health care finance. But the long-term effect was to spread this financial product throughout the economy and, ultimately, to transform the entire health care system.

The step was taken in the middle of the war. When America launched its war effort, it fully mobilized the economy. The country's industrial base was sent into overdrive to produce military goods, such as tanks and supplies for the troops. The shift in production away from consumer goods led to scarcities of many items, engendering fears of rampant price inflation. At the same time, many men who had been part of the workforce entered the armed forces, which reduced the supply of workers and led to fears of inflation in wages. In response, Congress imposed a national freeze on both. Increases in either prices or wages were only permitted with the permission of a federal board.[27]

Finding themselves unable to attract sufficient numbers of workers in a smaller labor force yet prohibited from offering higher wages as an inducement, a few large companies devised an alternative strategy. They would offer benefits, like health insurance, as an enhancement to wages to entice potential workers. However, they first had to convince the War Labor Board, which was charged with administering the wage freeze, that such add-ons to salary, commonly known as "fringe benefits," should be exempt from its restrictions. They succeeded in 1943, when the Board ruled that health insurance was distinct from wages and could therefore be added to employee compensation without violating the freeze.[28]

Blue Cross plans, which were the dominant health insurance providers at the time, reaped the greatest immediate benefits from the ruling. Their customer base grew almost fourfold during World War II, from seven million at the start to 26 million by the end.[29] However, all health insurance plans found bigger markets as large numbers of Americans were introduced to this new financial instrument and found it to their liking. In 1945, an estimated 30 million Americans were enrolled in a plan in some form.[30]

The wage freeze was repealed at the end of the war, but the growing popularity of health insurance as an employee benefit continued unabated.[31] Large companies began using it as a standard recruiting tool, and many workers came to expect it. Unions began to include it in their collective bargaining demands, and some ran insurance programs themselves. By the start of the 1950s, health insurance had become a standard component of employment relationships throughout much of American industry.

The Federal Wage Board ruling was intended to alleviate a short-term problem—the shortage of workers to staff key industries during World War II. As it turned out, the ruling exerted two profound effects on American health care finance that have continued to reverberate to the present day. The first was that it rapidly brought health insurance to millions of workers and their families who would not have thought to obtain it on their own. Although health coverage might have eventually grown in popularity without this boost, its spread would have been more gradual and its impact on the financial structure of the health care industry more muted. The second and perhaps more important effect was that it enshrined a link between health insurance and employment. As a widely offered fringe benefit, the workplace became the primary route for obtaining coverage. This stands in contrast to other forms of insurance that are most commonly obtained on an individual basis.

The linking of health insurance and employment has molded a key element of the financial base of health care in the United States. But its ramifications do not stop there. They extend throughout all aspects of the health care system. In particular, employer-based coverage has fostered an insurance paradigm that leaves large segments of the population without access to coverage. That has engendered the need for a set of government initiatives to fill the gap, with the ACA as the most ambitious. These programs, in turn, have exerted their own profound influence on the shape of American health care.

The World War II wage freeze exemption set the stage for the spread of private health insurance connected to employment, but it took a second federal action to cement the link. Since fringe benefits were not considered "wages" for purposes of the freeze, the Internal Revenue Service (IRS) had to decide whether their value constituted "income" for purposes of taxation. It took the position that benefit expenditures did not, meaning that health insurance could be provided to workers tax-free. This made health insurance even more attractive as an employee benefit because, unlike salary, a portion of its value would not be lost to taxes. Congress ratified this decision when it enacted a revision of the Internal Revenue Code in 1954.[32]

By exempting the cost of employer-paid health insurance premiums from income tax, the federal government forgoes a tremendous amount of potential revenue. Economists refer to this loss to government coffers as a "tax subsidy" because it funds an activity with a tax preference. In this case, the government is subsidizing the purchase of coverage by workers for themselves and their families. As health insurance spread as a common employment benefit, the aggregate cost of the subsidy grew with it. The amount is amplified by a shadow effect on state income tax because most states recognize federal tax exemptions in calculating their own assessments.

As employee health benefits have reached larger numbers of people, the size of the subsidy has grown dramatically. In 2010, about 155 million Americans were covered by employment-based health insurance, either directly or as dependents of covered workers. The revenue lost to federal and state governments from excluding its value from income tax stood at almost $250 billion.[33] The tax subsidy therefore constitutes the third-largest government health care finance program in the country after Medicare and Medicaid.[34] In 2006, it represented one-third of the cost of all private employment-based policies sold in the United States.[35] The government subsidizes the purchase of few other products on such a massive scale, and it does not provide a comparable inducement for the purchase of individual policies directly from insurance companies. It makes the purchase of coverage through employment a particularly good deal for workers and one that most readily accept.

TAX POLICY AND THE SHAPE OF MODERN HEALTH INSURANCE

The tax subsidy for employment-based health insurance has had two main consequences for the financing of American health care, one beneficial and one harmful. On the positive side, it has encouraged the widespread uptake of insurance and made the market more attractive for insurers. Four features of employment-based coverage are especially important in this regard. First, the tax break for purchasing coverage has made it affordable for many who otherwise might not have been able to come up with the cost. Second, the ability to obtain it through employment has made its acquisition more convenient than shopping in an open market. Third, the sale of insurance through employers to large numbers of workers is administratively easier for insurance companies because a single policy can cover a large number of people. Finally, employer groups form natural pools of beneficiaries for spreading the risk of claims. Insurance companies can review claims experience on an employer-by-employer basis to predict losses. Policies sold to individuals must be priced based on losses in entire communities, which are more difficult to estimate.

On the negative side, a system that bases coverage on employment status leaves many people behind. Two groups are of special particular concern. These are the elderly, many of whom have retired and are no longer part of the workforce, and the poor, many of whom have no employer through which to obtain benefits. The government addressed the needs of these groups in the mid-1960s with the enactment of Medicare for those over the age of 65 and Medicaid for those with very low incomes.

However, many people who lack access to employment-based health insurance are neither elderly nor poor. They include those who are unemployed, who work for themselves, and who work part-time and fail to qualify for their employer's benefits plan. Many others are employed by companies that do not offer coverage. A large number of mid-sized and smaller firms are unable either to afford the cost or to handle its administrative burden.[36] People in these circumstances lose not only the ability to obtain coverage for themselves but for their families, as well.

Those without access to employment-based health insurance must turn to the individual market to obtain it. However, before implementation of the ACA, the ability to purchase a policy directly from an insurance company was far from guaranteed. Many insurers avoided individuals as customers for two reasons. The administration of coverage is more burdensome when each individual has his or her own policy than when a single policy covers an entire employer group. And, perhaps more importantly, natural risk pools in employer groups, which make employment-based coverage attractive, are missing when each individual is insured separately.[37]

As a result, insurance companies often erected barriers to obtaining coverage in the individual market. In particular, they subjected applicants to individual underwriting, a process through which the likelihood of incurring claims is assessed based on factors such as medical history and results of a physical exam. Those considered at risk of running up high medical bills either because of preexisting conditions or advanced age were either denied policies outright or charged high prices that were often unaffordable.[38]

Compounding the challenges of obtaining coverage in the individual insurance market, those who find coverage must pay the full cost of premiums, with no employer assistance in paying the cost. To make matters worse, none of this expense is subject to the tax exemption that employment-based premiums receive.[39] This is the case even under the ACA. The policies that help millions of workers to obtain coverage thereby leave others with a combination of obstacles that make it difficult to enjoy the same benefits. In 2010, the year of the ACA's passage, an estimated 50 million Americans lacked coverage of any sort, many of whom would have obtained individual policies if they could.[40] Their ranks had been growing almost every year as an increasing number of employers dropped health benefits.[41]

Prior to the ACA, Congress had addressed the plight of some of those without access to employer-sponsored health coverage with two stopgap measures. The Comprehensive Omnibus Budget Reconciliation Act of 1986 (COBRA) allows many who lose their jobs to maintain coverage for a period of time.[42] However, after their employment ends, they must pay the entire cost, including the share that their employer had been contributing. The Health Insurance Portability and Accountability Act of 1996 (HIPAA) requires insurers to offer workers individual policies after employment coverage ends and requires that employment-based policies extend coverage to most new workers regardless of their health status.[43] However, the individual policy that is offered can be extremely expensive, and the provision for new workers provides no help to those who have no job at all. Therefore, although these laws have been lifesavers for many, their reach is limited.

In addition to biasing the market away from individual coverage, the tax subsidy for employment-based health insurance creates a significant inequity. Under America's progressive income tax structure, the value of a tax deduction increases with a taxpayer's marginal tax rate, which rises with income. As a result, its benefits are greater for those with higher earnings. Those at the bottom of the income spectrum, who need financial assistance the most, pay the lowest marginal tax rates and therefore benefit the least. Economists refer to programs like this that favor higher income over lower income beneficiaries as "regressive."

Despite these shortcomings, employment-based health insurance remains the foundation of America's system of health care finance. It is the largest single source of coverage, even under the market reforms implemented by the ACA. It holds this position not because the market demanded it but because a series of government policies created an environment conducive to its uptake and spread.

FOR-PROFIT HEALTH INSURANCE FINDS ITS NICHE

As the health insurance market expanded after World War II and through the 1950s, an important new player entered the scene. After leaving health coverage largely to nonprofit Blue Cross and Blue Shield plans though the 1930s and 1940s, for-profit insurance companies, known as *commercial insurers*, saw an opening. They realized that coverage for medical expenses could represent a profit center in itself, not just a payment vehicle for providers. Although their market share remained small, they added an important new element to the private coverage sector.[44]

Commercial insurers carved out a market niche by exploiting a key feature of employment-based insurance. Blue Cross and Blue Shield plans at the time considered the claims experience of all employer groups in their regions when setting rates, a process known as "community rating." Most states required them to use this approach as a condition of receiving special regulatory treatment. Commercial insurers, on the other hand, set rates according to the experience of each separate employer group that they covered, a process known as "experience rating." This allows them to offer lower prices to companies with healthier workers and thereby to skim this part of the market from Blue Cross and Blue Shield.[45] Moreover, if a company's claims experience turns adverse, a commercial insurer can drop coverage, leaving the firm to return to Blue Cross and Blue Shield, which were required by law to take it back.[46]

This business model turned out to be highly profitable. By cherry picking the healthiest employer groups, commercial insurers were able to significantly reduce their claims costs. Yet their products qualified for the same tax subsidy as those of the nonprofit Blue Cross and Blue Shield plans that were obliged to cover everyone.

Commercial insurers also reshaped the market in another important way. By regularly adding and dropping customers, they engendered instability, which was managed by another for-profit industry, insurance brokers. These businesses represent companies seeking to purchase insurance and serve as intermediaries between them and insurers seeking to sell it.[47] Without them, many smaller and mid-sized employers would find the process of obtaining commercial policies unmanageable. The business of brokering health insurance has grown into a major enterprise. Today, America has more than 100,000 insurance brokers, along with similar professionals who match corporate purchasers with insurance providers.[48] Their success represents another profitable private enterprise created as a consequence of government policies.

A NEW WRINKLE IN THE MARKET: SELF-INSURANCE

As workers came to expect health insurance as a part of their compensation during the 1960s and 1970s, companies increasingly found that it imposed significant expenses that they sought ways to reduce. One idea was to cut the administrative overhead and profit margins built into the premiums charged by insurance companies. Some large employers saw a way to accomplish this by insuring themselves for employee health benefits instead of purchasing coverage from a third party. For major corporations, this is a viable approach because they have the financial wherewithal to pay the medical claims of their employees on their own, without the need for a financial intermediary. By cutting out the middleman, they stood to realize significant savings.

However, multistate employers faced a regulatory hurdle to self-insuring their employee medical expenses. Under the McCarran-Ferguson Act, passed by Congress in 1945, primary authority to regulate insurance lies with the states.[49] Regulators in most states considered these arrangements to constitute insurance, which subjected them to governmental oversight. Among the regulations this brought to bear were requirements to obtain a license to operate as an insurance company and to maintain large financial reserves to protect against unexpected losses. Compliance would have been difficult if not impossible for companies that were not already in the insurance business.

Congress crafted a way around this obstacle in 1974 in the form of the Employee Retirement Income Security Act (ERISA).[50] The primary goal of that law was to shore up the solvency of pension plans, but it also addressed the barriers to self-insured health benefit arrangements by exempting them from most state regulations. In their place, it implemented a laxer set of federal standards. It also exempted employer plans that are not self-insured from some state requirements, thereby reducing the regulatory burden for all employment-based coverage.

ERISA's rules for employer-sponsored health insurance plans are extremely complex and have been the subject of much litigation. In essence, they accomplish two results. For plans that are not self-insured and for which an employer purchases coverage from a traditional insurance company, states are denied jurisdiction over plan management. With limited exceptions, they may not set terms for coverage or prices, and they may not oversee the process of claims administration and payment. For plans that are self-insured and for which an employer bears the financial risk of coverage itself, states are denied jurisdiction almost entirely. They may not impose requirements for maintaining reserves or for any other aspect of the financial arrangements involved.[51]

By limiting the oversight of employment-based health insurance, ERISA made the provision of coverage easier and cheaper for all companies. It freed insurers from the burden of complying with many expensive rules, and it permitted many employers to self-insure at substantial cost savings. By enacting the law, Congress had once again eased the path for health insurance with regulatory favors bestowed on no other kind of coverage.

However, the full impact of ERISA in molding health care finance was yet to come. The insurance plans available in 1974 were based predominantly on an "indemnity" model. Under it, the insurance company indemnifies beneficiaries for their medical expenses by reimbursing either them or their provider for a share of the cost. Under these arrangements, insurers do not actively intervene in the provision of care but rather respond to claims passively with payments after they have been incurred. Exemption from state regulations made the administration of these plans easier and less expensive for employers, but it had little effect on the nature of the medical care that was subject to coverage.

That changed dramatically about a decade after ERISA's enactment, when insurers increasingly turned to a managed care system of coverage under which they actively oversee the provision of health care services. Managed care plans allow insurers to direct the amount and kinds of care that patients receive, rather than passively paying the bills. Laxer state regulatory scrutiny is particularly helpful in implementing arrangements such as these. Under ERISA, the power of states to restrict the behavior of managed care companies is limited, and, even more significantly, beneficiaries are restricted in their ability to sue for improper denials of benefits.[52] Fewer regulations to contend with and a smaller chance of being sued for their actions meant an easier path for the spread of this form of coverage.

ERISA was only one of the ways in which the government promoted managed care. Other federal laws, regulations, and funding programs also served as key enablers of its rise. The result over the course of the late twentieth century was a transformation of the structure of private health care finance.

How the Government Created Managed Care

By the late 1960s, rising health care costs had become a significant national concern. Medicare and Medicaid, enacted in the middle of the decade, extended coverage to millions, but the greater demand for health care services that they engendered had caused spending to accelerate throughout the system. Some saw the answer in a universal insurance program similar to Medicare that extended coverage to all. Others looked instead to ways of improving the functioning of the private insurance market to make it more efficient.

In 1973, President Richard Nixon chose to try the latter approach. He latched onto the concept of managed care as a way to transform insurance companies from passive conduits for reimbursement into active guardians of the efficiency of the services for which they paid. This alternative approach to payment, he and his advisors hoped, would eliminate enough waste in the system to bring costs under control.[53]

THE MANAGED CARE MODEL

The concept of managed care as a financing vehicle was relatively new at the time. It had been developed four years earlier in 1969, by Dr. Paul Ellwood, a Minneapolis physician with a strong interest in health policy. He based it on the model of pre-paid plans, an alternative to traditional insurance that dated to the 1940s. Rather than reimbursing patients or providers for the cost of medical care, these entities provided health care services themselves. They maintained networks of designated providers for their members by hiring their own physicians and either owning or entering into contractual arrangements with hospitals and other facilities.[54]

The first such plans were created by a few large corporations in the middle of the twentieth century to cover workers and their dependents. They extended the model of the Northern Pacific Railway plan in the late nineteenth century.[55] The first to apply it on a large scale was the Kaiser Aluminum Company, which established a plan in 1942 for employees in its steel mills in Portland, Oregon and Oakland, California. It offered comprehensive coverage through employed physicians and owned hospitals. In 1945, it opened the plan to the general public under the name Kaiser-Permanente, and it grew rapidly, surviving to become a major health insurer today. In 1947, the City of New York launched a similar arrangement, the Health Insurance Plan (HIP), to provide physician services to municipal workers through physician practices that it organized.[56] Other plans that emerged at that time were Group Health Cooperative of Puget Sound in Seattle, Washington and Group Health Association in Washington, D.C.[57]

Dr. Ellwood designed the concept of managed care to mimic the structure of prepaid arrangements such as these and called the plans that implemented it "health maintenance organizations," or HMOs for short. However, unlike traditional prepaid plans, they do not directly hire physicians or own hospitals but instead provide care through providers that remain independent. This freed the plans from the expense of building facilities and managing clinical workforces. At the center of Dr. Ellwood's model is the primary care physician (PCP). Each beneficiary is assigned to one. The PCPs are charged with coordinating all care. In this role, they render all basic care themselves and must approve in advance most additional services, such as visits to specialists and diagnostic tests, before they can be eligible for reimbursement. The goal was to keep as much care as possible at the PCP level, where it is the least costly to provide.[58]

To encourage PCPs to be sparing in their recommendations for more advanced care, HMOs implemented an innovative compensation structure. Rather than paying for each service performed, they compensated PCPs with a fixed monthly fee for each patient assigned to their care, regardless of the amount of services actually rendered to them. Known as "capitation" payments, these sums were designed to recreate the incentive structure of salaries that staff physicians receive in prepaid plans. By paying practitioners for each patient cared for instead of each service provided, they eliminate the reward for rendering more care than is truly needed.

A second important cost control technique used by HMOs is a set of mechanisms that require patients to receive services beyond the primary care level from providers under contract with the plan. Visits to specialist physicians, hospitals, and providers of ancillary services are not eligible for reimbursement unless the provider is a member of the HMO's network. Membership in it requires acceptance of various restrictive terms, including a discounted schedule of fees and review of services provided to determine whether they are truly needed. Under the review process, physician specialists must receive approval before conducting or ordering expensive diagnostic tests or procedures, and hospitals must receive authorization before admitting patients or extending their stays for longer than a designated length of time.

A third important element of Dr. Ellwood's vision for HMOs was a focus on prevention. Unlike traditional indemnity insurers of the time, HMOs paid for preventive services such as checkups and immunizations. Dr. Ellwood also hoped that capitation payments would encourage PCPs to keep their patients as healthy as possible because they received no additional reimbursement for rendering additional care when their patients became ill.

Although the theory of HMOs held the promise of lower health care costs, the insurance market of the early 1970s was not yet ready to embrace it.[59] Initial uptake was extremely limited, and HMOs needed external assistance to gain a foothold. Two forms of help were particularly important for them. One was funding for start-up expenses. The other was a way to convince employers to offer their services to employees as a workplace benefit.

A LEGISLATIVE STIMULUS

The assistance came in the form of legislation supported by the Nixon Administration and passed by Congress in 1973 to give HMOs a jump-start. It was known as the Health Maintenance Organization Act (HMO Act).[60] The law offered regulatory relief and financial support to help this new form of prepaid plan realize Paul Ellwood's vision of networks of private providers rendering care under an altered economic paradigm. It may have seemed a fairly limited step at the time it was enacted, but the HMO Act marked a milestone in the government's involvement in health care finance. It was the first time that health insurance was directly regulated at the federal level. With ERISA following it one year later, the law began a new phase in the relationship between federal policy and the insurance industry that, over the coming decades, transformed the financial infrastructure of American health care.

Among its key provisions, the HMO Act required employers that offered health benefits to include an HMO among the coverage options, if the HMO met minimum standards and requested that it be included. The standards covered features such as the size of the provider network, the structure of reimbursement for preventive services, the ease of enrollment, and the nature of the grievance policy for patient complaints. They also required the use of community rating in setting premiums. HMOs that met these standards were classified as "federally qualified," and, in addition to gaining a tool for prying an opening into the market, they became eligible for subsidies and loan guarantees to help defray start-up costs. The HMO Act did not require employers to offer an HMO to their workers if they did not provide any health benefits at all, but if they did, HMOs had to be given the opportunity to compete against traditional insurance plans on an equal footing.[61]

The Act also granted managed care plans a number of regulatory advantages. It did this by requiring states, as a condition of receiving funding to support HMO development, to amend their laws to lift legal restrictions that could have stood in their way. Two kinds of laws could have posed particular obstacles. One was a rule imposed in many states that prevented corporations from employing physicians directly, known as the prohibition on the "corporate practice of medicine."[62] The other was a rule adopted in many states that prohibited insurance companies from limiting patients' choice of providers. Exemption from these restrictions gave HMOs advantages that no other insurance arrangements enjoyed.[63]

HMOs, with their aggressive cost control techniques, were able to limit the size of their premiums, but many of their members chafed at the restrictions they imposed on access to care. Insurance companies responded during the 1980s and 1990s by devising alternative forms of coverage with looser restrictions than traditional HMOs.[64] One took the form of preferred provider organizations (PPOs), which dispense with the requirement for PCP referrals before letting patients receive specialty or hospital care. Another was point of service (POS) plans, which permit patients to see any provider they choose, but with more generous coverage for those in the company's network. These alternative forms of managed care assuaged the concerns of many beneficiaries and enabled the market to expand more widely. Over time, they surpassed traditional HMOs in market share so that the concept of managed care came to encompass a variety of arrangements that differ in various details but share a core of common features.[65]

THE MARKET RESPONDS

The effect of the HMO Act on the health insurance market was limited at first. During the first few years after its passage, Congress revisited the law and tweaked it twice to address industry concerns.[66] In 1976, it passed amendments to reduce the number of mandatory benefits that HMOs were required to offer to maintain federally qualified status. In 1978, it increased the amount of federal financial support that the law provided. These changes had their desired effect. In the years immediately following their implementation, HMOs added 1.4 million new subscribers.[67]

Despite the uptick in the late 1970s, the market share of HMOs remained below 10 percent through the decade.[68] That low penetration rate began to change in the 1980s in response to a shift in health care's financial environment. The pace of increases in insurance premiums accelerated at the time, and many smaller employers found that their health benefit plans had become unaffordable. HMOs with their lower premiums offered a way to continue providing coverage.

With the rise in costs for conventional insurance, the number of managed care plans and of enrollees in them grew dramatically.[69] In January 1970, three years before Congress passed the HMO Act, 26 plans operated in the United States. The number had grown to 72 by 1973, the year of the law's enactment. It almost doubled during the following year to 142. By December 1984, the country had 337 plans and by June 1987, 662. The number of people enrolled in them grew from 6 million in 1976, three years after the Act's passage, to 29 million in 1987.

Along with increases in the number of plans and of enrollees, the share of the insurance market represented by HMOs and other forms of managed care rose precipitously during the 1980s and 1990s, as well. As a result, managed care grew to become the dominant form of health insurance in the United States. In 1988, it covered 27 percent of insured Americans.[70] The proportion reached 54 percent in 1993, 73 percent in 1996, and 92 percent in 2000.[71] In 2007, managed care plans served more than 97 percent of those with private health coverage. Of the total number of enrollees, traditional HMOs covered about one-fifth, with the rest in PPOs, POS plans, and similar arrangements. Many Americans today have never experienced health insurance in any form other than managed care.

Once they had become established, many HMOs, no longer in need of start-up funds or special regulatory advantages, chose to abandon their status as federally qualified and the restrictions that it involved. With the market for managed care established, Congress allowed the HMO Act to lapse in 1981. By that time, the law had clearly served its purpose. Managed care was well on its way to transforming the nature of American health insurance. Although controversy remains over the extent to which it has actually achieved its original goal of taming costs, there is little dispute about the importance of the federal role in fostering its ascent.[72] In this industry segment, as in health insurance overall, the government had served as the essential foundational force.

MANAGED CARE'S EFFECT ON THE LARGER HEALTH CARE INDUSTRY

When the HMO Act was passed in 1973, most of the prepayment plans then in existence operated under local control, and operation on a for-profit basis was rare.[73] As the market for HMOs grew and companies abandoned their initial nonprofit status, their attractiveness as acquisition targets for national insurance companies increased as well. More and larger corporations entered the market, and a spate of mergers and acquisitions followed. By 1980, the majority of HMOs had been swallowed up by regional or national networks operated by companies such as Kaiser Permanente, Prudential, and many Blue Cross plans. When the law expired in 1981, subsidies for start-up capital ended, and funding from corporate purchasers came to serve as the primary source of financing for market entrance and expansion. As the consolidation trend continued, HMOs became big business. When the industry matured during the late 1990s, it consolidated even further.[74] Large national firms gained even greater size while most of the smaller local ones disappeared.[75]

With larger HMO size came greater bargaining clout in negotiations with providers. Insurers that controlled large slices of the market held the power to direct significant numbers of patients to physicians and hospitals that agreed to their terms and to withhold patients from those that did not. This put managed care companies in a powerful position to extract price concessions.[76]

Many providers looked to join together into larger aggregations in response to try to match the insurers' bargaining power.[77] A consolidation trend followed on the physician and hospital side that swept through markets across the country over the course of the 1990s, as discussed in Chapters 4 and 5. Of particular importance to the structure of the overall health care system, many hospitals merged to form larger systems. Among the most significant of these were Partners Health Care in Boston, formed from the combination of Massachusetts General Hospital and Brigham and Women's Hospital; New York-Presbyterian Hospital in New York, formed from the combination of New York Hospital and Columbia Presbyterian; and the University of Pennsylvania Health System in Philadelphia, formed through the acquisition of several hospitals to operate as affiliates of the Hospital of the University of Pennsylvania.[78] Many physicians joined into large group practices, in some cases including hundreds of practitioners. In several instances, hospitals and physicians joined together into single enterprises, forming what came to be called "integrated delivery systems."[79]

By the end of the 1990s, much of American health care had crystallized into a more centralized enterprise.[80] Fewer hospitals continued to function as stand-alone entities, with the proportion that were part of multihospital systems increasing from 30 percent to 65 percent between 1995 and 2001.[81] Physicians increasingly practiced as employees of larger organizations, and many ancillary providers, such as clinical laboratories and radiology centers, became subsidiary components of larger systems. Many of these provider aggregations succeeded in gaining the bargaining strength with insurers they had sought.[82] But they did so at the loss of much of the autonomy that their individual components had previously enjoyed. Health care was no longer the cottage industry it had been for hundreds of years before the late twentieth century.

By creating the economic pressures that drove providers to consolidate, managed care had wrought an alteration of the structure of the entire health care industry.[83] Its transformative influence extended well beyond the structure of health care finance to the business model through which services are actually provided. The experiment with alternative payment arrangements that Congress had sanctioned with the HMO Act in 1973 thereby came to alter all aspects of American health care. Private businesses—insurance companies, hospitals, physicians, and many others—implemented the changes, and many of them prospered handsomely as a result. But the genesis of the transformation was in the government policies that created managed care and nurtured it into a powerful economic force.

Medicare, Medicaid, and the Steady Expansion of the Private Insurance Market

The government's role in shaping and sustaining private health insurance as we know it today, along with the managed care sector that now dominates it, did not stop with the formative programs that launched the industry. Public support for private insurance extends to the government-run coverage programs that supplement private plans. Far from serving as a competitor, direct government-provided health insurance in the form of Medicare and Medicaid has come to represent one of the industry's most reliable and lucrative business niches. The history of these programs and their indispensible support for American hospitals and for the medical profession of today are described in Chapters 4 and 5. They have also come to underlie much of the profitability of the private health insurance industry.

MEDICARE'S PRIVATE SECTOR BACKBONE

Medicare may seem on its surface to be the archetype of a single-payer government health care program. It is a national plan created by an act of Congress, and it is implemented through federal regulations. It is financed through tax revenue, some of which comes from a dedicated payroll tax and some from general government coffers. It is administered by a federal agency, the Centers for Medicare & Medicaid Services (CMS), a component of the Department of Health and Human Services.[84] These are certainly the trappings of a fully public initiative.

However, in Medicare's case, appearances are deceiving. In reality, the program functions as a huge public–private partnership. On multiple levels, it creates, both directly and indirectly, private market niches that are essential to its operations and that have sustained vast investor-owned enterprises.

New business opportunities for private insurance companies were built into the fabric of Medicare from the start. The most significant of these grew out of the political compromises that created the program. Medicare's gestation required a series of deals between its proponents and powerful industries that saw it as a threat to their business interests. One such industry with a large amount at stake was insurance.

Medicare's coverage for the elderly did not fill a complete void. Before its passage, a substantial proportion of elderly citizens, close to 60 percent, were able to obtain private insurance on an individual basis. The availability of public coverage promised to siphon away this business from the companies that provided it, most of which were Blue Cross and Blue Shield plans. To compensate for this loss of business, and to preempt insurance industry opposition to enactment of Medicare, Congress built two new lucrative business opportunities into the program's structure.[85]

The first was the chance to administer key aspects of Medicare under contract with the federal government. Beneath the surface of a unified single-payer, government-run program, much of Medicare's day-to-day management is conducted through private insurance companies.[86] Their role includes paying claims and making some coverage determinations. Under Part A of the program, which covers hospital and other inpatient services, insurers performing those functions are known as "intermediaries." Under Part B, which covers physician and other outpatient services, they are known as "carriers." Insurers have found these roles to be quite rewarding.[87]

The second business opportunity created by Medicare proved to be even more substantial. Although the program offers extensive coverage for most health care services, it requires beneficiaries to pay substantial co-payments and deductibles. It also omits coverage for some important items and services, such as eyeglasses and extended long-term care, and, under its original structure, prescription drugs and preventive care.[88] To fill these gaps, Congress permitted private insurers to sell policies, known as "Medicare supplement" or "Medigap," directly to beneficiaries.

After Medicare's implementation, between 80 and 85 percent of beneficiaries availed themselves of this fill-in coverage. This meant that rather than losing customers to Medicare, private insurers were able to gain large numbers of new ones. What made the market for these limited policies even more of a business bonanza for insurers was that they were able to charge premiums that were almost as high as those they had charged for full coverage prior to Medicare. The result was that, far from being crowded out, the market for private coverage of the elderly actually grew by almost 50 percent after Medicare took effect. Needless to say, the products were also less costly to provide because they merely filled the holes left by Medicare's extensive benefit structure. In facilitating the sale of this new kind of insurance product, the government created an especially profitable new business opportunity for the industry.[89]

Putting it all together, private insurers came away from the passage of Medicare with more customers who paid the same premiums for smaller benefits. They also gained a lucrative new line of business in administering claims that had not previously existed. This massive program was anything but a government takeover of the health insurance market. It substantially expanded the commercial opportunities available to private companies.

MANAGED CARE AND GOVERNMENT HEALTH INSURANCE

The private opportunities built into Medicare's initial structure were just the start. A second element of government support for the private health insurance industry bolstered the expansion of managed care in the 1980s and 1990s after the preferences of the HMO Act had expired. The government did this by becoming one of its main customers. Noting early signs of success in keeping premiums under control for private employers, government policymakers saw an opportunity to incorporate the managed care concept into public coverage programs. They did this by creating a new role for private companies in administering Medicare and Medicaid benefits, one that developed into a significant line of business for many of them.

The partnership between public insurance programs and private managed care companies began with limited state-level experiments under Medicaid. In 1981, Congress granted states the flexibility to test alternative arrangements for delivering services in the hope that they could find less costly approaches. To that end, it permitted states to request waivers from the federal government from rules governing administration of their Medicaid programs in order to try them out.[90]

The approach that generated the most interest was to place some beneficiaries in private HMOs that would be paid to administer their coverage and manage their care. The HMOs would limit costs by using the same techniques they applied for privately insured patients—directing care through PCPs, paying PCPs based on capitation, requiring prior approval for expensive tests and procedures, and limiting specialty and hospital care to providers in defined networks. The HMOs were still required to cover basic benefits, but they could use their set of management tools to try to avoid paying for unnecessary care.[91]

The initial trials of the concept were considered a success, and, over the next decade, a number of states requested waivers to implement it. Today, it is used in all states for at least some Medicaid beneficiaries. In some of them, it is now the norm.[92] As of 2010, almost 70 percent of the nation's 60 million Medicaid beneficiaries were enrolled in some form of managed care.[93]

With its adoption by states throughout the country, Medicaid managed care came to generate considerable business for the companies that provided it. Existing HMOs developed plans that were geared specifically to Medicaid patients, and new HMOs emerged to focus exclusively on this market. As this line of business grew, Medicaid managed care developed into its own industry.[94] Many of the arrangements have become quite complex, with separate companies covering narrow areas of service, such as behavioral health and prescription drugs. These are commonly known as "carve-outs," and the companies that provide them constitute yet another distinct industry, one for which the government, as the sole customer, provides all of the financing.[95]

With positive initial results from the use of private managed care in Medicaid, the federal government looked to incorporate it into Medicare in the mid-1980s. This was an easier challenge bureaucratically because Medicare is administered directly by the federal government as a single program. Separate waivers for individual states were not needed.

The first trial of private managed care in the delivery of Medicare benefits was launched in 1985. Under the arrangement, beneficiaries paid premiums to an HMO in lieu of the premiums they would otherwise have paid for coverage under Part B of the program, which is optional and requires a monthly contribution.[96] The premiums paid to the HMO were supplemented with additional payments from the government. Beneficiaries were offered two main enticements to accept coverage through the plans instead of through traditional Medicare. One was lower co-payments and deductibles than would have applied under the program's conventional coverage structure. The other was coverage of products and services that were excluded from Medicare, most notably outpatient prescription drugs, which were not added as a standard benefit until 2006.[97] Of course, beneficiaries faced some new limitations when they chose to receive Medicare benefits from a private HMO in the restrictions that managed care imposes to limit unnecessary care. However, for many the trade-off was worth it.

In 1997, Congress restructured these managed care arrangements as part of a larger set of revisions to Medicare contained in the Balanced Budget Act passed that year.[98] The managed care alternative was recognized as a separate Part C of the program and given a new name, Medicare + Choice. The revisions also permitted a wider range of managed care organizations to offer coverage, including PPOs and health plans organized by providers, and it set new formulas for determining the payments they received.[99]

In 2003, Congress modified Part C as part of the Medicare Prescription Drug, Improvement and Modernization Act (MMA), the law that added the prescription drug benefit.[100] Under that revision, payments to private managed care plans were enhanced considerably under an altered funding structure. The new arrangement reduced the financial risk that plans faced of encountering large claims expenses in a single year and allocated substantial federal subsidies as additional support.[101] It also permitted an even larger array of private payment arrangements to participate, including some that imposed very few restrictions on receiving care. With these changes, the Act gave the reinvigorated Part C another new name, Medicare Advantage.[102]

HMO enrollment by Medicare beneficiaries grew steadily, fortified by this steady stream of enhancements. In 1990, it attracted just 1.3 million of them, representing 3.8 percent of the total Medicare population. By 1998, those numbers had risen to 6.9 million representing 18.3 percent. By 2008, five years after passage of the MMA, the number of enrollees stood at 8.8 million, representing 19.7 percent.[103]

THE MEDICARE PRESCRIPTION DRUG BENEFIT

The expansion of support for private managed care coverage options through Medicare Advantage was only one of the private sector enhancements the MMA added to the program. In the magnitude of its generosity, the other was even more significant. That was a new prescription drug benefit.

Before the MMA, Medicare provided no coverage for prescription drugs that were taken on an outpatient basis. The program covered drugs administered in a hospital as part of an inpatient stay under Part A. It also covered drugs administered by a physician in his or her office, primarily injected medications, such as those used in oncology, under Part B. However, there was no provision for reimbursement of drugs that a patient obtained from a retail pharmacy under a prescription. That situation changed with the MMA's creation of a new Part D of Medicare. It permits beneficiaries to obtain prescription drug coverage on a voluntary basis as an additional benefit. Although they must pay a separate premium for it, much of the cost is subsidized.

The structure of the drug benefit was the subject of considerable debate when the MMA was passed. Some in Congress believed it should be administered directly by the government, along the lines of Medicare Parts A and B. Others favored reliance on a system of private plans in an arrangement comparable to Part C. With a conservative president in office at the time, George W. Bush, and a Republican majority in Congress, the political environment favored a private market approach, and the Part C model won out.[104]

Medicare Part D is administered through competing private plans known as prescription drug plans (PDPs). They operate in a similar manner to private managed care plans under Medicare Advantage. Each offers a set of benefits based on a standard design embodied in the law. Benefits vary between plans in the range of drugs covered, known as formularies, and in the premiums that are charged. Some PDPs stand alone as providers of coverage exclusively for prescription drugs. Others are incorporated into Medicare Advantage plans, which are authorized to include coverage for both medical care and pharmaceutical products in their offerings. Beneficiaries pay a premium for the coverage, but the Medicare program pays about 75 percent. Subsidies to cover some or all of the premiums are available for those with low incomes.[105]

In both the stand-alone and broader forms, PDPs have grown into a sizeable business niche.[106] In 2006, their first year of operation, they received $48.1 billion in revenue. Premiums paid by beneficiaries accounted for $3.5 billion of that amount, and the government paid $44.6 billion. Total enrollment was 25.4 million.[107] In 2011, they collected $67 billion, of which beneficiaries paid $7.7 billion and the government $52.5 billion.[108] Enrollment in 2012 reached 31.5 million.[109]

IS PRIVATE COVERAGE BETTER?

The use of private insurance plans to administer Medicare under both Parts C and D remains highly controversial. Opponents point to the overhead costs of private insurers, which are higher than those of traditional Medicare.[110] The insurance industry operates with a rate in the range of 10 to 15 percent, and the traditional Medicare program boasts a rate of only 2 percent. Analyses indicate that benefits under Medicare Advantage plans cost about 11 percent more per beneficiary than traditional Medicare benefits to deliver.[111]

Critics also charge that private plans realize much of their profitability by selecting the healthiest Medicare beneficiaries as customers. Insurers often direct the marketing of Medicare products to those who are most active, with enticements such as health club memberships that only the healthiest are likely to use. As commercial insurers in the 1950s found a market niche in selling policies to companies with the healthiest employees, Medicare managed care companies, it is claimed, specialize in serving patients who are the least likely to need significant amounts of care. In doing so, they skim the most profitable beneficiaries from the rest of the market, leaving the government to serve the needs of those who are seriously ill.[112] Supporters of private plans counter that market competition leads them to be more innovative than government-run programs and that beneficiaries tend to be quite satisfied with the service they receive.

Although debates continue over the actual efficiency of private insurers in delivering Medicare benefits, one point is clear. Regardless of whether they are more or less efficient than traditional government-administered coverage, their incorporation into the program has granted them tremendous business opportunities. They prosper in a significant market created and financed almost entirely by the government. Because of them, insurance companies join physicians, hospitals, ancillary care providers, and a host of other businesses as beneficiaries of Medicare. The program may have been designed with the elderly foremost in mind, but its largess also extends throughout the private insurance sector.

PRIVATE INSURANCE AND THE FUTURE OF MEDICARE

Medicare is widely championed as a public policy success. Polls show that more than 90 percent of its beneficiaries are satisfied, the highest rating for any insurance plan in the United States.[113] Because of its popularity, it has become entrenched in the political, social, and economic fabric of the country, and, in numerous contexts discussed in other chapters, as a mainstay of the entire health care system.

However, debates rage about the program's future direction. Medicare faces daunting economic challenges in the years ahead. The number of beneficiaries will increase markedly as the large cohort of Americans born during the "baby boom" years of 1946 to1964 reach the age of eligibility. Increasing life expectancies means that they will receive benefits for longer periods of time than beneficiaries in the past. And underlying health care costs that drive Medicare spending continue to rise relentlessly at a pace that is certain to accelerate as technology advances.[114]

One proposal for addressing the looming cost pressures is to restructure the entire program along the lines of Part C. A blue-ribbon commission recommended this approach in 2000.[115] Under it, the government would no longer operate the program directly but would instead give beneficiaries vouchers to purchase coverage from a private insurance company. Market-oriented politicians in both major political parties have endorsed similar proposals at various times.[116] Others advocate a modified version of the concept in which an enhanced Part C would compete with traditional Medicare for beneficiaries.[117]

The voucher approach, also known as "premium support," has its share of critics.[118] They point to the high overhead rate for private insurers under existing managed care arrangements and question whether a system that assigns all Medicare beneficiaries to private plans could truly save money.[119] They see the traditional structure, in which the government directly administers benefits, as the most viable one going forward. However, their opposition has not muted calls to expand the private sector role in one form or another.

The future structure of Medicare will likely inspire political debate for years to come. It will remain a central concern of policymakers because the inflationary effects of demographic changes and advances in medicine will only grow in intensity over time. The idea of placing greater reliance on the private market as a response is certain to remain a central part of those debates. It brings with it the prospect that the program will create yet more opportunities, perhaps with even greater profit potential, for private insurance companies down the road.

Regardless of whether private insurers come to play a dominant role in delivering services, the private market is likely to maintain an important position in Medicare's structure. Throughout the program's history, private insurers have performed key functions, from serving as carriers and intermediaries to selling Medicare supplement policies to delivering benefits through managed care plans to covering prescription drugs as PDPs. By creating business opportunities such as these, Medicare has served as an important pillar of the financial success of the private health insurance industry. It is certain to continue to do so in one form or another in the years ahead.

Two Case Studies in the Rise of Private Health Insurance

Many private insurance companies have thrived on the regulatory platforms and financial generosity of both the federal and state governments. On the road to the emergence of an industry with more than $300 billion in annual revenue, individual corporate success stories abound. Two of them, one of a for-profit and one of a nonprofit company, poignantly illustrate the path to prosperity.

THE TRANSFORMATION OF AETNA

Aetna, Inc. has been part of the bedrock of the insurance industry since its founding in 1853. It began in Connecticut as the Aetna Life Insurance Company, an affiliate of an existing insurer, Aetna Insurance Company, which provided fire coverage. The older company needed a new entity for its new line of business, because a law in New York State, where it planned to sell policies, prohibited a single company from offering both kinds of insurance.

The older Aetna took its name from Mt. Etna, a volcano in Sicily, to emphasize reliability in responding to disasters, particularly those of fiery origin. For much of the next 140 years, the company lived up to its image. It grew and diversified to become one of the largest and most stable insurance companies in the United States.[120]

Over the years, Aetna expanded its business into several new lines of insurance. In 1891, it added accident insurance; in 1899, liability insurance; in 1912, the first comprehensive automobile coverage; in 1913, group life insurance; and, in 1919, group disability insurance. The company was also a pioneer in health coverage. In 1899, it first experimented with this line, although without the expectation that it would be a significant revenue source. The policies were limited to customers of its accident and life insurance business in an effort to boost sales. In 1902, it moved further into health care when it opened an accident and liability department to provide workers' compensation coverage.

Aetna has traditionally taken a cautious approach to financial investments, which helped to protect it from significant losses during the Great Depression. As a result, it was able to expand its offerings yet again during that time. In 1930, it moved into pensions. And, in 1936, it first provided a new kind of protection that had been pioneered on a nonprofit basis seven years earlier—insurance for group hospitalization.

Through the decades that followed, the company saw its fortunes fluctuate, although it continued to grow and diversify. During World War II, it helped to cover the construction of seven aircraft carriers, and, toward the end of the War, it helped to insure the Manhattan Project, the huge government effort to develop the atomic bomb. It also expanded its coverage for employee group benefits, including life and health insurance, during that time. These steps helped it to build this business after the war as the market for commercial health insurance expanded. Innovations continued in the decades that followed, with entry into the international market in the 1960s.

The First Moves into Managed Care

In 1973, Aetna took a first tentative step into another new product line. The business potential was uncertain, but the opportunities seemed large. In retrospect, it turned out to be a seminal move that eventually set the course for the company's future. It was the year that Congress passed the HMO Act, and Aetna formed a subsidiary to operate an HMO.

The 1980s were a difficult time for the company. Earnings declined by 23 percent in 1988 from the previous year and by another 5 percent in 1989. The greatest challenges were in the property and casualty lines of business, especially liability coverage, which is insurance against losses stemming from lawsuits. Aetna encountered large claims from suits involving harm from asbestos and other hazardous products, as well as litigation involving environmental pollution. Over the next several years, the company withdrew from a number of lines of liability coverage. It abandoned the personal automobile market in several states and curtailed its business in personal mortgage insurance.[121]

Although its property and casualty lines of insurance were showing losses, the opposite trend held for Aetna's growing HMO business. As that trend accelerated in early 1990s, the company began to reorient its focus to health care. It divested much of its non–health care business, selling its reinsurance line (coverage for large losses by other insurance companies) to American Re Corporation in 1992 and its entire property and casualty subsidiary to Travelers Group in 1996. It continued the divestment process in the years that followed, selling its personal life insurance business to Lincoln National Corporation in 1998 and, through a complicated set of transactions, its financial services operations to ING in 2000.

Piggybacking on One of the First HMOs—US Healthcare

The watershed year for Aetna's transformation into a health care–focused insurer was 1996. In April of that year, it announced the surprise acquisition of US Healthcare, Inc., a major HMO in the northeastern United States, for $8.9 billion. Overnight, the company became the country's largest managed care provider.[122] To cement its new identity, the name of the corporate parent of Aetna's operations was shortened from Aetna Life & Casualty to Aetna, Inc., to jettison the link to the company's former businesses, and the existing health care operations were merged with those of US Healthcare into a subsidiary that was renamed Aetna US Healthcare, Inc.

US Healthcare at the time was the poster child for success in the managed care industry. By 1996, it had acquired significant expertise in administering HMOs that Aetna lacked. It also had a track record of aggressively negotiating frugal contracts with physicians and hospitals.[123] The acquisition was, in effect, an admission on Aetna's part that if it wanted to enter the health care field in a serious way, it could no longer rely on the same indemnity model that it had worked with so proficiently for 150 years. It needed to gain a different kind of expertise to navigate the new world of health insurance.

The company Aetna acquired was the brainchild of Leonard Abramson, one of the first entrepreneurs to appreciate the business potential of the new market that government policy, in the form of the HMO Act, had created.[124] Abramson was a pharmacist by training. In the early 1970s, he left a position as a retail pharmacist to work for R. H. Medical, Inc., a hospital management company based in the suburbs of Philadelphia. There, he ran a secretive project to lay the groundwork for a plan to develop an HMO, based on the model laid out in the Act. Abramson quickly came to realize the concept's possibilities and the opportunities that federal grants and loans opened for new market entrants. He left R. H. Medical in 1975 to start his own HMO on a nonprofit basis, which he named HMO of Pennsylvania. The following year, the new company obtained a license from the Commonwealth of Pennsylvania to begin selling policies.[125]

Abramson's vision was to earn profits by cutting unnecessary medical expenses. To that end, his company employed aggressive strategies to encourage providers to economize. One technique was to financially penalize PCPs each time they referred a patient to a specialist.[126] Another was to emphasize prevention in the structure of coverage with free mammograms and other screening tests to catch diseases early, when they can be treated most efficiently.[127] The strategy of focusing on cost control paid off. Although US Healthcare perennially lagged behind its competitors in revenues, it consistently outpaced them in profits.[128]

However, an array of obstacles stood in the company's way. For one, it had very little money for start-up capital. For another, physicians and hospitals resisted participating, seeing little reason to accept the lower rates and oversight of care that HMOs imposed. Perhaps most importantly, the Philadelphia market, where US Healthcare began operations, was dominated at the time by Blue Cross, which worked tenaciously to hold onto its customers.[129]

However, HMO of Pennsylvania also had several important advantages in the market. Among the most significant was $3 million in loans from the federal government issued under the HMO Act. Abramson was also relentless in his commitment to the business and had a keen sense of marketing. And his company benefitted from its largest competitor's shortsightedness. Blue Cross dismissed the possibility that it could pose a serious threat and ignored the HMO market altogether at the time, believing that the concept would never catch on.[130]

US Healthcare's biggest advantage of all was a shift in the health insurance market that began in the early 1980s. During that time, many employers saw double-digit increases in their health insurance premiums. With an HMO structure in place, the company was able to offer them a product with significantly lower costs. HMO prices rose by about 13 percent annually in the late 1980s, compared to 20 percent for traditional indemnity insurance plans.[131] With this price differential, US Healthcare's customer base began to increase, and it was able to begin making inroads into Blue Cross's market share.

With a larger market share and a greater complement of members, many providers that had initially declined to participate began to reconsider. Growing numbers of them acceded to HMO of Pennsylvania's demands for lower reimbursement rates, especially when confronted with its hard-line negotiating style. The company continually sought out new opportunities and, in 1985, was one the first HMOs to test the waters of the new market for coverage under Medicare.[132]

In the run-up to this growth spurt, the company had taken a series of steps to convert itself into a for-profit enterprise. In 1981, with the end of start-up support from the federal government, it formally abandoned its nonprofit status, and, in 1983, it went public, raising $34 million in two stock offerings.[133] It also expanded its geographic scope beyond its original base in the Philadelphia area to include New York and much of the northeast. In 1982, in recognition of its broader geographic market, it changed its name from HMO of Pennsylvania to United States Healthcare Systems, Inc. and was popularly known as US Healthcare from then on.[134]

Once it was on a for-profit footing, the company's growth was explosive. Between 1982 and 1986, it averaged 85 percent a year.[135] Between 1985 and 1986 alone, earnings jumped 127 percent to $24.5 million.[136] Between 1989 and 1992, US Healthcare's membership grew by almost 50 percent to 1.33 million, and between 1991 and 1992, its profits increased by 95 percent.[137] Between September 1991 and March 1992, its share price more than doubled from $21 to just under $56. By 1996, when it was acquired by Aetna, the company was anything but nonprofit, generating more than $3 billion in revenue a year.[138]

When he negotiated the sale of US Healthcare, Abramson owned 1.3 percent of the company's stock. After the deal, he owned 2.5 percent of Aetna's stock. Its value turned him into one of the richest men in America almost overnight.[139]

In acquiring US Healthcare, Aetna gained a business that had grown and flourished because of the drive and vision of an inventive entrepreneur. Leonard Abramson saw the potential of HMOs before most others in the health insurance industry. However, that early vision was not of a business opportunity that arose from a natural evolution of market forces. It was of an opening that, like much of the rest of the health insurance industry, was crafted and nurtured by deliberate federal policy.

Aetna Redefined as a Managed Care Company

With the US Healthcare deal behind it, a refocused Aetna continued to expand its HMO operations through additional acquisitions. In 1998, it bought the health care business of New York Life Insurance Company for $1 billion.[140] That move added 2.5 million members to the 13.7 million it had at the time and gave the company a larger HMO presence in several important markets around the country, including Illinois, Maine, New Jersey, New York, and Washington. In 1999, Aetna paid another $1 billion for the health care operations of Prudential Insurance Company of America. That deal caused membership in Aetna's health plans to grow from 16 million to 22 million and its dental insurance business to almost double in size to 15 million.[141]

Aetna's move to a predominant focus on health care, and on managed care in particular, faced rough sledding at first. It had inherited from US Healthcare an aggressive bargaining style with physicians and a stingy approach to approving benefits for patients, both of which it continued. This engendered considerable animosity from both groups. Moreover, soon after the acquisition, Aetna discovered that it had purchased US Healthcare at the peak of the market, and it tried to squeeze physicians and patients even further to make up for its poor judgment. A series of class action lawsuits ensued. Other challenges arose from logistical difficulties in integrating US Healthcare's operations and from heavy losses for the business the company had acquired from Prudential.

Aetna's financial fortunes changed in the early 2000s, with a renewed commitment to its new health care identity. In 2000, it brought on a new senior executive team with a different approach. Among its first steps was to repair relations with physicians and patients by loosening many of its restrictive payment and coverage policies, speeding up payments, and reducing its bureaucracy. In 2003, it settled its share of a large class action lawsuit that had been brought against all of the country's managed care providers. It also expanded its offering of alternative managed care arrangements such as PPOs and POS plans.[142] By emphasizing plans that did less to constrain patient choice, Aetna hoped to burnish its image further as a customer-friendly company. These arrangements came to represent more than half of Aetna's portfolio of product offerings.[143]

The company also dropped some unprofitable markets and unprofitable products. Its customer base shrank as a result, from 19 million to 13 million, bumping it from its position as the nation's largest managed care company and reducing its revenues. However, its profits improved, as did its share price.

Despite the diminution in size during the early 2000s, Aetna today is one of the largest health insurance companies in the United States. It provides coverage for more than 18 million members through contracts with 597,000 physicians and 5,400 hospitals.[144] A total of 35,000 people earn their livelihoods as Aetna employees, and the company generates annual revenues of $35.54 billion.[145]

Aetna and Government Policy

Without question, Aetna would look quite different today had the government not molded the health insurance market the way it did over the past 75 years. Health care coverage would be more expensive for most beneficiaries without the tax subsidy for employment-based policies, which would mean fewer customers and a smaller revenue base. Without the tilt toward employment coverage fostered by government policies, the company would almost certainly have placed greater emphasis on selling individual rather than employer products. More importantly, had the government not created and nurtured the managed care market, it is highly unlikely that Aetna would have delved into this line of business at the expense of its 150 years of experience selling traditional indemnity coverage.

Aetna's series of strategic moves since the mid-1990s, like most corporate actions in the health care industry over the past half-century, were driven by a business environment shaped largely by the government. A business model constructed by federal policy today defines the company's very identity. This large and successful player in the lucrative health insurance market did not emerge in its present form by responding independently to changes in market demand. It did so as a collaborator in an elaborate public–private partnership.

KAISER PERMANENTE

Kaiser Permanente is the largest nonprofit HMO in the United States and the third largest overall behind UnitedHealth Group and Wellpoint.[146] It serves more than 9 million members nationally, although more than two-thirds are located in its home state of California. The company owns 36 hospitals, employs 533 physicians who practice in 15,853 offices, and employs more than 167,000 people overall. In 2010, its operating revenue exceeded $44 billion.[147]

The company dates its founding to 1945 and attributes its genesis to the challenge of providing health insurance during the Great Depression and World War II.[148] It was an innovator from the start. Kaiser was the first insurance plan to offer prepaid care on a large scale, the first to cultivate physician group practice, and the first to build an organized integrated delivery system.[149]

The groundwork for Kaiser Permanente's business model predated its emergence in 1945 as an insurer for the general public. It was born of necessity, with a gestation in the late 1930s and early 1940s as an innovation by a group of companies owned by Henry J. Kaiser that needed an efficient way to treat the illnesses and injuries of their workers. These companies engaged in heavy manufacturing activities—large-scale construction, shipbuilding, and steel mills—that were rife with the potential for worker injuries.

The Genesis of the Kaiser Model

The concept of prepaid care that Kaiser built on originated with the work of a young surgeon named Sidney Garfield, in the 1930s.[150] Dr. Garfield was an entrepreneur who sought ways to improve the delivery of health care. To apply new approaches, he built a small hospital near Los Angeles that was dedicated to treating the thousands of workers employed in constructing the city's aqueduct. It was a 12-bed facility located six miles from the city in the town of Desert Center. However, the project encountered financial difficulties from the start. Many of the workers it treated lacked insurance and had no other means of payment for the services they received. Even when patients did have coverage, insurance companies were often slow to pay. It was not long before expenses were far outstripping revenue.[151]

An acquaintance of Dr. Garfield, an engineer turned insurance agent named Harold Hatch, offered a solution. He suggested that, in lieu of payment for each service rendered, the hospital accept a fixed amount per day for each covered worker that would be paid in advance. The primary purpose of this approach was to guarantee a steady flow of funds, but it also had the effect of changing the financial paradigm under which the hospital operated. The facility would now have an incentive to promote worker health and safety to reduce the risk of having to treat maladies after they occurred. Dr. Garfield adopted Hatch's idea, setting the payment at five cents per day. For an additional nickel, workers could also receive coverage for nonoccupational medical needs.

The plan worked and, before long, the hospital had become a financial success. However, the implications of the turnaround extended more broadly than the fortunes of a small rural medical facility. Without realizing it, the two men had created the model for a new form of general health insurance coverage—prepaid health care.

News of Dr. Garfield's success soon spread. As the Los Angeles aqueduct project neared completion, he was sought out by another construction firm, this time to provide health care for 6,500 workers employed in building the Grand Coulee Dam, along with their families. It was the largest construction project in American history up to that point. He approached the assignment by turning an existing marginal hospital into a modern facility and hiring a complement of physicians to form a group practice to render services in association with it. The plan worked, and Dr. Garfield was able to replicate his initial financial success. What is more, the covered workers and family members reported high levels of satisfaction with the arrangement.[152]

Kaiser's Growth During World War II

With two successes behind him, Dr. Garfield's accomplishments began to receive wider notice. In 1941, he was recruited to apply his approach on the largest scale yet. Kaiser Shipyards in Richmond, California had been commissioned by the US Navy to build warships as the country entered World War II. It was assembling a workforce of 30,000 for the task. Its president, Henry Kaiser, asked Dr. Garfield to take responsibility for the health care needs of this huge contingent of employees by applying the prepaid model he had pioneered.[153]

Kaiser found that availing himself of Dr. Garfield's services was not easy. He had to request a special accommodation from President Franklin Roosevelt to release the physician from active military duty. The request emphasized the unique nature of Dr. Garfield's expertise and the large potential value of his services. Such appeals were granted sparingly, but this one proved persuasive, and Roosevelt acquiesced. With Dr. Garfield at the helm of the initiative, Kaiser's company was about to take the concept of the prepaid health plan to a new level.[154]

Once again, Dr. Garfield's approach was a success. At its peak during the war, Kaiser Shipyards employed 90,000 workers who, along with their families, were all covered by his plan. All told, the size of the covered population reached 200,000.[155] To provide physician services in conjunction with hospital care, the company set up two separate foundations in 1942, one for the Pacific Northwest and one for California, under the name Permanente.[156] These entities retained a complement of 75 physicians. The cost to employees for coverage was $25 a year.[157]

A New Business Model and National Prominence After the War

After the war ended, the Kaiser shipyard operations shrank rapidly. The number of employees fell within a few months to 13,000, and only 12 members of the physician corps remained. However, recognizing that the health plan had served its purpose well, both Henry Kaiser and Dr. Garfield sought to keep it in operation. In late 1945, they restructured it and opened membership to the public beyond the Kaiser workforce under the name Permanente Health Plan. Over the course of the next 10 years, it grew to 300,000 members, mostly in northern California. Much of Kaiser's growth stemmed from the support of large unions, which also encouraged the plan's geographical expansion to the Los Angeles area. Union health plans had risen in popularity after the war and benefitted from the same favorable tax treatment that employer-based health insurance enjoyed.[158]

Kaiser's model of prepaid care rendered by closed panels of physicians also engendered fierce opposition from many in the medical profession. In particular, the American Medical Association (AMA) tried vigorously to halt its spread. The AMA was then, and still is, a powerful force in American health care, and it had the ability to create significant impediments. However, its effort to do so in this case was derailed by a series of lawsuits alleging that its opposition constituted an illegal attempt to stifle competition with traditional physician practices.[159]

In 1952, the plan and its hospitals took the name Kaiser, which was more recognizable to the public. The medical group, which was structured as an independent entity, kept the Permanente name. The result is an organization that functions as a collaboration between two partners and operates under the name "Kaiser Permanente." Its success eventually attracted the interest of policymakers across the country, including Paul Ellwood, who modeled his concept of HMOs on it. Kaiser's paradigm thereby came to serve as the basis for the federal HMO Act and, consequently, for the entire HMO industry.[160]

With its new identity and substantial presence in California, Kaiser set its sights further east.[161] Its growth was especially rapid during the 1970s, after passage of the HMO Act. In 1976, its membership surpassed 3 million. In 1977, it obtained federally qualified status under the Act, enabling it to more aggressively pursue a larger market share. In 1980, it expanded into the mid-Atlantic region, opening plans in Maryland, Virginia, and the District of Columbia.[162] In 1985, it expanded again, this time to Georgia. Through the 1980s and 1990s, it entered into a series of partnerships both with other prepaid plans, including Group Health Cooperative of Puget Sound, and with employers, including state governments. A venture launched in 1997 with the AFL-CIO marked the first formal collaboration between a prepaid plan and organized labor.[163]

Kaiser has had its share of ups and downs since then. Some ventures into new terrain did not succeed, and the company has had to retrench several times. In 1997, it sustained its first negative financial returns, losing $266 million. However, it was able to return to the black four years later after a series of rate increases.[164] Despite these setbacks during a period of market volatility for managed care during the 1990s, over the long-term, its financial position has remained relatively stable. Kaiser remains the dominant HMO in its home state of California and a significant force nationally.

Kaiser and American Health Care

Kaiser's story embodies the history of managed care in the United States. It did not represent the first attempt to create a prepaid plan. Smaller ones had been launched decades earlier. Neither was it the only plan to emerge during the 1940s.[165] Health Insurance Plan in New York and Group Health Cooperative of Puget Sound began operating at about the same time. However, it was the first plan to apply the model of prepaid health care coverage across a broad geographic region and the first to offer it nationally.

Kaiser's success demonstrated how health care could be delivered more efficiently by changing the structure of financial incentives. It served as the model for federal policy that promoted the growth of HMOs nationwide and then benefitted itself from those policies. It is also distinctive for retaining its nonprofit status while most of the rest of the managed care industry joined the world of for-profit corporate enterprise. Its survival in nonprofit form serves as proof that health care finance can function under more than one economic paradigm.

As with the other corporate success stories in American health care, Kaiser did not achieve its success alone. It benefitted from the same set of federal initiatives that nurtured the rest of the managed care industry. The policy of allowing employers to add worker health benefits without violating the World War II wage freeze provided its first big boost. It established the legal grounding that permitted Kaiser shipyards to contribute financial support for the coverage of employees and their families at a time when an outright increase in wages was prohibited. Federal tax policy after the war provided a second boost by exempting health benefits from income tax. That rule enabled Kaiser to expand as an independent operation after the war by offering employment-based coverage to other employers and to unions. The HMO Act contributed a third boost by providing direct financial support for expansion, which enabled Kaiser to pursue its national strategy. Finally, the federal Medicare program contributed significant amounts of revenue by serving as a customer when it let beneficiaries choose coverage through private plans such as Kaiser's while picking up the lion's share of the premiums.

Kaiser's story shows what can come of ingenuity and innovation with the right kind of outside support. Sidney Garfield and Harold Hatch tried out an idea in the 1930s for financing health care in an unconventional way, and it ended up transforming American health care finance. Kaiser Industries liked the idea and provided the backing to bring it to fruition. However, it was the support of an additional partner that turned it into a national economic force. Kaiser became a dominant player in managed care by taking advantage of a foundation that was laid by the government.

The Government and Private Health Insurance

With this background on the growth and development of private health insurance, we can ask, as we have for other key sectors, what this aspect of American health care would look like in the absence of government support. However, the answer for health insurance is somewhat different than it is for the components of health care's provider side. Those sectors had all existed for thousands of years before the American government intervened in the health care system. Health insurance, in contrast, is a relatively recent phenomenon. It came into being less than a century ago. Without government support, it might not even exist as a distinct industry. If it did, it would bear little resemblance to the financial powerhouse we know today.

Most importantly, it is unlikely that the link between health insurance and employment would be as close as it is had the federal government not forged it during World War II and sustained it with a huge tax subsidy afterward. As the employment basis of health insurance gained favor in the wake of these federal policies, individual coverage received short shrift. Today, the health insurance bond with employment is entrenched in the fabric of the health care system.

Had the industry developed along the lines of other kinds of insurance coverage, the market for policies that individuals purchase and maintain as they move from job to job would likely be more robust. Those who are unemployed or work for a firm that does not offer coverage would not have needed the assistance of the ACA to obtain coverage on their own. Even with this help, individual policies are still less desirable than employer-sponsored coverage. Employment benefits enjoy favored tax treatment, and a company usually pays part of the cost.

As discussed in Chapter 8, the ACA creates a major new market for insurance companies. It brings them an estimated 12 million additional customers for coverage. What is more, those new customers who have low incomes receive subsidies from the federal government to help them purchase policies. Those who decline to obtain insurance in any form are subject to a financial penalty, a provision that guarantees that this new market will perpetually remain strong. Few, if any, other industries enjoy government assistance on a comparable scale in creating and maintaining their customer base. The result is an influx of additional premium revenue that is predicted to reach $55 billion a year.[166]

Another effect of the tax subsidy is that it lets insurers charge higher rates than they would otherwise be able to. Without it, premiums would have to be lower to attract the same customer base, leaving insurance companies with fewer financial resources for paying claims. One result would be lower reimbursement levels for providers. That would result in less money entering the health care system, which would mean lower earnings for physicians and other practitioners and smaller revenues for hospitals and pharmaceutical firms. That, in turn, would leave fewer resources in the hands of providers and product manufacturers to support innovation and technological advance.

Were health insurance not based on coverage for employer groups, the industry's pricing structure also would be quite different. Insurers would find it difficult to apply experience rating because their customers would not fall into natural risk pools. As a result, community rating, in which costs are spread among all covered individuals in a region, would likely dominate. This would lead to higher rates for those who are healthy and lower rates for those who are ill.

Without the ability to use experience rating and to sell their products through employers, commercial insurers that today compete by selecting the healthiest employer groups might never have found the insurance market attractive. That would have left health insurance predominantly in the hands of nonprofits such as Blue Cross and Blue Shield, and, without the pressure of commercial competitors, these companies might never have found the motivation or resources to develop their operations into regional or national enterprises. Health insurance could have remained a small-scale nonprofit industry into the latter part of the twentieth century or even beyond.

Moreover, the structure of coverage would look quite different. Managed care would likely play a minor role, if it played any role at all. The HMO Act jump-started this alternative form of finance and launched it as an industry in its own right. Whatever shape the private health insurance market would have taken in the absence of that law, the underlying business model would look nothing like that of the corporate financial giants that dominate private health care finance today. Several huge publicly traded companies that earn billions of dollars a year in revenue by providing managed care coverage would not exist. Others, like Aetna, would operate in very different forms. Managed care, if it survived at all, would have remained confined to nonprofit prepaid plans that function on a local or regional basis.

Perhaps such outcomes would have been preferable. Critics charge that a financing system composed of large private payers generates excess costs and inefficiency. They point to expenses for advertising, sales, and claims review as unnecessary expenditures that burden the system. Smaller regional companies operating on a nonprofit basis might spend less in these regards. The profits that private companies earn, as well as the high salaries of some executives, similarly impose costs unrelated to the actual provision of care. They represent large sums that leak out of the health care system and help to make it the most expensive in the world.

Others question whether a system based on employer sponsorship of coverage is desirable. The burden of administering health benefits weighs heavily on the companies that provide them. Another line of criticism concerns the oversight of medical services through managed care, which is often characterized as cumbersome and ineffective. It adds bureaucratic layers that may cost as much as any savings they achieve. And the political prowess of the industry in shaping government health care initiatives, such as the ACA, is a cause of widespread dismay.

Had the government not intervened to shape American health care finance as it did, the system might have followed a dramatically different course. The rising cost of health care might have led it to create a single public payment mechanism, in essence a Medicare program for all. Advocates of such an approach feel it would be more efficient and leave fewer people without coverage.

Nevertheless, regardless of whether it is as efficient as it could be, the health insurance industry fulfills the coverage needs of a large number of Americans. It has been a significant force in expanding access to the services of hospitals, physicians, and many other providers and in enabling them to grow and prosper. Moreover, it has pioneered numerous innovations in health care finance and continues to play a key role in fostering the system's evolution. America's system of private health care finance might have been crafted more wisely, but it still represents a powerful force that lends financial support to much of the country's health care enterprise.

Hundreds of billions of dollars trade hands through the system of private health insurance every year. Businesses rise and fall, investors gain and lose fortunes, and the health care system responds to the financial incentives that the industry creates. Had health insurance not emerged in its present form, large sums of money would still move through American health care. However, without federal support, there would be less of it, and it would be distributed in very different ways. And most Americans would encounter a vastly different financial apparatus when they access care.

7

The Distinctively American System that the Government Created

> The significant difference in real health care spending per capita between the United States and other wealthy nations is consumed largely by monopoly profits generated by providers—and quasi-providers such as consultants.
>
> —BRUCE V. VLADECK AND THOMAS RICE, *HEALTH AFFAIRS*[1]

For the past hundred years, the federal government has been hard at work creating the American health care system. Some of its efforts have been deliberate, like establishing the National Institutes of Health (NIH) to support basic research that pharmaceutical companies use to develop new drugs. Others have been inadvertent, like exempting employment-based health insurance premiums from income tax, which tilted the coverage system toward job-based policies. However, regardless of the planning and design reflected in each, a vast web of laws, regulations, and funding programs stands behind every aspect of American health care.

The government today funds more than half the cost of health care in the United States.[2] Its contribution totals close to $1.5 trillion a year in a $2.5 trillion industry.[3] Every sector of the industry reaps the benefits of this largess, along with every participant in the system, from providers to payers to patients.

Yet despite the huge regulatory infrastructure and financial contribution, the government's foundational role in American health care remains obscure to many. The policies and programs that created and sustain the medical goods and services that Americans receive are largely invisible to those outside the industry. Instead of seeing the seminal force in establishing and nurturing the health care system, many people perceive an external intruder that stands in its way.

The government's central role in American health care is concealed from view because it stands largely hidden behind the vast private sector it supports. The health care that most Americans receive is provided not by the massive government infrastructure but by private entities. Investor-owned pharmaceutical companies sell medications. Private hospitals, both nonprofit and for-profit, provide facilities for inpatient care. Physicians in private practice render professional services. Private insurance companies serve as the primary conduits for the system's finance. And countless other private entities render an array of services and sell an endless assortment of products.

A typical encounter with the health care system puts an American patient in contact with this private domain. Even when the government's role is more visible, as when Medicare pays the bill for an elderly beneficiary, the role of private providers is the one that is most directly apparent. For those receiving care, and even for many who provide it, the government's presence remains opaque.

However, the huge private sector that is so visible in the health care system did not arise on its own. The private entities that constitute this huge swath of the American economy, many of them giant corporations, did not grow out of the interplay of conventional market forces and consumer demand. They were, and continue to be, shaped, funded, and often invented by government policy.

The intertwined relationship of the government and the private sectors in the functioning of American health care is unique. The private role is larger than in any other developed country, both when measured as a percentage of overall system expenditures and in absolute terms.[4] Yet the private role has not grown at the expense of the public one. Health care is not a zero-sum game in which the expansion of one sector necessarily crowds out the other. The size of the public role in American health care is also among the largest in the world. The amount the government spends per capita on health care in the United States exceeds that in most other developed countries.[5]

In health care's public–private partnership, the contributions of both sides have grown in tandem. New government programs perennially mean greater, not fewer, opportunities for the private side. The system keeps expanding and making more room for both. It has given America the largest and most expensive health care sector on Earth.[6] In good economic times and bad, it just keeps growing.

The Government and the Pillars of Market-Based Health Care

The previous chapters have shown how a public–private interplay created and sustains four key sectors of American health care. In each of them, a market-based system in which private entities compete with one another in the pursuit of revenues and profits thrives. Some even point to these systems as examples of the "free market." However, if the term is meant to signify markets that arise of their own accord, independent of government actions, then, in reality, American health care is anything but. It is rather a market-based system formed in the same manner as many other major components of the economy—as an outgrowth of government policy.

To distill the highlights of the story, the pharmaceutical industry thrives as one of the most profitable in the United States.[7] That is a very different position than the one it held before the start of the twentieth century, when unproven potions and home remedies were sold alongside effective medications.[8] Congress altered that set of affairs with a series drug safety laws, the first enacted in 1906, that enforced regulatory oversight through the Food and Drug Administration (FDA), thereby building public confidence in pharmaceutical products. Starting in the middle of the twentieth century, it underwrote the foundation of a stunning era of industry innovation through the NIH, which spends $30 billion a year on biomedical research, the intellectual fuel for pharmaceutical progress.[9] Pharmaceuticals have been part of health care for thousands of years, and companies that manufacture them have existed for hundreds. However, it took an intricate web of regulatory oversight and significant government funding to turn the pharmaceutical industry into the pillar of market-based health care that it has become.

America's 5,000 hospitals continue to serve as the institutional hubs of the health care system, even in the face of significant changes in medicine.[10] Their modernization into marvels of high technology began just after World War II, when the federal government injected billions of dollars into the construction and renovation of facilities under the Hill-Burton Act.[11] In the mid-1960s, an even larger government initiative reinforced and expanded the industry's financial foundation in the form of Medicare, which provides the single largest source of reimbursement for most facilities. Hospitals have existed for hundreds of years in various parts of the world and for more than 250 years in the United States. However, before the government entered the financial picture, the industry was comprised primarily of stand-alone facilities, many of which were of limited size and capabilities. Today, thanks to a half-century of government support, hospitals serve not only as centers of advanced care but also as engines of economic growth and employment for cities and towns across the country.

Medicine is today one of the most respected and lucrative professions, but it was not always that way. The profession initiated its own change in fortune through the actions the American Medical Association, which brought consistency and accountability to medical training during the late nineteenth and early twentieth century and worked in partnership with state governments to implement licensing programs that enforce quality standards. The trajectory of medicine's rise took a major leap in the mid-twentieth century with the launch of government programs that expanded the profession's size, thereby enhancing its influence. More importantly, starting at about the same time, Medicare injected billions of dollars into reimbursement for physician services as it did for hospital care, significantly increasing the earning potential of practitioners, especially those in specialties that treat large numbers of elderly patients with technologically complex procedures.

Physicians have treated patients for millennia.[12] However, for most of that time, they lacked the earning potential and social standing they enjoy in the United States today. Hundreds of billions of dollars of government support built medicine into a paradigm of professional stature.

With advances in pharmaceuticals, hospital care, and physician capabilities, modern health care has become too expensive to function without sophisticated financing. Most Americans receive insurance to cover the cost from one of hundreds of private insurance plans, most operated by large national companies. Government support nurtured the growth of these financial giants from the start, with special regulatory treatment granted by states for the first Blue Cross and Blue Shield plans in the 1930s.[13] The federal government established these and similar plans as a mainstay of American health care with a combination of policy decisions during the 1940s. One of them let employers offer health benefits during World War II despite a freeze on underlying wages, and the other exempted the premiums that employers paid on behalf of workers from income tax, creating a huge indirect subsidy for its purchase.[14] When Medicare and Medicaid were enacted in the mid-1960s, opportunities for private insurers grew even further with the chance to offer special policies to supplement Medicare coverage, to administer Medicare benefits on behalf of the government, and to offer private plans to beneficiaries under both programs. The government placed a further stamp on the structure of health insurance in 1973 through the Health Maintenance Organization Act, which jump-started the market for managed care.[15] Over time, this form of payment fundamentally transformed relationships among patients, providers, and payers.

The health insurance industry today is highly profitable, but, as with other key sectors of American health care, it did not get that way entirely on its own.[16] The hand of government provided essential support. To be sure, had the government not intervened, an alternative system of funding would undoubtedly have developed as technology pushed health care costs ever higher. However, that system would almost certainly bear little resemblance to the distinctive structure of private finance that patients, providers, and investors know today.

The Health Care Industry Without the Government

We know what the American health care industry looks like today, and we know the nature of the government initiatives that have served to fund and shape it. However, demonstrating the role of public policy in creating today's private health care system begs the question of what it would have looked like had it been left on its own. Of course, we can never know for sure, but reasoned conjectures are possible.

Let us, for a moment, entertain an alternative hypothesis. Perhaps the parallel rise of market-based health care and government initiatives was a coincidence. Maybe government programs did not facilitate the expansion of the private health care but merely overlapped with them in time. Possibly, they even impeded the burst of private health care enterprise over the course of the late twentieth century. Was the government really necessary to the creation of American "free-market" health care as a robust enterprise? Could the explosive growth of private health care in America have been even more extensive had the government not intervened?

MIGHT THE GOVERNMENT ACTUALLY BE A DRAG ON PRIVATE HEALTH CARE?

Critics of regulation assert that government involvement in health care has actually been a drag that has prevented the system from reaching its full potential.[17] They see an industry that would be more, not less robust if left entirely in private hands. It would be freed from a heavy hand that imposes costs and delays on innovative activities, thereby dampening the entrepreneurial spirit.

An initial observation in support of this perspective is an obvious one. Not all government health care programs have supported private sector growth. Quite to the contrary, many have, in fact, stood in the way. Previous chapters have focused on public policies that have promoted the expansion of private markets.

Unquestionably, they have injected large amounts of money into the system and cleared many logistical hurdles out of the way. However, some aspects of these and other programs have just as clearly had the opposite effect. These are the elements of government intervention to which critics of the regulatory process often point.

Examples abound of regulatory labyrinths that can hold back the health care market. One that is frequently cited is the set of rules governing the exchange of patient medical information under the Health Insurance Portability and Accountability Act, commonly known as HIPAA.[18] The laudable goal of the law is to protect patient privacy. However, it is effectuated through a web of complex regulations that can make routine exchanges of patient data cumbersome and impede promising avenues of research.

Another is the bureaucracy that surrounds the Medicare and Medicaid reimbursement process. Providers often face burdensome paperwork demands and delays in receiving payments, particularly under state Medicaid programs. They must also abide by voluminous sets of rules to qualify for participation. Violations of even minor regulations can sometimes result in criminal charges of fraud. And even after navigating the system, the payments they receive are often quite low, in some cases less than the cost of providing care.

NIH funding for research comes with numerous strings attached. Moreover, its budget priorities sometimes respond more to political considerations than to scientific merit. Congress has at times allocated funding to investigations into specific diseases in response to the demands of articulate interest groups rather than to the conclusions of informed scientific judgments. Once funding is obtained, investigators must comply with various sets of complex rules. Some address accounting procedures for grants. Others seek to protect human subjects by requiring that investigators receive approval for their research from regulatory bodies within their home institutions known as Institutional Review Boards (IRBs). The approval process can be time-consuming, and over vigilant IRBs may impede valuable investigations.

Critics of regulation also point to the liability system as imposing significant costs.[19] Physicians, hospitals, and other providers face the prospect of costly malpractice claims when patients are harmed or treatments fail to produce desired results. Even frivolous lawsuits can impose substantial burdens to defend. Many physicians contend that they order excessive amounts of diagnostic testing to protect against potential claims, a practice known as "defensive medicine." Although most of the costs for legal defense and plaintiff compensation are covered by insurance, the amounts expended nevertheless increase the nation's overall health care bill.

Without question, much government regulation is inefficient. Regulatory mechanisms add costs and delays to whatever they are overseeing. The line between appropriate and excessive costs can be difficult to draw. However, the same is true for all administrative processes. Professional self-regulation, such as the accreditation process for hospitals administered by the Joint Commission, or the specialty certification process for physicians administered by medical societies, imposes costs and inefficiencies that are comparable to those imposed by the government. Internal quality controls used by manufacturing firms in other industries are no different. Assuring quality is seldom cost-free.

The question is not whether regulatory oversight imposes costs and inefficiencies but whether they outweigh its benefits. Harms such as patient injuries, ineffective care, and substandard treatment engender considerable inefficiency, usually dwarfing that of the mechanisms designed to avert them. It does not matter whether the mechanism is administered publicly or privately; the calculus of costs and benefits is the same. Regulatory costs are often necessary and are not unique to government programs.

The presence of inefficiencies may be reason to improve the manner of regulation, but it is not an indication that regulation is fundamentally counterproductive. Whatever flaws lie in the drug vetting process of the FDA, pharmaceutical firms would have difficulty instilling confidence in their products without it. Frequent tales of dangerous drugs reaching patients, like elixir of sulfanilamide and thalidomide, would significantly dampen the enthusiasm of physicians and patients for trying new products. Medicare and Medicaid might be more effective if they streamlined their reimbursement rules and raised their payment rates, but the programs in their present form still serve as financial mainstays for many physicians and for most hospitals. NIH funding might produce an even greater array of scientific breakthroughs if the oversight of studies were less burdensome, but its support is nevertheless responsible for countless discoveries, including the basic biomedical knowledge that lies behind most prescription drugs on the market today.

There are few who contend that the liability system is efficient. By some estimates, less than half of the amount spent on malpractice litigation actually reaches injured plaintiffs.[20] Most of the rest goes to overhead expenses and attorneys' fees. Certainly, it contains ample room for improvement. Reforms could make it more efficient and more effective at compensating those who are injured through the fault of others. However, it is not an example of regulatory overreach. It evolved not from a specific set of policy decisions but from a web of case law stretching back centuries. The liability system did not create the regulatory programs that built American health care but rather responds to them.

Combining estimates of the net costs of these and other examples of regulatory inefficiency, one strident critic of the regulatory process, the libertarian Cato Institute, has asserted that it imposes a net burden of $169 billion on American health care.[21] This estimate is questionable on several counts, but even if one were to accept it, the costs it purports to measure are not imposed in a vacuum.[22] The amount the government injects into the system each year through reimbursement, research funding, and other programs totals more than $1 trillion. Even under this draconian projection, the net gain to the health care market from government initiatives is still overwhelming.

COULD THE PRIVATE MARKET HAVE DONE IT ALONE?

Nevertheless, it is one thing to argue that government intervention has not impeded private health care. It is another to contend that the government actually fostered the market's growth. Perhaps the private health care sector could have reached its present size and vitality on its own. Regulatory and funding incentives might have been superfluous.

It is impossible to prove what would have happened had American health care policy over the course of the twentieth century been different. However, we can ask whether the industry could have obtained the resources that were essential for its growth from alternative sources. For the four segments examined in previous chapters, we can ask where such sources might have been found.

Could a private entity assure the safety of prescription drugs as the government does? If such an entity took the form of an industry-sponsored organization, it would be inherently suspect. Were it to function as an independent consumer organization, it would have difficulty obtaining sufficient funds to do the job. The FDA spends billions of dollars a year on its mission.[23] It is difficult to imagine that anyone but the government could have the resources and impartiality needed to instill public confidence in the drug supply.

Could a nongovernmental body have lent support for basic science research on a scale comparable to the NIH? Many nonprofit foundations today fund biomedical investigations.[24] Might they have stepped up their role had the NIH not been created or had it not grown to its present size? Such a turn of events seems highly unlikely. The support supplied by all nonprofit medical research foundations combined is a fraction of the $30 billion that the NIH spends.[25] No private organization could afford such largess. Even the Bill and Melinda Gates Foundation, the largest private funder of health-related research in the world, allocates far less than this amount to investigations, about $2.47 million a year.[26] Moreover, no privately owned pharmaceutical firm could risk the same level of investment in the speculative process of generating basic scientific knowledge. In other words, there is no obvious candidate that could have filled the gap had the government not provided this assistance.

Could a private finance mechanism cover the health care needs of the elderly, disabled, and poor as do Medicare and Medicaid? These are the groups most difficult for private insurers to cover because they are the most likely to become ill and incur medical expenses. From the industry's perspective, insuring them would be akin to providing fire insurance for a burning house. It would be almost impossible to set an affordable premium.

The government is the only entity with both an interest in the nation's overall well-being and the resources needed to address that interest. If a segment of the market for insurance is unprofitable, the government will not exit to move on to greener financial pastures. It would be difficult to imagine a private insurance system evolving on its own that would be continually available to everyone, even those in a state of perennial need.

Having established a reimbursement system for those most likely to become ill, the government also created the financial base for the practices of many physicians and the operation of most hospitals. Providers could expect patients to pay them out of their own pockets a century ago when medical care was much simpler and less technologically sophisticated. Today, when advanced health care can cost more than most people's annual incomes, insurance provides the only means with which most can afford medical services. If Medicare and Medicaid were abolished, the number of insured Americans would drop precipitously and with it the customer base of most providers. The opportunities that these providers enjoy to generate revenues would then decrease dramatically.

Moreover, it is unlikely that private insurance companies could have achieved their present size and profitability without the support of a huge tax subsidy. Perhaps the insurance market would function more effectively without this support, but, undeniably, it would be different. The tax subsidy for employment-based insurance increased the affordability of coverage for millions and molded the present system into one containing tremendous business opportunities in providing workforce coverage.

A common theme in these government programs is that many of them provide what economists call a public good.[27] These are products and services with benefits that are widespread and that cannot be restricted to those willing to pay, even though they may be essential for commerce. Private companies are therefore ill-suited to provide them.

Scientific knowledge is such a product. It benefits everyone, and once a discovery has been made, it is difficult to restrict its spread. Moreover, the fundamental workings of nature are not patentable, so others are free to use findings concerning them. Private firms can charge for inventions based on this knowledge, but it is difficult to profit from the raw knowledge itself.

Access to health care by the most vulnerable is another public good. It benefits everyone, either directly or indirectly, because those who are not needy today may become so in the future. A strong safety net therefore represents insurance for all citizens. The enhanced financial security that it provides makes the overall economy and society itself more stable, but it would be difficult to limit that effect based on payment.

The tax subsidy for employer-sponsored health insurance has helped countless enterprises attract and retain stable workforces. The premiums that are paid have helped to create the financial base on which much of the health care system rests. Only the government could have provided the substantial incentives on a national scale that were needed to entice companies to adopt this benefit and thereby solidify the backbone for much of American health care finance.

Once a government intervention is in place to provide a public good, private enterprises can build on it to create new markets. Just as natural environments contain the infrastructure on which species can survive and thrive, government-provided public goods create resources that are needed to sustain private businesses. We have seen this dynamic at work throughout the economy. It enabled the expansion of the computer industry based on the Internet, of the automobile industry based on the Interstate highway system, of the telecommunications industry based on satellites, and of the construction industry based on mortgage support.

The private health care industry is no different. It could not have produced on its own the public goods on which much of it relies. However, once the government supplied them, it was able to use these resources to expand and thrive. The production of key public infrastructure by the government contemporaneously with the industry's remarkable growth could have been a coincidence. However, history and logic suggest otherwise. There was no source of fuel other than the government that could have propelled the industry's engine of growth.

What Has the Government Wrought? Has It Been for the Best?

In building the public infrastructure on which American health care rests, how good a job did the government do? To call the system less than perfect is to engage in extreme understatement. Along the three dimensions that health policy experts commonly measure in assessing system performance—cost, quality, and access—American health care is woefully deficient.[28] It is by far the most expensive system in the world. Thousands die every year because of preventable medical errors. And millions lack the financial means to access care, even under the ACA.

Is the government's role to blame for these and other shortcomings? The preceding chapters have shown how a public–private partnership created a robust and highly profitable private health care sector. However, has it been for the best? Might American health care have been better served had the government led the system to develop in another way?

THE BENEFITS OF PUBLIC–PRIVATE HEALTH CARE

By constructing a private market on a government foundation, health care in the United States has enjoyed substantial benefits that stem from the distinctive mission of each sector. The government takes a national perspective. Its mission is to look out for the entire population, not just the segment that represents a particular customer base. Private companies, which face competitive market pressures, can serve as engines of innovation.

The benefits of our public–private health care system are reflected in many of its accomplishments. On the public side, the NIH leads the world in promoting basic biomedical research. Its support has generated findings that have transformed our understanding of biology and led to 107 Nobel prizes.[29] It has spearheaded the successful initiative to decode the entire human genome.[30] Most of the pharmacological armamentarium of modern medicine is an outgrowth of its efforts. The health of the entire world benefits from this public investment.

America's elderly enjoy one of the best health coverage plans available in the United States in the form of Medicare.[31] It is comprehensive in scope and ensures access to the most technologically advanced care available. The private insurance market could not provide coverage at affordable rates to such a high-risk population.

On the private side, market incentives have promoted innovation on several fronts. They have led pharmaceutical companies to develop troves of lifesaving medications. Statins, oncology drugs, wide-spectrum antibiotics, and vaccines are but a few examples. They have encouraged hospitals to equip themselves with cutting-edge technological tools. They have led insurers to experiment with financing innovations, such as the prepaid plans of the post-World War II era. Many of these advances are controversial, but they all expand the horizons and possibilities of medical care.

THE BURDENS OF PUBLIC–PRIVATE CARE

Nevertheless, many of the shortcomings of American health care also may be traced to the public–private paradigm. The system lacks important elements of coordination, leaving gaping holes in key attributes. For example, private insurers focus principally on markets that are likely to generate profits. These are employer groups and individuals who can afford the premiums and are unlikely to engender extensive medical expenses. Market pressures do not leave room for private insurers to direct their concern to those who are left behind.

Hospitals have historically faced relatively few financial incentives for vigilance in patient safety.[32] In fact, they can sometimes profit when their care causes harm by gaining additional reimbursement for the added care needed to remedy it.[33] Until the Institute of Medicine warned of an epidemic of medical errors in 2000, neither the public nor the private sector directed much attention to the problem.[34]

Perhaps the greatest downside of the public–private partnership is its effect on costs. As technology advances, medical care becomes increasingly unaffordable, but neither the public nor the private side has the wherewithal to bring the bills under control. With the assurance of government payment, hospitals and physicians continue to run up the Medicare tab, but political fallout from proposals to reduce Medicare's generosity has stymied numerous attempts to more effectively manage costs.[35] Private insurers are no more effective than Medicare.[36] Their incentive to be efficient is diminished by their ability to pass escalating medical expenses along to customers in the form of higher premiums.

America spends almost twice as much on health care as most other developed countries.[37] The public and private components of spending each on its own comes close to the typical aggregate national health care budget for a developed country on a per capita basis. By maintaining both, and giving neither one the tools to effectively control costs, we have the equivalent of two health care systems, along with the bills to show for it.

This disjointed system and the gaps it leaves led the World Health Organization (WHO) to place the United States as 37th in a ranking of national health systems in 2000.[38] America spends the most on health care of any country in the world but does not receive a commensurate return on the investment in terms of better health or better health care services. The public–private partnership has given us a system that is distinctive in its size rather than in its effectiveness.

A SILVER LINING IN AMERICA'S EXCESSIVE HEALTH CARE SPENDING

Nevertheless, our system can boast one clear return for our higher costs: the level of respect for individual patients. In contrast to its overall assessment, WHO ranked the United States as first in the world in concern for patient autonomy and privacy.[39] American patients also enjoy the best amenities when they receive care, as reflected in the quality of medical facilities, efforts to enhance comfort, and amount of personal attention.

Providers bestow amenities on patients in response to market forces.[40] In a competitive environment, these serve as enticements to generate business. The actual quality of care rendered in a hospital or by a physician is difficult to measure, but the nature of the care experience is readily discerned. Patients can easily tell if a facility is modern and clean. They notice whether nurses and other staff members are attentive and courteous. They know whether a hospital room comes equipped with a television and can judge the quality of the food. The private market may not have given us the most accessible or affordable health care in the world, but it has helped to enhance the experience of using it.

Whether American health care's position as the paragon of patient amenities is worth the cost is open to debate. Some would argue that amenities contribute little to better health. Others would respond that we are getting what we value most. Whatever its ultimate worth, a more patient-centered environment does serve to increase the inclination of people to use the system, and greater use adds to its costs. Perhaps that is why America's costs are not just higher than those in any other country but perennially rise at a faster pace.

THE INSIDIOUS SIDE OF PUBLIC–PRIVATE CARE

However, behind these shortcomings of public–private health care in America lurks a more insidious corrupting force. As private entities gain size and resources in the market that the government created for them, they obtain the ability to nurture, sustain, and influence the hand that feeds them. Health care companies have used their robust financial state to shape and, in some cases control for their own benefit, the government programs on which they rely.

When regulated entities come to dominate the agencies that oversee them, political scientists apply the term "regulatory capture."[41] The regulators have been captured by the regulated. Health care companies may not have succeeded in capturing their entire complement of overseers, but they exert a powerful influence at all levels of government.

The private health care sector has evolved into a lobbying powerhouse. It outpaces all other industries in the amounts it spends trying to influence legislation.[42] In particular, the American Medical Association (AMA), representing physicians, and the Pharmaceutical Research and Manufacturers of America (PhRMA), representing pharmaceutical companies, repeatedly rank in the top tier of organizations in terms of lobbying expenditures.[43]

The influence of health care lobbying can be seen at all levels of government policy. On a microlevel, medical societies and similar organizations shape reimbursement policies under Medicare and Medicaid. Their lobbyists focus on minute details of payment formulas that can have huge impacts on the revenues of individual specialties and industry segments. The financial fortunes of some providers are tied almost entirely to the generosity of Medicare. Renal dialysis centers, home health agencies, and rehabilitation hospitals, for example, live and die based on Medicare reimbursement. They lobby to ensure continued eligibility of their services for coverage at levels that are sufficient to assure ongoing profitability.

On a macrolevel, health care industry influence has been instrumental in determining the fate of federal health reform efforts. The initiative of President Bill Clinton to reform the system in the mid-1990s, along with the model of managed competition on which it was based, engendered fierce opposition from some industry segments that stood to suffer financially.[44] These included traditional health insurance companies, insurance brokers, and pharmaceutical firms. They lobbied intensively against the plan and sponsored advertisements to sway public opinion. Largely because of these efforts, Clinton failed to advance his initiative even as far as the floor of either house of Congress.

President Barack Obama took the lesson of the Clinton plan to heart in devising the political strategy behind his reform efforts in 2009 and 2010.[45] As discussed in more detail in Chapter 8, he worked closely with key sectors of the private health care industry in crafting his approach. The plan's mandate that all Americans maintain health insurance served as an enticement for private insurers to support it, or at least to mute their opposition. Various elements were included to meet objectives of the pharmaceutical industry in return for political backing and financing for communication efforts to build public support. The plan's predicted outcome of adding more than 30 million Americans to insurance rolls solidified support from the hospital industry even as it limited some elements of their Medicare reimbursement, and it garnered the support of the AMA.

Congress enacted Obama's plan in 2010. It has faced a difficult road both politically and in the courts since then, but it still stands as a significant political achievement as the first federal initiative to guarantee widespread health coverage for the entire population. It was possible only because Obama was able to obtain the backing of key segments of the private health care industry.

Other examples abound of the power of industry and professional interests to shape government health care policy. Pharmaceutical firms successfully fought for passage of the Prescription Drug User Fee Act in 1992, which sped up the process of FDA new drug approvals.[46] The industry also lent key support to the Medicare Improvement, Prescription Drug and Modernization Act, which was enacted in 2003 to establish a prescription drug plan under Medicare.[47] That law substantially expanded the number of beneficiaries eligible to receive reimbursement for purchasing its products. The managed care industry has fought to maintain subsidies for private plans under the Medicare Advantage program.[48] Hospitals have fought to maintain funding for residency training.[49] And medical schools have championed increases in NIH funding for biomedical research.[50]

Within the parameters of legislation already on the books, health care companies exert a powerful influence on the decisions of regulators charged with implementation. Renal dialysis centers fight for coverage for expensive medications used in dialysis and kidney transplantation under Medicare.[51] Physicians seek Medicare coverage for new technologies and procedures.[52] Pharmaceutical firms routinely push the FDA to approve their applications to market new drugs.[53]

Beyond efforts to shape the laws and regulations under which it operates, the health care industry has proven itself quite adept at gaming the system as it exists. Hospitals have learned to identify the most remunerative diagnosis for each inpatient under the diagnosis-related group reimbursement system.[54] Physicians have learned to increase the volume of patient visits to compensate for reductions in payment for individual services.[55] Pharmaceutical companies have used regulatory preferences for orphan drugs to gain approval for expensive new medications that treat rare diseases and then marketed them more broadly for relatively common ailments.[56]

In essence, in giving private health care companies the power to shape and manipulate public policy, the government has created its own master. It built the pillars of modern health care as we know it today and then sustained it with ongoing sources of funding. The private entities that enjoy this beneficence thereby gain strength and resources, which they use to ensure that the public generosity continues. As the government maintains its supporting role, their influence expands even further.

This cycle forms a kind of feedback loop, in which new government initiatives add to public spending, which promotes higher levels of expenditures in the private sector. A larger private industry then exerts pressure for greater spending on those initiatives and for the creation of new ones, which allows them to expand once again. The result is more health care, regardless of the amount we actually need or even want.

Another effect of some government regulatory policies is to dampen competitive forces that can control prices. In health care, this effect is seen, for example, in restrictive licensing rules for professionals that increase the latitude of established practitioners to raise their fees. Programs that guarantee generous reimbursement for health care goods and services, such as some parts of Medicare, similarly enable providers to charge more than the market would bear on its own. As described in Chapter 1, economists apply the term "rents" to the excess prices that can be charged as a result of such a favorable economic position. When rents are extracted, resources are diverted from more productive uses.

Beyond the effect in increasing system costs, the power of private interests may work at cross-purposes with the regulatory mission of the government in other ways. Critics claim that key consumer protections across health care are diluted because of industry pressure.[57] They see compromises in regulatory spheres ranging from FDA drug safety vigilance to state protection of insurance beneficiaries to physician discipline. Whatever the validity of these criticisms in individual instances, it is clear that private enterprises are extremely effective at using their government-granted resources to ensure that their interests are consistently well represented.

DOES GOVERNMENT-CREATED HEALTH CARE SERVE THE PUBLIC INTEREST?

The American brand of government-created health care has produced its share of winners and losers. Among the most apparent winners are the firms and professionals that comprise the private market for health care products, services, and finance. The government has been very good for their businesses. Among the losers are those left without coverage because they are not eligible for public programs and are unable to afford a private policy, even under the ACA. The losers also include those with illnesses that are unprofitable to treat, such as patients with rare diseases that have yet to interest a pharmaceutical firm in developing an orphan drug.

Perhaps the most widespread group of losers is composed of those who bear the cost of the most expensive health care system in the world. They include employers that pay ever-higher insurance premiums to cover their workers, patients who face larger gaps in coverage under their policies, and taxpayers who ultimately pay the bill for cost escalations in government programs. To a greater or lesser extent, that group of losers includes everyone in America.

Under even the most optimistic scenario, America's health care system leaves ample room for improvement. This description of its underlying dynamics is not meant as a blanket endorsement. It is rather an explication of the complex relationship between the public and private sectors that shape it. Neither the successes nor the failings of the health care system can be traced exclusively to the actions of either one. Both have made contributions, and both have left gaps. Therefore, the only way to improve the system is to accurately appreciate the role of each. The greatest danger is that we misconstrue those roles and pursue reforms based on misperceptions.

The market-based character of American health care emerged from a crucible of government. Its fate continues to rest in the hands of public programs that created the private side of the system, for better or worse. Those programs may introduce inefficiencies, and some of them may lead to outcomes that are counterproductive to their stated goals. The private industry that they engendered may include an ample share of inefficiency and waste. However, without them, the kind of health care we take for granted would not exist.

Health Care in the Rest of the World—Is America Different?

This book recounts the story of health care in America. It is the most expensive system in the world, and it has the largest private sector of any developed country.[58] But is this underlying structure unique? Is this the story of an exceptional set of dynamics or of a common theme that is simply different in size but not in kind? Every national health care system has its own distinctive structure and history. In the developed world, all health systems support both public and private health care enterprise to at least some extent. How different is the United States?

A comparison with other major health care systems suggests that health care in the United States is, in fact, exceptional. It is not exceptional in having both strong public and private sectors that interact in complex ways, but rather in the size, influence, and visibility of the private side. In no other country is the private health care industry as powerful, and in none does its power obscure the formative role of the government.

In all other developed countries, the public role in guiding and funding health care is clearly apparent. Private providers and payers function within explicit parameters set by government policy. Of course, they do so in the United States, as well, but many of the largest and most influential of America's government health care programs operate behind the scenes, with effects that are hidden from public view. In that regard, the United States stands apart from the rest of the world.

One way to understand the nature of different health care systems in developed countries is to order them along a continuum according to the tilt of the public–private balance. On this spectrum, Great Britain stands at one end. The government provides all aspects of health care directly to its citizens.[59] This includes not only coverage for the cost, but also medical care itself. The system is administered by a government agency known as the National Health Service (NHS), which operates a network of hospitals located throughout the country that provide inpatient care. A set of nonprofit organizations established by the government and known as primary care trusts employ physicians who render outpatient care. Prescription drug prices are set according to a formula. The cost of all services is covered through tax revenue, and citizens have no need to obtain insurance on their own, although they can if they wish.

Although the care provided by the NHS is comprehensive, many citizens still choose alternative sources of treatment in the private market.[60] Some do so to avoid waiting lists for various services, while others believe they can obtain higher quality care. A bustling market of private physicians and hospitals fulfills the demand for nongovernmental care, and private insurance can be purchased to cover some of the cost. The private market is a fraction of the size of the NHS, but it is nonetheless significant.[61]

The British government did not create the "free-market" health care sector that functions alongside the NHS. It arose as a parallel system outside of the public program. Moreover, without government support, it is dwarfed by the government's health care presence. In those regards, the British system presents the clearest contrast with the American public–private partnership.

Another system toward the same end of the continuum is that of Canada. Under its model, publicly funded insurance covers all citizens. However, in contrast to the British system, the government role is limited to financing, rather than actually delivering, care. Hospitals function as independent nonprofit entities, and physicians render care in private practices. Reimbursement rates are negotiated annually between funds in each of the country's 11 provinces and their hospitals and medical societies. The insurance funds also set prices for prescription drugs.[62]

By letting them hold the purse strings directly, the Canadian system puts the provincial governments in a dominant position. They control the financial state of the country's health care providers. Reimbursement is set at a level that supports the operating costs of facilities and the basic income needs of professionals, and it leaves little room for entities that also seek to realize substantial profits. The

Canadian system thereby discourages the development of a robust American-style private health care sector.

At the other end of the continuum lie the systems of Switzerland and the Netherlands. Both of those countries adopted reforms to place a larger share of responsibility for health care finance on the private market.[63] The model they follow is similar to the one embodied in the ACA. It encourages the development of a market for insurance comprised of competing plans. All citizens face a mandate to obtain coverage in some form. If an employer does not make it available to them, and they are not eligible for a public program because of age or income, they must purchase a plan directly from an insurance company on their own.[64]

The Swiss and Dutch systems echo the American model in that the governments of these countries have created a foundation for private markets within the health care sector.[65] The goal of this approach is to harness the incentives for innovation and efficiency that arise from market-based competition while structuring the parameters within which companies function to meet public needs. The two countries hope that these public–private partnerships can bring the best of both worlds, public and private, to bear on meeting their health care needs.

These systems incorporate elements of the American approach but leave the government in a much more dominant position. Costs are controlled through the imposition of stringent fee schedules for provider reimbursement.[66] Insurance rates are heavily regulated, and substantial financial assistance is available for those unable to afford coverage. Most institutional providers function on a nonprofit basis. The Swiss and Dutch governments have created islands of market-based health care, and their private health care sectors are larger than those of most other developed countries.[67] However, they have not encouraged the same expansive private enterprise that pervades American health care.

In the middle of the continuum lie the systems of most other developed countries, including those of France, Germany, and Japan. These systems evolved at different times, but their structures contain common elements that define similar roles for the contributions of the public and private sides. In these countries, the governments facilitated the creation of insurance funds that finance care and cover all, or almost all, citizens. The governments operate some of these funds directly, but many are administered by nonprofit organizations and in some cases by unions. Participation in the funds is principally arranged through employment, with both the worker and the company contributing part of the cost. Those who are self-employed or unemployed can join a fund directly. Those who are elderly or poor receive coverage through government programs that subsidize much of the cost.[68]

These countries facilitate payment for health care for virtually all of their citizens, but they do not provide it directly. Hospitals, as in most of the developed world, are independent entities, most of which operate on a nonprofit basis. Physicians function either in private practices or as hospital employees. Government rate-setting programs determine the prices of prescription drugs.

Once again, these systems leave room for the private sector, but the nongovernmental role is predominantly filled by nonprofit organizations rather than by for-profit, investor-owned entities. They rely, for the most part, on reimbursement from government-controlled or government-facilitated payment arrangements and therefore include little opportunity to generate substantial profits. The key elements of an American-style market of investor-owned health care companies are missing.

In comparison to these other countries, the public–private paradigm of American health care is, indeed, distinctive. In no other country is the private sector as large or as important to the system's functioning, and in no other do private entities enjoy as much leeway to explore new business opportunities and strategies. The private sector's position is so large and visible in the United States that it obscures the pervasive and foundational role of the government, as important as it is. That is not the case anywhere else.

Market-based health care in America is distinctive not only for its economic strength, but also, as discussed, for the political clout that its financial position confers. The private health care industry is unique in the size and power of its lobbying operations at both the legislative and regulatory levels. Health care interests are key political players in several developed countries, but they are no match for the massive political operations of America's multi-trillion-dollar health care industry.

When the government created "free-market" health care in the United States, it built a system unlike any other in the world. The government did not cede its central role when it implemented the numerous programs that built and sustain private health care. Rather, it overlaid that role with a market-based structure. The result is a complex system in which separate public and private spheres build on one another, maintaining large measures of independence while at the same time remaining inextricably intertwined.

America's Government-Run System

Without the government's active role, health care in the United States would look nothing like it does today. Most significantly, the industry would be substantially smaller. In maintaining its numerous regulatory and funding programs, the government has not stifled private health care, nor has it crowded out private companies from business opportunities. Quite to the contrary, it has built the foundation on which private health care rests.

Some critics characterize the system as a "medical-industrial complex" that renders large amounts of unnecessary care, significantly inflating America's health care bill.[69] The opportunities that this private sector juggernaut enjoys are largely funded at taxpayer expense, and they help to make our bloated system the most expensive in world.[70] Nevertheless, the point remains that the system, for all of its accomplishments and failings, is chiefly a creation of the government. It does not, and could not, exist independently of its public benefactor. Government programs have not grabbed a share of the pie from private entrepreneurs. They have enlarged the entire pie so that everyone can have a bigger slice. If they can be faulted, it is not for stunting the system's growth but for allowing it to become too large.

Health care in the rest of the developed world is often referred to as government-run care. In some regards, this characterization is accurate. England has a fully socialized system, and Canada has a system of socialized health care finance. In much of Europe, private entities provide care, but the government plays the dominant role in guiding its provision.

However, in important ways, this characterization can be applied to the American system, as well. Over a third of the United States population receives care that is directly financed by government programs—an example of socialized insurance as clear as that of the system in Canada. Over half receives care funded by employer-sponsored plans that are heavily subsidized by the government through a tax preference and heavily shaped by layers of regulation. Some of these arrangements, especially those administered by unions, bear striking similarities to some of the insurance funds of Europe. And under the ACA, much of the rest of the population purchases individual policies from private companies in a regulated market along the model of the systems in Switzerland and the Netherlands.

In light of this structure, America does not face the risk that the government could take over health care, since for all intents and purposes, it took over the system decades ago. The mechanism through which it exerts its influence may be different from that employed elsewhere in the developed world in the room it leaves for private businesses, but the public role is as pervasive and entrenched as it is anywhere else. It is just more difficult to see.

Health care reflects the same dynamic that drives much of the rest of our modern complex economy. What we see as the "free market" is often a manifestation of arrays of government policies. Those policies are far from perfect, and we can certainly strive to improve them. However, we cannot eliminate the government's role without undermining the entire system. And in health care, the system's demise would reverberate not only among the patients who rely on it for lifesaving goods and services. It would devastate countless private entities that depend on the government, both directly and indirectly, for their very existence.

8

Health Reform, Government Initiative, and the Future of American Health Care

> In US health policy, the status quo is deeply entrenched and, despite all its failings, the system is remarkably resistant to change, in part because many constituencies profit from it.
>
> —JONATHAN OBERLANDER, *NEW ENGLAND JOURNAL OF MEDICINE*[1]

We have seen how a paradigm of public–private partnership created the distinctive American health care system we have today. Let us now take the analysis one step further. Looking ahead, what can we expect as health care in the United States continues to evolve?

A seminal step in that evolution unfolded in the passage and implementation of President Barack Obama's health reform plan, which followed passionate political debates. The core of the plan is an effort to ensure that all citizens are able to obtain coverage. Although many of its key elements are novel, the road to its enactment and the structure of its mechanisms to expand coverage follow a well-trodden path in important regards. The law represents a supreme collaboration of private and public enterprise. Few aspects of American health policy better illustrate the development of the country's government-created, market-based system than this initiative, which stands as the culmination of repeated attempts over the course of a century to achieve universal health care coverage.

The Push for Universal Coverage: Origins and Obstacles

The Obama plan grew out of a long history of health reform initiatives. For almost a century, the goal of granting coverage to all Americans had been a siren for politicians. The first to hear the call was Theodore Roosevelt, who proposed a universal coverage plan in 1912, as part of his campaign for president under the banner of the Bull Moose Party. He saw universal coverage as a natural extension of Progressive Era reforms he had championed four years earlier as president, including the creation of the US Food and Drug Administration (FDA) in 1906 and standards for meatpacking enacted the same year. The Bull Moose Party went down to defeat, and Roosevelt's proposal soon disappeared from public view along with it. However, Roosevelt had succeeded in giving the issue new visibility on the American political agenda.[2]

Universal coverage as a national cause lost traction with Roosevelt's defeat, but supporters moved their advocacy to the states.[3] During the period between 1915 and 1919, numerous proposals were introduced in several of them. None was enacted; however, the goal retained widespread notice. The failure of these efforts stemmed in large part from the strident opposition of organized medicine in the form of the American Medical Association (AMA). It leveled the charge that government-guaranteed insurance represented a form of socialism and framed it in a way that would recur in all future health reform campaigns by calling it "socialized medicine."

The move to overhaul the health care payment system faded in the 1920s and remained largely dormant during the next decade, waiting to be revived by President Franklin Roosevelt in the 1930s. He was the first president to consider the notion of universal coverage while in the White House. As elements of Roosevelt's New Deal reforms fell into place, he sought to add a national health insurance plan to its list of programs. The approach would have been similar to Social Security, which guaranteed every working American a pension.[4]

Roosevelt's initial preference was to include a health plan in the legislation he proposed to create Social Security in 1935. However, he changed course out of concern over its political sensitivity. A new proposal for universal health coverage seemed certain to resurrect the AMA's charges of socialized medicine. Opponents could then paint the entire package as too radical for the public to accept. He therefore proposed and achieved enactment of Social Security as a stand-alone initiative. In 1937, with that program in place, Roosevelt considered sending Congress a stand-alone health care plan as a supplement, but he relented again for fear of the intense opposition it might provoke. Soon thereafter, World War II began, and the issue had to be set aside, with the intention of reviving it after the war.[5]

In the meantime, several members of Congress kept the cause of universal coverage alive. Bills to create a plan were introduced almost every year starting in 1939. None came close to passage, but these efforts kept the issue in public view.

Roosevelt did not live to see the end of World War II, and the task of completing a vision of the New Deal that included universal health care fell to his successor in the White House, Harry Truman. The cause was dear to Truman, who pursued it passionately. He proposed it as a cornerstone of a set of reforms he labeled the "Fair Deal." However, he faced an opposition that was equally passionate, and the effort proved to be an uphill struggle.[6]

Truman first tried to enact a universal coverage plan in 1946, but even with his fellow Democrats in charge of Congress at the time, he made little headway. Truman did gain a consolation prize in passage of the Hill-Burton Act to fund hospital expansion and construction.[7] However, proposals for national health insurance to provide guaranteed access to those facilities went nowhere. Their fate was the same between 1947 and 1949, when Republicans held control of Congress. In 1949, with Democrats back in charge, Truman's plan was resurrected in the form of legislation known as the Murray, Wagner, Dingell Bill.[8] In an attempt to gain the support of physicians, the law explicitly granted patients the freedom to choose their physician and physicians the right to choose their patients. However, the AMA was not placated, and it waged a vigorous campaign in opposition, including, yet again, charges of "socialized medicine."[9]

In the face of this intense opposition, the Truman administration changed course in 1951. It was a tactical move that turned out to have profound consequences. Truman dropped the call for universal coverage to target instead the needs of a particularly sympathetic subset of the population—the elderly. Most Americans at the time who were past retirement age were poor and therefore in particular need of help in paying medical bills. The plan was known as the Ewing proposal, after Oscar R. Ewing, a presidential adviser who led the effort to develop it. Truman hoped that a more incremental reform such as this would reduce some of the opposition to government-run health insurance and make it easier to enact a more comprehensive plan down the road.[10]

However, the AMA remained opposed to public coverage, even in this more limited form, and the plan did not pass. Truman left office without a major health reform initiative to show for his efforts. Nevertheless, the Ewing proposal set the stage for a new health reform push a decade later.

THE FIRST STRANDS OF SUCCESS

In 1960, the last year of the Eisenhower administration, Congress finally enacted a federal health coverage program, although one of limited scope. The plan took the form of the Kerr-Mills Act, which subsidized care for some categories of the poor.[11] Although the law's focus was narrow, it was significant in marking the first entrée of the federal government into the business of directly covering health expenses for a segment of the general population after 50 years of attempts.

The following year, John F. Kennedy took office, and he made the extension of government health coverage a priority. His approach was to build on Truman's plan to target the needs of the elderly, and he incorporated it into a proposed program called Medicare. The concept was embodied in the Anderson-King bill, which was introduced in 1961.[12] However, once again, opposition from the AMA and some business groups brought about its defeat.[13]

Lyndon Johnson assumed the presidency after Kennedy's assassination, and he took upon himself the mission of enacting much of the social agenda that remained unfinished, including passage of Medicare. He saw his chance after the 1964 election. Johnson won the presidency in a landslide, and Democrats made huge gains in Congress, claiming 69 seats in the Senate and two-thirds of the House of Representatives.[14] Johnson also gained momentum for his efforts from public sympathy for Kennedy's unfinished legacy.[15]

The year 1965 was a seminal one for American health policy. No sooner had the new Congress taken office in January, but Johnson began maneuvering for passage of Medicare. As with past efforts, his were met with vehement opposition from the AMA, including charges that Medicare represented not only "socialized medicine," but also the first step toward establishment of an entire Soviet-style economy. However, Johnson was a skilled legislative tactician, having served many years in his party's leadership in the Senate, and he was able to use that skill to fashion a series of legislative compromises that eased the path to passage.[16]

To entice members of Congress to support Medicare, Johnson promised favors on other issues in return.[17] To woo business interests, he offered financial inducements.[18] As discussed in Chapter 6, he agreed to a structure for the program that gave private insurance companies the chance to play a major role in administering it as carriers and intermediaries in each state. It also gave them the opportunity to sell policies that supplemented Medicare's coverage and to charge ample prices for them. As discussed in Chapter 4, Medicare gave hospitals assurance that the bills of their elderly patients would be paid. And, as discussed in Chapter 5, physicians gained a reimbursement scheme that perpetuated generous payment levels.

Johnson's deal making succeeded. By the end of June, Congress had passed two new major health care coverage programs. Medicare covered the elderly and totally disabled, and Medicaid covered the poor.

The passage of Medicare and Medicaid were watershed events in American health care. Previous chapters have described how they transformed not only the care of millions of vulnerable citizens but also the financial fortunes of the providers whose services were eligible for coverage. Their enactment also represented a defining moment politically. With them, government health insurance entered the country's economic and social fabric.

THE PUSH TO COVER EVERYONE

Despite their importance to American health care and political discourse, Medicare and Medicaid still fell short of the dream of universal coverage. They met the needs of targeted segments of the population but left most people without guaranteed access to care. Truman had promoted a precursor of Medicare as a stalking horse for a broader program that would cover everyone. Johnson and the architects of Medicare and Medicaid saw these programs in the same light. With their passage, the battle for the next step, health insurance for the entire population, had begun.

The extension of Medicare and Medicaid into a comprehensive program did not come as quickly or as easily as supporters of universal coverage had hoped. In part, the social upheaval of the 1960s initially stood in the way. The country was preoccupied with a host of other pressing concerns at the time, such as civil rights, the Vietnam War, environmental protection, and women's rights. Health care remained a significant social concern, but it faced fierce competition for a top spot on the nation's political agenda.

After the 1960s, a series of new political roadblocks arose. Another 45 years would pass before a universal coverage plan came to fruition. And the program that finally emerged would be radically different from the concept that the architects of Medicare and Medicaid had envisioned.

PRIVATE MARKET SOLUTIONS COME TO THE FORE

The focus of the debate over national health insurance changed markedly at the start of the 1970s. For President Richard Nixon, who came to office in 1969, a new government health care program held little appeal. However, shortcomings in the country's health care system were becoming increasingly apparent and could not easily be ignored. Costs started to rise precipitously in the wake of Medicare's implementation, and a sizeable and growing portion of the nonelderly population remained uninsured. Advocates for reform remained vocal, leaving Nixon no choice but to focus attention on health care, but he adopted an approach that differed fundamentally from that of his predecessors. By the end of his administration in 1974, he had caused much of the political thinking on how to achieve universal coverage to veer in a new direction.[19]

Nixon's conservatism led him to prefer private market approaches to solving health care challenges over direct government solutions. His market orientation led him to support the Health Maintenance Organization (HMO) Act in 1973 as a response to rising health care costs.[20] As discussed in Chapter 6, it is not clear whether that law actually succeeded in lowering the nation's overall health care bill, but it was instrumental in creating a new segment of the private health care industry—managed care.

The same year that the HMO Act passed, Nixon entertained a novel approach to increasing the availability of coverage. His goal was to find a solution based on the private market rather than on a new or expanded government program. The challenge he faced was to induce private insurance companies to cover all comers regardless of health status. Companies balked at the idea out of concern that only those who were sick would apply. They feared that potential applicants who were healthy would wait until they became ill to join the ranks of premium-paying customers, which would make it impossible to spread the risk. This would lead to the phenomenon of "adverse selection," in which only those who are likely to incur claims obtain coverage, a situation that is financially unsustainable for a private insurance market.

A viable private market for individual health insurance that offers coverage to everyone can only function if all potential customers, both healthy and sick, participate. The challenge for policymakers was to find a way to bring a broad range of people under the insurance umbrella. Nixon's approach was to mandate coverage. All citizens would be required to maintain health insurance of some sort. They could obtain it through a government program if they were eligible, through an employer if it offered health benefits, or directly from an insurance company. Individuals who failed to avail themselves of one of these options would face a penalty.[21]

Nixon found the concept of an individual mandate appealing not just on its own merits. It also represented an alternative to an approach that was finding increasing favor among some Democrats, who supported a mandate not on individuals to obtain coverage for themselves but on businesses to offer it to their workers. Although this would not have produced universal coverage, it would have helped some of those left uninsured because their employers declined to provide health benefits. Nixon preferred a directive aimed at individuals to one that would have targeted private industry.[22]

However, Nixon never had the chance to develop the individual mandate approach into an actual legislative proposal. In mid-1973, the Watergate scandal began to capture the country's attention. He spent the rest of his presidency responding to a cascade of charges involving the activities of campaign operatives during his 1972 reelection bid and White House efforts to cover them up. The scandal forced him to resign in 1974. Were it not for Watergate, health reform based on an individual mandate might have become law by the middle of the 1970s.[23]

Nevertheless, the notion of structuring a universal access system around the private insurance market did not fall off the political agenda with Nixon's demise. To the contrary, it formed the basis for numerous proposals over the next several decades. In particular, the approach of reforming the market for individual policies based on a mandate that everyone obtain coverage underwent several embellishments and refinements over the years. Attention to it grew steadily, and it became the central focus of the health reform plan that Congress eventually enacted in 2010.

The fight for universal health coverage lost some of its immediacy during the 1970s and 1980s. It was kept alive largely through the efforts of Massachusetts Senator Edward Kennedy, who devoted much of his 40-year political career to the cause.[24] Despite his passion, he failed to convince fellow-Democrat Jimmy Carter to take on the issue during his presidency in the late 1970s. During the 1980s, the Republican administrations of Ronald Reagan and George H. W. Bush maintained even less interest in the issue than Carter's had. By the start of the 1990s, Senator Kennedy and other advocates of national health insurance found themselves largely adrift.[25]

CLINTON'S FAILED ATTEMPT AT A PRIVATE-MARKET SOLUTION

Bill Clinton won the presidency in 1992, at a time when the country was mired in a recession. The economy was forefront on voters' minds, but one economic concern generated particular public interest—the cost of health care. It was rising rapidly, along with the insurance premiums paid by individuals and their employers. Growing numbers of companies found coverage for their workers unaffordable and chose to drop it, thus swelling the ranks of the uninsured. With the public eager for a solution, Clinton resurrected the issue of health reform and promised to pursue a universal coverage plan, if elected.[26]

Once in office, Clinton set about to make good on his promise. To craft a plan, he set in motion a complex and controversial process. He put his wife, Hillary, in charge of the effort and constituted a collection of task forces and working groups to formulate individual elements. These bodies conducted their planning work in secret, hidden from public view, to try to insulate themselves from the influence of lobbyists who might dominate the discussions before a plan had even been devised. However, the secretive nature of the process served to engender public skepticism from the start.[27]

The proposal that emerged relied heavily on the private sector to broaden the availability of health insurance. A direct government program was never seriously considered. The planning process focused on crafting a public–private partnership in line with attitudes toward health reform that had solidified over the previous two decades.

At the core of the Clinton plan was a requirement that all employers provide coverage for their workers. They would have purchased it not through the system of insurance brokers that existed at the time but through new nonprofit entities that served as insurance clearinghouses, which would have overseen the sale of policies and standardized coverage terms. It was expected that most plans sold by the clearinghouses would provide coverage through managed care arrangements. The managed care plans, in turn, would purchase health care services for their beneficiaries from networks of hospitals, physicians, and other providers that would band together to integrate care to improve quality and efficiency. The networks were known as integrated delivery systems (IDSs).[28]

The Clinton plan did not include a mandate that all individuals obtain coverage. Those without access to employment-based insurance would have been able to purchase a policy through a clearinghouse, if they wished to obtain one. However, they would not have been required to do so.

Had it been enacted, the Clinton plan would have been a boon for some segments of the health care industry. HMOs stood to gain new prominence in the market for private coverage. Some larger hospitals would have been able to spearhead the creation of IDSs and thereby to assume new influence over the provision of services. However, numerous other industry segments stood to see their business fortunes decline. Traditional indemnity insurance companies, which at the time dominated the market for health care finance, feared the eradication of their business model. The AMA anticipated that a finance system based on managed care would discourage the use of specialty physician services. Pharmaceutical companies foresaw tougher price negotiations with managed care plans. And insurance brokers who earned commissions by helping employers find coverage could have been rendered obsolete by the clearinghouses.

The industry sectors that stood to gain under the plan that emerged were not among the most influential and well funded at the time, but the sectors that stood to lose were. As a result, instead of engendering support from the health care business world, the plan produced powerful enemies that ultimately orchestrated its political doom. When combined with strident political resistance from Republicans, the obstacles to passage grew almost daily.[29]

Opponents characterized the Clinton plan as overly complex and an unwarranted government intrusion into America's free-market health care system. Familiar charges of "social medicine" were heard. One well-financed business group, the Health Insurance Association of America, which represented traditional insurance companies, sponsored a widely aired television commercial that played a key part in shaping public attitudes. In it, a young couple named Harry and Louise reviewed the plan and found it bewildering and threatening to their existing health coverage.[30]

As public and political opposition mounted, Congressional support began to evaporate. Even with Democrats in control of both houses of Congress, the plan failed to gain the approval of any of the committees that considered it. The Clinton health reform plan died without ever making it to the floor of either chamber. Along with it went the political momentum that had moved the universal coverage cause to the center of the political agenda.

Democrats suffered major defeats in the mid-term Congressional elections in 1994. Observers attributed part of the reason to Clinton's failure to enact any form of health legislation after promising to usher in major reforms. Republicans were able to cast his party as ineffectual. Chastened by the experience, Clinton steered clear of major health reform efforts for the remainder of his presidency.[31]

Although universal health coverage remained short of fruition at the end of the twentieth century, a number of significant, although less ambitious, health reform measures were enacted during this time. These incremental laws addressed some of the more glaring gaps in the coverage net. Taken as a whole, they functioned as a series of Band-Aids for aspects of the system that were particularly frayed.

Among the more significant of these, the Comprehensive Omnibus Budget Reconciliation Act of 1986, commonly known as COBRA, implemented a rule enabling those who lose employer-sponsored insurance because their employment is terminated to retain coverage for an additional period of time.[32] The Health Insurance Portability and Affordability Act, passed in 1996 and known popularly as HIPAA, restricted the ability of insurers to limit coverage based on preexisting conditions for newly hired workers under employer plans.[33] The Children's Health Insurance Program, commonly known as CHIP, enacted the same year, provided federal funding for new state initiatives to cover children in low-income families who lacked insurance but were not poor enough to qualify for Medicaid.[34] And the Medicare Prescription Drug, Improvement and Modernization Act (MMA) of 2003 added a prescription drug benefit to Medicare.[35]

THE "FREE-MARKET" ANTECEDENTS OF THE OBAMA PLAN

Although they had balked at the scope and complexity of the Clinton plan, many conservative policy analysts and Republican politicians remained open to the notion of harnessing market forces to extend health coverage to everyone. They were especially attracted to the individual mandate approach that had first been considered by Richard Nixon in the early 1970s. In 1989 and again in 1990, the Heritage Foundation, a conservative think-tank that promotes private sector solutions for public concerns, fleshed out the idea into a detailed policy proposal.[36]

In its analysis, the Heritage Foundation outlined a three-part mechanism to enable the individual health insurance market to cover all applicants regardless of income or health status. First, the federal government would provide subsidies toward the purchase of policies in the form of tax credits to those whose earnings fell below specified levels. Second, insurers would be obliged to offer coverage to all who applied for it, regardless of health status. And third, to enable insurers to spread the risk over a large enough pool of insureds to avoid the threat of adverse selection, every citizen would be mandated to maintain coverage. This would be enforced with a penalty for noncompliance that would be collected by the Internal

Revenue Service along with income taxes. The Heritage Foundation termed this a "personal responsibility" requirement because it discouraged individuals from behaving as free riders. These are people who would avail themselves of insurance to cover the expense of care when they became ill or injured without contributing their fair share of the overall cost by maintaining coverage when they were well.

In 1993, a group of Republican senators led by John Chafee of Rhode Island proposed a plan based on the Heritage Foundation approach as an alternative to the Clinton proposal.[37] It included a mechanism based on an individual mandate to extend coverage, and they embodied it in a bill that attracted 19 co-sponsors, including then-Senate majority leader Bob Dole. They dropped their proposal after the Clinton effort met its demise, but the initiative established the concept of an individual insurance mandate as a Republican-endorsed approach to market-based health reform.[38]

A decade later, a mandate-based plan reached fruition at the state level. In 2006, the legislature of Massachusetts, with the support and encouragement of the state's Republican governor, Mitt Romney, enacted a measure based largely on the outline proposed in 1990 by the Heritage Foundation. Under it, private policies are brokered through a nonprofit organization known as the Connector Authority, which helps applicants find suitable coverage. For those whose incomes fall below or near the poverty level, eligibility is expanded under the state's Medicaid program.[39] Large employers face a penalty if they do not offer health benefits. And every state resident must maintain coverage or pay a penalty.

The Heritage Foundation lent strong support to the initiative. It released policy pronouncements encouraging passage and provided technical advice during the legislative debates leading up to the proposal's enactment.[40] With implementation of the plan, the market-based approach to health reform was about to receive a real-world test.

By most accounts, the Massachusetts experiment in health reform has been a success.[41] Within a few years of its launch, the state's uninsured rate fell by half to about 4 percent, the lowest of any state in the nation.[42] Initial public unease with the mandate dissipated fairly quickly. In 2012, six years after its passage, the plan enjoyed the support of almost 70 percent of the population and of a sizeable majority of physicians.[43] Large numbers of residents sought primary care services that had previously been unavailable to them, and hospitals saw large declines in the amount of uncompensated care they were forced to provide.[44] The increase in demand for health care services led to long waiting times for some primary care providers, but the backlogs gradually shrank over time.[45]

OBAMA'S HARD-WON VICTORY

Two years after Massachusetts acted, Barack Obama was elected president. Like Bill Clinton before him, he made health care a focus of his campaign. When he took office, the country was in the middle of a major financial crisis, and he faced calls for reform on several fronts. Yet of all the concerns demanding attention, he chose to place health reform at the top of his agenda.[46]

Obama let Democratic leaders in Congress take the lead in crafting a plan, but lent support and guidance to their efforts. Nevertheless, his name was ultimately linked to the result. Although officially known as the Patient Protection and Affordable Care Act[47] (ACA for short), it is widely identified as the Obama health reform plan. Opponents attached the name "Obamacare" to it as a derogatory reference, but the title came to stick with the broader public, and some supporters, even including Obama himself, began to adopt it.[48]

The Obama plan closely tracked the Massachusetts reform in restructuring the market for individual policies according to the Heritage model. It established new bodies, known as "insurance exchanges," in each state to facilitate the sale of policies along the lines of the Massachusetts Connector Authority. It expanded Medicaid in all states to cover all people with incomes up to 133 percent of the federal poverty level.[49] To induce companies to retain worker health benefits, it imposed penalties on larger employers that failed to offer coverage to their workers. It also implemented new regulatory protections for consumers, including restrictions on the ability of insurers to rescind policies once they are in force and to impose annual and lifetime caps on coverage.[50]

In pursuing a health reform plan that would guarantee coverage to all Americans, Obama sought to avoid some of the political missteps of the Clinton efforts. One lesson he took from the Clinton plan's demise was to act quickly, before opposition had a chance to build. The slow pace of Hillary Clinton's working groups had given opponents time to sow public unease. Speed had also been a key part of Johnson's strategy in securing passage of Medicare and Medicaid in 1965.[51] Another lesson was to try to build bipartisan support. Endorsement by at least some Republicans seemed likely at first because the plan tracked an approach that had been favored by their party for several decades. Congressional deliberations over the plan included a period of intense negotiations involving several prominent Republican senators.[52]

However, Obama was thwarted on both of these fronts. Republican leaders eventually adopted a strategy of opposing all health reform efforts, even those based on their own party's precepts. They feared that the public would perceive passage of an Obama-supported plan in any form as a legislative triumph for the president that he could tout in future elections. As tactics in their resistance, they tried to prolong the process to permit time for public skepticism to build, delaying ultimate action for almost a year. They declined to endorse any compromise measures or to sanction further negotiations after the initial round in the Senate dissolved without reaching an agreement. They leveled charges that the plan represented a "government takeover" of health care and, in a familiar refrain, that it represented "socialized medicine." The opposition strategy they pursued was concerted and relentless.[53]

Nonetheless, Obama had learned one lesson from the Clinton effort that proved invaluable to him in overcoming political resistance. It was the power of the private sector to shape public health care policy. Acting on this knowledge, Obama set about to forge a set of alliances, both implicit and explicit, with health industry sectors. The accommodations that he reached ultimately paved the way for his plan's passage. As Johnson had done before him, he preempted powerful sources of potential resistance by including them in the framework of his reforms.

OVERTURES TO BUSINESS

Four sources of business support were key to the success of Obama's health reform effort. One came from the insurance industry. Although private insurers remained cautious about elements of the plan that added new consumer protections and limited their ability to raise rates, they were tantalized by the prospect of gaining millions of new customers who would be mandated to purchase their products. The mandate also assured them of the ability to spread the risk of covering sick individuals across a broader population. In the expansion of Medicaid, private insurers could also expect significant new opportunities to administer the programs in many states.[54]

As part of his political strategy, Obama vilified the insurance industry for raising rates and denying coverage to needy applicants. However, insurers did not respond with the kind of public relations and advertising campaign that had helped to sink the Clinton effort. Instead, they largely stood back and let the legislative process proceed.

A second source of support came from the pharmaceutical industry. Drug companies were initially concerned about a plan that could give greater bargaining leverage to insurance companies in negotiations over prices. To head off their opposition, the Obama administration entered into a series of agreements to grant the industry favors in other regards. Most prominently, he promised to oppose the efforts of many in his own party to permit large-scale reimportation of prescription products from Canada, where prices are lower than in the United States, and to permit the government to purchase drugs directly under the Medicare prescription drug plan. In return, they agreed to make price concessions and to contribute funding to an advertising campaign in support of the health reform effort.[55]

A third key source of support came from the hospital industry. Hospitals were natural allies for health reform. They stood to realize substantial financial benefits from a plan that would dramatically decrease the number of customers unable to pay their bills. In return for this benefit, they accepted a part of the plan that reduced some elements of their reimbursement under Medicare for providing charity care.[56]

Finally, Obama succeeded in garnering support from one of the most unlikely sources of all. Because it would relieve the burden of uncompensated care for many physicians, the AMA endorsed the plan. This marked the first time the organization had backed universal health coverage legislation since the early 1920s. The AMA's stance proved to be extremely controversial and provoked intense protests from within its membership. However, after almost a century of opposition, the most influential medical organization in the country had finally returned to the cause of universal health insurance, which it had once embraced.[57]

THE HOME STRETCH TO PASSAGE

The health reform plan that emerged from the political bargaining was extremely complex. In addition to the provisions that increase the availability of insurance coverage, it contains initiatives in a number of other areas. These include efforts to reduce medical errors, to better coordinate care and control costs, and to vet expensive new medical technologies for effectiveness. With these and other elements, one printing of the bill reached 2,700 pages in length.[58]

Nevertheless, the core of the Obama plan remained the mechanism to realize the hundred-year dream of guaranteeing health care coverage to every American who wants it. For all its intricacies and compromises, it largely accomplished that goal. Teddy Roosevelt's vision of 1912 did not come to fruition through a direct government effort, as many of his successors had anticipated. It came about through a complex interplay of public and private interests. In the politics of American health care at the beginning of the twenty-first century, there was no other viable way.

Congress passed the ACA by the narrowest of margins. Not a single Republican voted for it. When Ted Kennedy died in late 2009, his seat was filled by a Republican, which denied Democrats the 60 Senate votes needed to avoid a potentially lethal filibuster. A parliamentary maneuver enabled them to circumvent that obstacle, but it required careful procedural planning. Nevertheless, the Democrats ultimately succeeded in gaining passage for their health reform plan, and Obama signed it into law on March 23, 2010.

The ACA faced a rough road even after its enactment. Opponents continued to wage a bitter fight to build public sentiment against it. The effort achieved a considerable measure of success as polls consistently showed the public deeply divided over the law's merits.[59] Republicans repeatedly promised to repeal all or part of it or, if unable to do so, to block as much of its implementation as they could.[60] A series of lawsuits were brought to challenge the constitutionality of two key components of the plan—the individual insurance mandate and the expansion of Medicaid. The Supreme Court resolved them in June 2012, in a ruling that permitted the mandate to take effect as written and the Medicaid expansion to proceed in a modified form.[61]

In the end, the Obama plan endured. With it, the landscape of health insurance in the United States stands to be transformed. Obama owed his success in no small part to the alliances he forged, both explicit and implicit, that induced much of the private health care industry to stand behind it.

Obama's health reform plan is a true public–private partnership in the mold of the longstanding American paradigm. The government created a new regulatory infrastructure within which private health care finance can function. It contributes considerable financial support, estimated at more than $1 trillion over the first 10 years, to subsidize the public's use of the new finance mechanisms.[62] Built on this new foundation, private companies can sell products to a vastly expanded customer base.

The ACA set the stage for a financial boon for the health care industry in numerous ways. It enables millions of new customers to purchase individual policies. It permits Medicaid programs in many states to retain more managed care companies to administer benefits. It helps hospitals and many physicians to realize increased revenues by giving more of their patients access to the financial resources needed to pay for care. And, over time, countless other businesses will emerge and thrive under the ACA's government-created structure as the ingenuity of the private sector finds ways to thrive off its new public base.

From the public's perspective, the most visible aspect of the Obama plan is the reinvigorated private insurance sector. People can clearly see the marketing efforts of companies to promote policies on the insurance exchanges and competition among providers for newly insured patients. However, the public may miss an even more important aspect. As a massive new infusion of government funding leads many industry segments to grow even larger, their increased size will bring greater political influence. The historical pattern will certainly repeat as they use this influence to maintain and expand the programs that sustain them.

The result will enlarge the American health care system yet again. The government sector will grow as it pours money into subsidizing coverage through the insurance exchanges and into expanding Medicaid. The private sector will grow at least as much, with millions of new customers obtaining health care financing and medical services. And it will expand in new directions as the array of available services increases. Some may point to the enlarged health care industry as the "free market" in action. However, once again, it will be the government, this time in the form of the Obama health reform plan, that created and sustained the engine of market growth.

Beyond the Obama Plan: The Government and the Future of American Health Care

Health care systems are not static because health care is not static. The practice of medicine changes almost daily. New technologies continually transform the landscape, and the pace of their advance steadily accelerates. Technological progress invariably brings higher costs, so, as clinical care evolves, the economics of health care undergoes a steady transformation along with it.

A few major challenges lie on health care's immediate horizon. Costs continue to rise at an unsustainable rate. In their wake, employee coverage is becoming unaffordable for a growing legion of companies.[63] The Medicare program faces a cost explosion as the number of beneficiaries increases over the next several decades with the aging of the baby boom cohort and the ratio of taxpaying workers to program beneficiaries shrinks.[64] The plague of medical errors continues to afflict thousands each year.[65] And a means of financial access to the system remains difficult for millions, even under the ACA.[66]

Looking further down the road, the underlying nature of medical care stands on the verge of entirely new terrain. Genomics has already begun to change the basis of care, with new diagnostic tests that can predict each patient's likely reaction to medications and new techniques for manipulating the genetic makeup of individuals to eliminate disease risks. An era of personalized medicine that tailors treatments to each patient's physiology is fast emerging. However, along with tremendous therapeutic possibilities, it brings novel risks, both medical and social—not to mention even higher costs.

Medicine is also undergoing a transformation into more of an information-based enterprise. Electronic medical records facilitate both the exchange of patient data and new capabilities to analyze it. Genetic findings will expand the possibilities of information-based diagnosis and treatment even further.

As health care evolves further in its scientific and technological capacities, the history of the last century teaches how the economic and political forces that govern it will adapt. The government, as the only entity with sufficient resources, national perspective, and legal authority to supply foundational support will always play the leading role. Health care cannot function without a solid infrastructure of regulation and financing that only it can provide.

At the same time, a substantial private sector role will always pervade the system. Two forces will keep it in the forefront. The first is the nation's temperament. Americans are inherently uncomfortable relying too much on the government to meet their needs. Even as the popularity of programs like Medicare and Social Security stays at extremely high levels, the public remains suspicious of new initiatives. Obama's health reform plan has faced considerable public skepticism based on this widespread apprehension, even though it relies heavily on the private market for its implementation.

The second is political. The private health care sector is a power to be reckoned with. The vast resources of many industry segments confer tremendous influence in the political sphere. Hospitals, medical societies, pharmaceutical firms, insurance companies, and many others wield the clout needed to guarantee a role in any future public initiatives that affect their interests as they did in the debates that determined the ultimate shape of the Obama health reform plan.

A number of recent policy initiatives in addition to the ACA have followed the pattern of public–private collaboration and demonstrate the extent to which that paradigm remains the norm. As an example, the relatively slow pace of commercialization of genomic medicine has raised concerns at the National Institutes of Health (NIH). The agency has sought to address them by playing a more active and direct role in promoting the translation of basic research findings into medical products through the new National Center for Advancing Translational Sciences.[67] The Center will directly support the development of promising clinical applications based on findings in genetics and other cutting-edge areas of research, in the hope of enticing private partners to bring products to market.

Another example is the approach adopted by federal policymakers to promote wider use of information technology in medicine. The uptake of computer technology by much of the health care industry has been frustratingly slow. To address this concern, Congress passed the Health Information Technology for Economic and Clinical Health (HITECH) Act in 2009, which implements financial incentives to induce hospitals and physicians to adopt new computerized systems and imposes penalties on those that do not.[68] That law does not supply the technology to providers or even specify the systems they must use but rather promotes the provision of computerized systems by private vendors, which operate in a robust and expanding market for medical technology services.[69]

And the ACA applies the model on a grand scale.[70] To expand the availability of health care coverage, it relies on a restructuring of the market for private insurance, with the goal of making private policies more accessible and affordable. It also expands Medicaid in many states, which is administered to a large extent through private managed care companies. With all of these reforms operating together, market-based health care has never had it so good.

The Next Steps for Health Policy

The past teaches that American health care will not advance unless the government remains actively involved. Medical treatment is not a consumer product that the private sector can produce entirely on its own. There are too many ways in which the market is incapable of producing it effectively.

Among the more obvious elements that distinguish health care from other goods and services is that its use is not discretionary. Everyone needs it. A market system that relies on price to determine allocation leaves out many potential buyers with limited means. That may be acceptable for television sets or designer clothing but not for a lifesaving service. Moreover, health care has become so expensive that it is not just those with limited means who would be locked out of a conventional market. Only the very rich can afford most complex treatments, which can cost hundreds of thousands of dollars.

The industry is also distinctive in its reliance on explorations into basic science to advance. New treatments require better understanding of human biology. This knowledge is a public good that is available to all. The private sector is extremely adept at translating it into products and services once it has been generated but not at creating it in the first place. The payoff from contributing to the body of human knowledge is too speculative for entities concerned about short-term profits and too difficult to charge for; yet, without this resource, they cannot thrive and grow.

A third distinguishing element is health care's highly technical nature. Most consumers have limited ability to understand what services they need or why. They must rely on highly trained practitioners, who spend as much as 10 years, and often more, learning the field. Consumers can judge for themselves which brand of television produces the clearest image, but few patients can assess the meaning of their symptoms or the appropriate treatment once a condition is diagnosed. The market paradigm of comparison shopping does not work, so a system to oversee the providers of care is needed in its place.

The government has addressed these areas of mismatch between health care and the functioning of conventional markets in various ways. It directly provides insurance for some vulnerable groups, facilitates access to private coverage for many others, supports basic biomedical research, and oversees the practice of physicians and the operation of hospitals. However, in none of these endeavors does it act alone. It creates and maintains large private industries to do much of the work and then collaborates with them to meet public health care needs. This arrangement has produced a gigantic health care enterprise that provides high-quality care to most citizens and an economic juggernaut that now represents more than one-sixth of the country's economy.

A Blueprint for New Rounds of Reform

Beyond the massive changes wrought by the ACA, further reforms will be needed in the years ahead to address the failings in the health care system that remain. The next order of business for health policy should be to contain the excesses that the public–private partnership has engendered. The most consequential change would be to move the reimbursement paradigm away from one in which a separate fee is paid for each service rendered. The system that currently prevails under most reimbursement arrangements strongly encourages physicians to render as much care as they can, regardless of its value. It pays them when care is inefficient and even when it is ineffective. Commentators ranging from academic researchers to analysts in the popular press have noted the consequences of this payment structure for the cost of American health care.[71]

An alternative arrangement with several decades of experience behind it is payment by capitation. This approach pays a physician or hospital a predetermined fee to provide all services that a patient needs during a set period of time. It has been used by HMOs since the early 1970s to compensate primary care providers in their networks. However, it is not the only feasible alternative. Both the public sector through Medicare and the private sector through insurance plans have been testing other possibilities for several years. These include combining payments for a range of related services into a single bundled amount and paying a set fee to alliances of providers for treating each episode of care. Some payers are also taking the tentative first steps toward a radically different approach of paying providers based on actual patient outcomes. This rewards them for producing greater amounts of health rather than greater numbers of services. The ACA explicitly encourages experiments along all of these lines.[72]

Beyond changing the reimbursement paradigm, four areas stand out as candidates for public policy attention. Initiatives regarding them would simplify the maze of administrative complexity, reverse the specialty domination of the medical profession, halt the overcommercialization of medical care, and control the proliferation of excessively expensive technology. Each stems from the unintended consequences of government programs of the past, and they cry out for new government efforts to provide remedies. The ACA contains limited steps with regard to some of them, but for the most part, these are only a start.

Taming Administrative Complexity

The administrative complexity of health care reimbursement has become overwhelming. The private health insurance industry, which emerged from a series of government policies implemented over the course of decades, contains dozens of companies that offer hundreds of different plans. Each has its own network of providers and distinctive coverage rules. Teams of workers at insurance companies administer these arrangements, and additional teams at hospitals, physicians' offices, and other providers navigate the process to obtain payment. This disjointed system adds considerable costs, not to mention delays in treatment while reimbursement approvals are sought. It also engenders considerable frustration for all involved.[73]

The ACA does little to address this problem. In fact, it may make the situation worse. By funneling additional millions of patients through hundreds of new insurance plans, administrative complexity stands to grow even further.

The government has taken a few steps to ease some of the burden. For one, the HIPAA privacy law, among its numerous provisions, includes a directive that the Department of Health and Human Services promulgate uniform standards for electronic transmission of health care claims data.[74] The Department has issued those rules, and they have succeeded in facilitating the efficient flow of billing data through computerized systems. For another, the ACA standardized health insurance policies that are sold to individuals on exchanges into four types, each with a defined level of coverage.[75] Consumers can choose between platinum, gold, silver, and bronze policies according to the generosity of reimbursement they desire. The law also empowered the Department to prescribe the format and content of informational material that insurers issue to describe each of their offerings.

However, more needs to be done. Policies of all sorts, including those offered through employers, could be standardized according to categories of generosity. All Americans would then know what to expect from their coverage, regardless of where they work. Reimbursement processes could be standardized so providers can follow the same procedures regardless of which company covers a patient. And provider networks could be coordinated so that patients are assured of continuous coverage across different insurers and through different levels of care.

The private sector has failed to produce such coordination on its own. To the contrary, it has largely resisted harmonization. That is not surprising, since no market forces encourage it. The government policies that subsidize and structure the private insurance industry could be redirected to promote needed efficiency in the absence of adequate market incentives.

Righting the Tilt Toward Medical Specialization

The heavy tilt toward specialization in the medical profession has left American health care with an abundance of highly trained and generously compensated specialists and a relative dearth of primary care practitioners. These specialists treat many ailments for which care can be provided just as well by generalists. They rely heavily on expensive tests and procedures at the expense of cognitive interventions and prevention. The result is care that is often overly costly and inefficient.

Once again, it was the public–private partnership that created the imbalance. In particular, Medicare reimbursement policy has consistently favored specialty services, and private insurance tends to follow Medicare's lead. Paradoxically, while the government rewards physicians for specializing, policymakers continually bemoan the detrimental effects on costs that result.

The government has several levers at its disposal to reverse the trend through the Medicare program. First, Medicare supplies the funding for most of the residency training that new physicians receive after finishing medical school. It could more aggressively dedicate slots to primary care and limit the funding of training for specialties. Second, the Medicare process for determining reimbursement for physician services could be revised to reverse its favorable treatment of procedures and tests over counseling and preventive care. A shift in the balance between the two would make primary care more attractive to new practitioners, and private insurers would almost certainly follow that lead.

Finally, and most importantly, Medicare could change the underlying paradigm for reimbursement from payment for each service rendered to bundled payments for overall courses of treatment. Providers will naturally render as much care as possible when each unit adds to their income. Under a bundled payment system, a group of providers involved in treating a patient receives one payment for all care that is needed, and the providers decide on their own how to divvy it up. Their incentive then is to treat the patient efficiently and to focus on achieving the best clinical outcome rather than the maximum number of discrete services. This makes it financially rewarding to coordinate care more effectively, rather than leaving each provider to function in a silo. The ACA contains provisions intended to test new approaches along these lines, but they are fairly modest. Medicare could build on those experiments that are successful to create new models that can be used throughout the health care system.

Reversing Overcommercialization

Many physician practices have taken on the attributes of general commercial enterprises that aggressively seek to enhance revenues through complex business arrangements. This often leads to unnecessary care and excessive referrals to affiliated providers for needless and duplicative tests and procedures. Numerous studies have documented the effects on costs and on care when physicians function as entrepreneurs. A 2009 analysis by Atul Gawande, a physician and health policy analyst, compared two cities in south Texas.[76] Midland, in which physicians tended to focus on private practice, generated considerably lower costs than McAllen, where business ventures had become the norm. However, the differences in spending produced no discernible differences in outcomes for patients.

When physicians maintain ownership stakes in related ventures like clinical laboratories and specialty hospitals, they have an interest in seeing that the facilities have a steady stream of business. Through their medical practices, they are in a position to make that happen by referring patients. Numerous studies have shown that physicians who invest in medical facilities refer patients to them more readily than physicians with no investment interests.[77] Those referrals generate costs for services that are often unnecessary.

Laws have been in place for more than 30 years to discourage these practices. The anti-kickback provisions of the Medicare statute were reinforced in 1977 and again in 1987 to classify payments for referrals as a felony.[78] The Stark Amendments, passed 1991 and 1994, prohibit the referral of patients for certain designated health care services to providers with which a referring physician has a financial relationship.[79] The ACA added funds to reinvigorate enforcement of these laws; however, the temptation remains too great for many physicians to resist. Payments for referrals and overprescription of tests and procedures remain widespread and generate tremendous costs for the health care system.[80]

The government-created structure of the system is, once again, largely responsible for this form of abuse. Medicare can represent a bonanza for providers able to devise creative ways to access its trove of funds. It is a system ripe to be gamed. Having created it, the government is the natural instigator for reforms to change the elements that led to this dysfunction. The ACA includes an initial step with regard to specialty hospitals by banning their construction and expansion, except in limited circumstances.[81]

The most effective strategy would be to promote more extensive integration among providers. America's system of private physicians and hospitals does not have to function under an incentive structure that rewards disorganization and inefficiency. A system in which providers function as components of larger entities would discourage much of the gamesmanship that can corrupt medical judgment and encourage the provision of excessive care.

In an integrated system, especially one that accepts bundled payments, payers can more easily structure incentives to reward good clinical outcomes, coordination of care, and efficiency in treatment. Examples of such systems have operated for decades around the country. One example is the Kaiser Health Plan, which, as described in Chapter 6, began operation in northern California as a prepaid health plan in the 1940s. Several others are controlled by large hospitals, including the Mayo Clinic in Minnesota, the Cleveland Clinic in Ohio, Geisinger Health System in Pennsylvania, and Intermountain Health Care in Utah. They all serve as national leaders in health care innovation, rendering high quality care within efficient frameworks.

Health care has experienced a trend toward greater integration for some time. The percentage of physicians who work as employees, particularly of hospitals and health systems, has risen especially dramatically over the past decade.[82] However, a tremendous amount of system fragmentation and private practice entrepreneurship remains.

The ACA takes some steps toward encouraging providers to integrate their operations. In particular, it encourages them to band together into alliances that work in concert to coordinate care. These are the entities that the law describes as accountable care organizations (ACOs). Experience with them may suggest additional ways to promote similar kinds of ventures. However, an even stronger policy response is also possible. Reimbursement reforms that place greater emphasis on bundled payments under Medicare along with higher reimbursement rates for care that is coordinated could further reduce the incentives for providers to create the kinds of ventures that run up medical bills.

Physicians have functioned as entrepreneurs purchasing investment interests in medical facilities largely because the existing structure of Medicare encourages them to do so. It lets them share in payments both for their own services and for those rendered in facilities that they own. If Medicare can create a system that encourages this dysfunctional arrangement, it can also forge a new one that incentivizes physicians and other providers to make clinical decisions based on desired patient outcomes without regard to reimbursement potential.

Controlling the Proliferation of Technology

Many of medicine's technological advances have produced miraculous results. However, some lead to outcomes no better than those achieved with conventional treatments. And most of these new kinds of care, both those with clear therapeutic benefits and those of dubious value, come with a large price tag.

The cost of some new technologies is staggering. Two treatments for prostate cancer illustrate the point. The biotechnology drug Provenge costs $70,000 for a year's supply.[83] Proton beam accelerators require an investment of $100 million for hospitals to build.[84] In both cases, there is scant evidence of better effectiveness than cheaper preexisting therapies.[85] As technologies like these proliferate, the expense is spread throughout society through higher insurance premiums and larger budgets for public payment programs.

If technologies like these were truly superior to older and cheaper techniques, few would dispute their value. However, when this kind of expenditure renders little or no improvement in clinical outcomes, the drain on the country's resources is difficult to justify. We as a society tend to give medical treatments the benefit of the doubt. We would rather take a chance that money will be wasted on a futile treatment than that patients will lose a chance for a cure. As a result, Medicare and private insurers tend to cover the cost of most new technologies, as long as there are clinicians willing to use them. Without a way to separate the wheat from the chaff, the financial burden on the system will eventually become unsustainable.

Fortunately, a new science is emerging to assess the value of medical treatments. It is known as comparative effectiveness research (CER), and it compares the outcomes of different treatments for the same condition. CER seeks to determine, for example, whether a new technology such as a proton beam accelerator differs in effectiveness from older forms of radiation therapy and, if it is more effective, by how much. Based on the findings, patients, clinicians, and payers can decide which they prefer. Well-designed CER studies can thereby help to tame the most formidable threat to cost containment. They can also help patients to avoid treatments that seem superior because they are new but that are, in reality, of limited value.

Once again, the ACA makes a start at encouraging the use of CER. It created a new independent body known as the Patient-Centered Outcomes Research Institute (PCORI) that funds and promotes CER studies and disseminates the results. However, the law prohibits Medicare from using these findings to decide which new technologies to cover. This significantly compromises its capacity to contain runaway costs.

In virtually every instance, the research behind the development of new medical technologies is funded at least in part by the federal government, usually in the form of NIH research grants. Often, the process of clinical trials and the path to commercialization relies on a partnership with the NIH, as well. Of particular importance going forward, all genomic therapies stem from the work of the Human Genome Project, which decoded the entire human genome at government expense.

The public–private partnerships described in Chapter 3 that bring new drugs and devices from concept to market have served us well. However, it should not be too much to ask the private firms that benefit from these collaborations to prove the value of their inventions before expecting government sanction and public payment for their use. The regulatory approval process for new medical technologies offers an opportunity to vet expensive new technologies more stringently for value. The FDA looks only at whether a new product is safe and whether it is incrementally more effective than the one currently in use. More should be expected of products that emerge from the crucible of public funding. Manufacturers should be obliged to demonstrate true clinical value before taxpayers and premium payers are asked to underwrite their cost. This kind of oversight may not fit within the traditional mission of the FDA, but a new regulatory body could work in coordination with it to house the expertise for such reviews.

In this regard, as in the others, the problem is of the government's own making. It provides the financial underpinning for new product development by private companies, and it creates a guaranteed market through Medicare, Medicaid, and other public insurance programs. If the government can create these products and enrich the companies that manufacture them, it can also vet more vigorously their entry into the market. More widespread use of CER and more stringent requirements for positive results prior to marketing and eligibility for reimbursement would protect the health care system from a financial burden it can ill afford to bear.

WHAT PUBLIC POLICY CAN LEARN FROM THE PAST

The cost pressures that arise from each of these failings may soon lead the system to collapse of its own weight. We have fed and nurtured a private health care sector that has grown so large we may soon be unable to sustain it. Government policies have enabled it to reach this point, but they have proven themselves increasingly ill equipped to contain what they have created.

Were the government to back away from its activist health care role, the challenges would not go away. To the contrary, many of them would almost certainly become much worse. Public policy therefore faces a bind. If existing programs remain in place, the health care juggernaut will continue to grow unsustainably. If they are scaled back indiscriminately, the system will shrivel, taking much of the economy with it.

The answer is to refine the public policies that guide American health care so that the system can continue to grow but at a pace commensurate with our true health care needs and with our capacity to support it. We know how to create public–private collaborations to expand health care. We can apply what we have learned to the task of crafting a system that is viable in the long term. It will not be easy, and it will not be quick. It has taken more than 100 years to build the system we have today. However, we know what the challenges are, and we know how to harness the private sector to address them. By recognizing what we have created and how, we can begin the process of bringing it into balance.

Debates over whether the government should intrude on American health care accomplish nothing. If we want to maintain a strong and effective health care system, the only alternative to what we have now would be a system that is fully government-run, something the American temperament would never accept. The question is not whether the government should be involved. It is how that involvement can be channeled most wisely. The most effective role for public policy is to build on its history of activism so it can move beyond the excesses it has created to craft a future for health care that is robust and sustainable.

Over the coming decades, medicine will be transformed through genomics, information science, and technologies that are yet to be developed. Fifty years from now, it will surely be unrecognizable from what it is today. New health care sectors will arise, and new markets will allocate the goods and services they produce. With the help of the government, they are likely to comprise an even greater force than the health care industry of today for enhancing our well-being, both physical and financial.

American Health Care in the Years Ahead

In the years ahead, the pattern of government health care policy is certain to repeat. Public programs will initiate responses to challenges while carving out central roles for the private sector to implement them. Existing markets for health care goods and services will expand, and new ones will emerge based on new regulatory structures that the government creates. Whether the public role is transparent or hidden, direct or indirect, targeted or broad, it will continue to be the foundational force in shaping American health care.

At the same time, the private sector will remain the system's most visible component. It will continue to serve as the primary point of contact for most Americans when they receive and when they pay for care. Much of the government apparatus that stands behind it will remain difficult to spot for those outside the industry, unless they know where to look.

Every day in the United States, millions of patients receive treatments that relieve their suffering and extend their lives. Millions of health care workers, from highly trained clinicians to support staff, earn paychecks at steady jobs. And millions of investors gain financial rewards from interests in profitable private medical enterprises. They all reap the benefits of a huge market-based system, one often cited as a shining example of the "free market" in action. However, whether they realize it or not, that system relies on the support of an essential benefactor that makes its very existence possible—the government. The market's sponsor may not always lend its assistance in the wisest or most effective ways. But, without it, we would never have come to know the behemoth economic engine that we recognize today as American health care.

NOTES

Chapter 1

1. Adam Smith, *An Inquiry into the Nature and Causes of the Wealth of Nations* (New York: PF Collier & Son, 1909), 473–74.

2. Barry Cohen, "Pfizer Pushes to Keep Lipitor Profits Flowing," *Investor Place*, November 11, 2012, http://investorplace.com/2011/11/pfizer-lipitor-generics-ranbaxy/.

3. Mark Lennihan, "Pfizer, Inc.: 2012 Earnings," *New York Times*, August 8, 2012, http://topics.nytimes.com/top/news/business/companies/pfizer_inc/index.html.

4. "HCA Holdings Inc.," *New York Times*, August 7, 2012, http://topics.nytimes.com/topics/news/business/companies/hca-holdings-inc/index.html.

5. "UnitedHealth Group Inc.," *New York Times*, November 11, 2012, http://topics.nytimes.com/top/news/business/companies/united_health_group_inc/index.html.

6. National Center for Health Statistics, *Health, United States, 2011* (Hyattsville, MD: US Government Printing Office, 2012), 374, table 128, http://www.cdc.gov/nchs/data/hus/hus11.pdf. In 2009, the last year for which data are available, physician services cost $505.9 billion.

7. The number of cardiologists is reported in George Rodgers, "Cardiology Workforce Crisis: Shortage or Surplus? Reply," *Journal of the American College of Cardiology* 55, no. 8 (2010): 834–38. Average cardiologist salaries are reported in Medscape News, "Cardiologist Compensation Report 2012," http://www.medscape.com/features/slideshow/compensation/2012/cardiology. The incomes of the highest earning cardiologists are reported in Larry Husten, "Top New York City Interventional Cardiologists Now Making $3 Million a Year," *Cardiobrief*, October 22, 2010, http://cardiobrief.org/2010/10/22/top-new-york-city-interventional-cardiologists-now-making-3-million-a-year/.

8. Sean Keehan et al., "Health Spending Projections Through 2017: The Baby-Boom Generation Is Coming to Medicare," *Health Affairs* 27, no. 2 (March 2008): w145–w155; Karen Davis et al., *Slowing the Growth of U.S. Health Care Expenditures: What Are the Options?* (The Commonwealth Fund, 2007), http://www.cmwf.org/publications/publications_show.htm?doc_id=449510.

9. Ibid.

10. Leonard E. Burman, Sarah Goodell, and Surachai Khitatrakun, *Tax Subsidies for Private Health Insurance: Who Benefits and at What Cost?* (Robert Wood Johnson Foundation, 2009), http://www.urban.org/UploadedPDF/1001297_tax_subsidies.pdf.

11. Congressional Budget Office, "Nonprofit Hospitals and the Provision of Community Benefits" (2006), 3, http://www.cbo.gov/ftpdocs/76xx/doc7695/12-06-Nonprofit.pdf.

12. Steffie Woolhandler and David U. Himmelstein, "Paying for National Health Insurance—And Not Getting It," *Health Affairs* 21, no. 4 (July 2002): 88–98.

13. Centers for Medicare and Medicaid Services, "National Health Expenditure Projections 2011–2021: Forecast Summary," http://www.cms.gov/Research-Statistics-Data-and-Systems/Statistics-Trends-and-Reports/NationalHealthExpendData/Downloads/Proj2011PDF.pdf.

14. From 1980 to 2006, the number of home health agencies increased from 2,924 to 8,618, outpatient physical therapy providers from 419 to 3,009, and portable x-ray providers from 216 to 549. Between 1985 and 2004, the number of ambulatory surgery centers certified to provide services under Medicare grew from 336 to 4,136, of home health agencies from 5,679 to 7,519, of outpatient physical therapy providers from 854 to 2,971, of portable x-ray services from 308 to 608, and of hospice providers from 164 to 2,645. National Center for Health Statistics, Health, "Health, United States 2011," table 118.

15. An example of the view that government oversight and private enterprise represent a dichotomy composed of opposing sides is an analysis of the regulation of prescription drugs by the Food and Drug Administration by Richard Epstein, who believes that overregulation is stifling innovation. Richard A. Epstein, *Overdose: How Excessive Government Regulation Stifles Pharmaceutical Innovation* (New Haven, CT: Yale University Press, 2008).

16. The view that government intervention is a force external to the market that holds back the health care industry is presented by Michael F. Cannon. Michael F. Cannon, *Health Competition: What's Holding Back Health Care and How to Free It* (Washington, DC: Cato Institute, 2005).

17. Jennifer Jenson, *Government Spending on Health Care Benefits and Programs: A Data Brief* (Congressional Research Service, 2008), 2.

18. Congressional Budget Office, "The Health Care System for Veterans: An Interim Report" (2007), http://www.cbo.gov/sites/default/files/cbofiles/ftpdocs/88xx/doc8892/12-21-va_healthcare.pdf.

19. Lloyd J. Mercer, *Railroads and Land Grant Policy: A Study in Government Intervention* (Washington, DC: Beard Books 1982).

20. Ibid.

21. A comprehensive account of the railroad land grant program describes the government's role this way: "The nineteenth-century railroad land grants are frequently viewed and evaluated as a simple matter of governmental gifts to business. In fact, the railroad land grant policy is a good example of active government intervention in the operation of the market. What happened in the economy and to particular railroads was determined to a significant extent by this intervention, rather than simply by the working of the market. The rate of growth achieved by the national economy and by particular regions, and the very existence of some railroads, was to some extent a product of the railroad land grants". Ibid., 2.

22. Janet Abbate, *Inventing the Internet* (Cambridge, MA: MIT Press, 2000). The history of the Internet is also presented as a timeline on various websites. For example, see Dave Kristula, "The History of the Internet," http://www.davesite.com/webstation/net-history.shtml.

23. Dave Kristula, "The History of the Internet."

24. Miniwatts Marketing Group, "Internet Growth Statistics," January 2008, http://www.internetworldstats.com/emarketing.htm.

25. BNEt Business Network, "Computer Industry Almanac: 25-Years PC Anniversary Statistics; IBM-Compatible PC Sales Have Topped 1.5B Units with $B 3,100 Value," August 14, 2006, http://www.thefreelibrary.com/Computer+Industry+Almanac%3A+25-Years+PC+Anniversary+Statistics%3B...-a0149450229.

26. Betty W. Su, "Monthly Labor Review, The U.S. Economy to 2010" (US Department of Labor, 2001), http://www.bls.gov/opub/mlr/2001/11/art1full.pdf.

27. "Automobile Popularity: Crowds View the Horseless Vehicles in the Big Garden," *New York Times*, January 21, 1903, 10 (reporting on the tremendous and growing public interest in automobiles).

28. "The Automobile Shapes the Suburbs," America on the Move, http://amhistory. si.edu/onthemove/exhibition/exhibition_15_2.html.

29. "Urbanization of America, Move to Suburbia," Countries Quest, http://www. countriesquest.com/north_america/usa/people/urbanization_of_america/move_to_suburbia.htm.

30. American Association of State Highway and Transportation Officials, "The Interstate is 50," http://www.interstate50th.org/index.shtml.

31. American Association of State Highway and Transportation Officials, "The Interstate is 50—History," http://www.interstate50th.org/history.shtml.

32. Ibid.

33. Ibid.

34. US Department of Transportation, "Research and Innovative Technology Administration, Bureau of Transportation Statistics, National Transportation Statistics 2000" (April 2000), Table 1–9—Number of US Aircraft, Vehicles, Vessels, and Other Conveyances, http://www.rita.dot.gov/bts/sites/rita.dot.gov.bts/files/publications/national_transportation_statistics/2000/index.html.

35. "Making the Long Haul: A History of the Truck and Trucking Industry," July 14, 2008, http://www.randomhistory.com/2008/07/14_truck.html.

36. University of California at Berkeley Traffic Safety Center, "From the Battlefield to the Soccer Field: The History of the SUV as a Tragedy of the Commons," *Traffic Safety Center Newsletter* 2, no. 4 (2005); Stacey C. Davis and Lorena F. Truett, *An Analysis of the Impact of the Sport Utility Vehicles in the United States* (Oak Ridge, TN: Oak Ridge National Laboratory, 2000).

37. US Department of Transportation, "Research and Innovative Technology Administration, Bureau of Transportation Statistics," National Transportation Statistics 2007, http://www.rita.dot.gov/bts/sites/rita.dot.gov.bts/files/publications/national_transportation_statistics/2007/index.html, table 2-1 Transportation Fatalities by Mode and table 2-3 Transportation Accidents by Mode.

38. The early history of the telecommunications industry is described in Paul Starr, *The Creation of the Media* (New York: Basic Books, 2004).

39. US Census Bureau, *Statistical Abstract of the United States: 1891 edition* (1891; reprint, *Statistical Abstract of the United States: 2006*, Washington, DC: US Government Printing Office, 2006), 730.

40. Helen Gavaghan, *Something New Under the Sun: Satellites and the Beginning of the Space Age* (New York: Springer, 1998).

41. "Electronics: The Room-Size World," *Time*, May 14, 1965, http://www.time.com/time/magazine/article/0,9171,898835,00.html.

42. Benjamin M. Compaine, *Size and Growth Trends of the Information Industry, 1970–1983*, Program on Information Resources Policy, Center for Information Policy Research, Harvard University (Cambridge, MA, 1986).

43. US Census Bureau, *Annual Survey of Communication Services—1998* (Washington, DC: US Government Printing Office, 1999), 1.

44. US Census Bureau. *Statistical Abstract of the United States: 1999* (Washington, DC: US Government Printing Office, 1999), 581.

45. David Wessel, "Housing Passes a Milestone," *Wall Street Journal*, July 11, 2012, http://online.wsj.com/article/SB10001424052702303644004577520414196790098.html.

46. "What Are the Origins of Freddie Mac and Fannie Mae?" George Mason University's History News Network, September 18, 2008, http://hnn.us/articles/1849.html.

47. James R. Hagerty, "Fannie Mae Reports Drop in Mortgage Holdings," *The Wall Street Journal*, December 5, 2007, http://online.wsj.com/article/SB119686009925114403.html.

48. Ibid.

49. "Our Mission," Freddie Mac, http://www.freddiemac.com/corporate/company_profile/.

50. "Making Home Possible in the United States," Freddie Mac, 2009, http://www.freddiemac.com/corporate/about/pdf/United_States.pdf.

51. Ibid.

52. Roger Lowenstein, "Who Needs the Mortgage-Interest Deduction?" *New York Times*, March 5, 2006, http://www.nytimes.com/2006/03/05/magazine/305deduction.1.html?pagewanted=print&_r=0. The tax deduction for mortgage interest was never crafted as an explicit policy. It grew out of the structure of the federal income tax code, which dates to 1913. Interest on loans was considered a legitimate business expense that could be deducted from earnings, and this principle was applied to interest paid by individuals, as well. At the time, few Americans owned homes, and interest on consumer loans was rare, so the deduction was worth very little to most people. However, as home ownership and the use of mortgages as a financing vehicle grew over subsequent decades, it became an important, and expensive, economic incentive program.

53. US Census Bureau, "The 2009 Statistical Abstract," table 927—New Privately Owned Housing Units Started—Selected Characteristics, http://www.census.gov/compendia/statab/cats/construction_housing.html.

54. Ibid., table 940—Total Housing Inventory for the United States, http://www.census.gov/compendia/statab/cats/construction_housing.html.

55. Ibid., table 964—Value of Private Construction Put in Place: 2000 to 2010, http://www.census.gov/compendia/statab/cats/construction_housing.html.

56. Karl E. Case, Ray C. Fair, and Sharon C. Oster, *Principles of Economics*, 10th ed. (New York: Prentice Hall, 2011), 40.

57. N. Gregory Mankiw, *Principles of Economics*, 6th ed. (Mason, OH: South-Western Cengage Learning, 2011), 10.

58. Paul Krugman and Robin Wells, *Microeconomics*, 3rd ed. (New York: Worth Publishers, Inc., 2012), 2.

59. Oxford English Dictionary, http://oxforddictionaries.com/us/definition/american_english/free%2Bmarket?q=free+market.

60. Merriam-Webster Dictionary, http://www.merriam-webster.com/dictionary/free%20market.

61. Smith, *An Inquiry*.

62. Robert B. Ekelund, Rand W. Ressler, and Robert D. Tollison, *Economics: Private Markets and Public Choice* (New York: Pearson, 2006), 108.

63. Gavin Kennedy, "Adam Smith and the Role of Government," *Economist's View*, 2010, http://economistsview.typepad.com/economistsview/2010/03/adam-smith-and-the-role-of-government.html.

64. United States Constitution, article I, section 8.

65. Milton Friedman, *Capitalism and Freedom* (Chicago: University of Chicago Press, 2002), 15. Friedman also saw the judicial system as essential to maintaining an orderly market. It enforces standards of fair dealing, which ensures trust in the system that makes business transactions possible, for example by penalizing, and thereby deterring, practices such as deceptive advertising, manufacture of defective products, and provision of deficient services.

66. Daniel Carpenter, *Reputation and Power: Organizational Image and Pharmaceutical Regulation at the FDA* (Princeton, NJ: Princeton University Press, 2010), 12.

67. Lucy Madison, "Elizabeth Warren: 'There Is Nobody in this Country Who Got Rich on His Own,'" *CBS News*, September 22, 2011, http://www.cbsnews.com/8301-503544_162-20110042-503544.html.

68. Stephen Breyer, *Regulation and Its Reform* (Cambridge, MA: Harvard University Press, 1984).

69. Joseph E. Stiglitz, *Globalization and Its Discontents* (New York: W.W. Norton, 2003), 54.

Chapter 2

1. Paul Starr, *The Social Transformation of American Medicine* (New York: Basic Books, 1982), 8.

2. Data on relative profitability is available at "Fortune 500, Top Industries: Most Profitable (2008)," *CNN Money*, http://money.cnn.com/magazines/fortune/fortune500/2008/performers/industries/profits/. Data on the rate of return is discussed in Uwe E. Reinhardt, "Perspectives on the Pharmaceutical Industry," *Health Affairs* 20, No. 5 (2001): 136–49.

3. National Institutes of Health, "About NIH," http://www.nih.gov/about/.

4. Victoria A. Harden, "A Short History of the National Institutes of Health," National Institutes of Health Office of NIH History, http://history.nih.gov/exhibits/history/index.html.

5. National Institutes of Health, "NIH Budget," September 18, 2012, http://www.nih.gov/about/budget.htm.

6. National Institutes of Health, "The NIH Almanac—Appropriations," June 6, 2008, http://www.nih.gov/about/almanac/appropriations/part2.htm.

7. National Institutes of Health, "About NIH," http://www.nih.gov/about/.

8. Government Patent Policy Act of 1980, 35 U.S.C. §§202, 210.

9. National Research Act of 1974, 42 U.S.C. §§201, 218.

10. The effects of NIH funding on medical progress in the United States are discussed in National Institutes of Health, "About NIH," http://www.nih.gov/about/.

11. Although overall life expectancy in the United States increased dramatically over the course of the twentieth century, it is still lower than that in several other industrialized countries, including France, Japan, and Iceland. This has led to speculation that the health care delivery system in each country may play an important role in determining life expectancy, in addition to the role of scientific progress. Comparative trends in life expectancy across countries are discussed in World Health Organization, *World Health Report 2000—Health Systems: Improving Performance* (Geneva: World Health Organization, 2000).

12. US Government Accountability Office, "New Drug Development: Science, Business, Regulatory, and Intellectual Property Issues Cited as Hampering Drug Development Efforts," Report GAO 07-49, 2006, http://www.gao.gov/new.items/d0749.pdf.

13. Pharmaceutical Research and Manufacturers of America, "Medicines in Development," http://www.phrma.org/research/new-medicines.

14. Orphan Drug Act, 21 U.S.C. §§360aa et seq.

15. The Act authorized grants, tax credits, and seven years of additional market exclusivity beyond a patent's expiration for drugs that are developed for rare conditions. Food and Drug Administration, "Orphan Products: New Hope for People with Rare Disorders," http://www.fda.gov/Drugs/ResourcesForYou/Consumers/ucm143563.htm. These are defined as ailments that afflict 200,000 people or fewer in the United States. This includes more than 7,000 conditions that together affect more than 25 million people. National Organization for Rare Diseases, "Research Grant Policy," http://www.rarediseases.org/medical-professionals/research-grants/policy.

16. Food and Drug Administration, "Developing Orphan Products: FDA and Rare Disease Day" (February 27, 2009), http://www.fda.gov/downloads/ForConsumers/ConsumerUpdates/ucm107301.pdf.

17. See Carpenter, *Reputation and Power*.

18. It is possible that, in the absence of government drug safety regulation, the industry might have developed its own standard-setting and enforcement mechanism. There is precedent for this in the American National Standards Institute (ANSI), which sets standards for manufacturing and production in a range of industries, and Underwriters Laboratories, which sets safety standards for products and tests them for compliance. However, legal sanctions are not available to private bodies such as these to enforce compliance, such as levying fines, impounding defective products, and prohibiting the sale of unsafe goods. With dangerous drugs presenting clear risks to life and health, it is therefore unlikely that a nongovernmental oversight mechanism could function as effectively as a government agency and thereby engender the same level of public trust in the industry's products.

19. Pure Food and Drug Act of 1906, Ch. 3915, 34 Stat. 768 (1906).

20. Food, Drug and Cosmetic Act of 1938, 21 U.S.C. §355(c) (1938).

21. Kefauver-Harris Amendments of 1962, P.L. 87–781, 76 Stat. 780 (1962).

22. Food and Drug Amendments Act of 2007, P.L. 110–85 (2007) (codified at 21 U.S.C. §§301 et seq.).

23. The cumulative effect of these laws is that new drugs often take more than 10 years to reach market from the time they are first developed in a laboratory. Beginning with in vitro testing in test tubes and petri dishes, therapeutic candidates must be tried in animals before they reach even their first human subjects. Once approval to administer a drug to humans is obtained from the FDA in the form of an investigational new drug exemption (IND), it is tested in three phases involving progressively more subjects and more detailed analyses of effects. At the end of this process, data from all of these studies are submitted to the FDA in the form of a new drug application (NDA). If approved, the drug can only be marketed for specified conditions and symptoms, with clear warnings of possible risks. Publicity material is also subject to prior approval. After marketing, the FDA continues to compile data on drug safety with an eye to requiring stricter warnings or even withdrawal from the market if unacceptable hazards are found.

24. Janet Lundy, "Prescription Drug Trends" (Kaiser Family Foundation, 2010), 4, http://www.kff.org/rxdrugs/upload/3057-08.pdf.

25. IMS Health, "IMS Health Reports U.S. Prescription Sales Grew 5.1 Percent in 2009, to $300.3 Billion," *Bloomberg*, April 1, 2010, http://www.bloomberg.com/apps/news?pid=newsarchive&sid=au5OPQhtu2bI.

26. IMS Health, "IMS Forecasts Global Pharmaceutical Market Growth of 5–8% Annually through 2014; Maintains Expectations of 4–6% Growth in 2010," April 20, 2010, http://www.imshealth.com/portal/site/ims/menuitem.d248e29c86589c9c30e81c033208c2 2a/?vgnextoid=4b8c410b6c718210VgnVCM100000ed152ca2RCRD.

27. Paul Starr, *The Social Transformation*, 150.

28. The formal name of the law is the Hospital Survey and Construction Act of 1946, P.L. 79–725, 42 U.S.C. §§ 291 et seq. (1946).

29. Starr, *The Social Transformation*, 350.

30. Claudia Haglund and William Dowling, "The Hospital," in *Introduction to Health Services*, 4th ed., eds. Stephen J. Williams and Paul R. Torrens (New York: Delmar Publishers, 1993), 135–76.

31. Although the Hill-Burton Act outlawed racial discrimination by hospitals that received funds, until 1963, hospitals in the South were permitted to meet the nondiscrimination requirement by providing racially segregated services that were of equal quality. This was a vestige of the doctrine of "separate but equal" that had permitted states to maintain segregated public facilities, including schools, but that was overturned by the Supreme Court in 1954 in the case of *Brown v. Board of Education*, 347 U.S. 483 (1954).

32. Congressional Budget Office, "Medicare—March 2012 Baseline" (March 13, 2012), http://www.cbo.gov/sites/default/files/cbofiles/attachments/43060_Medicare.pdf.

33. Ibid.

34. National Center for Health Statistics, "Health, United States, 2011," 376, table 129.

35. Brian M. Kinkead, "Medicare Payment and Hospital Capital: The Evolution of Policy," *Health Affairs* 3, no. 3 (Fall 1984): 49–74.

36. In some states, such as Pennsylvania and Utah, extension of the federal tax exemption to state and local taxes, such as real estate and sale taxes, is not automatic. Hospitals must prove that they actually serve a charitable function in their communities. However, most nonprofit hospitals are successfully able to prove their case, thereby qualifying for the full range of tax-exempt benefits.

37. Internal Revenue Service, "Requirements for Exemption," http://www.irs.gov/ Charities-&-Non-Profits/Other-Non-Profits/Requirements-for-Exemption. See also the discussion in Robert Field, *Health Care Regulation in America: Complexity, Confrontation and Compromise* (New York: Oxford University Press, 2007), 189–97.

38. Congressional Budget Office, "Nonprofit Hospitals and the Provision of Community Benefits" (December 6, 2006), 3, http://www.cbo.gov/ftpdocs/76xx/doc7695/12-06-Nonprofit.pdf.

39. National Center for Health Statistics, "Health, United States, 2006" (Washington, DC: US Government Printing Office, 2006), 392, table 130—Hospital expenses, by type of ownership and size of hospital: United States, selected years, http://www.cdc.gov/nchs/ data/hus/hus06.pdf.

40. Kinkead, "Medicare Payment and Hospital Capital."

41. Ibid.

42. The federal law mandating that states adopt certificate-of-need programs was the National Health Planning and Resources Development Act of 1974, P.L. 93–641, 88 Stat. 2225 (1975), codified at 42 U.S.C. subchapter XII sec. 300K et seq. and 42 U.S.C. subchapter XIV sec. 3000 et seq.

43. Patrick John McGinley, "Beyond Health Care Reform: Reconsidering Certificate of Need Laws in a Managed Competition System," *Florida State University Law Review* 23, no. 1 (1995): 141–88.

44. The evolution of the status of the medical profession is discussed in Starr, *The Social Transformation*, 60–144.

45. Abraham Flexner, *Medical Education in the United States and Canada: A Report to the Carnegie Foundation for the Advancement of Teaching* (New York: Carnegie Foundation for the Advancement of Teaching, 1910).

46. See discussion in Starr, *The Social Transformation*, 102–12.

47. See discussion in Field, *Health Care Regulation*, 26.

48. The law that implemented this funding was the Higher Education Act of 1965, P.L. 89–329, 79 Stat. 1219 (1965), portions codified at 20 U.S.C. §1088.

49. Starr, *The Social Transformation*, 421.

50. Robert L. Phillips, Jr. et al., "COGME's 16th Report to Congress: Too Many Physicians Could Be Worse Than Wasted," *Annals of Family Medicine* 3 (2005): 268–70.

51. Aaron Young et al., "A Census of Actively Licensed Physicians in the United States, 2010," *Journal of Medical Regulation* 96, no. 4 (2011): 10–20.

52. Richard A. Cooper, "Medical Schools and Their Applicants: An Analysis," *Health Affairs* 22, no. 4 (July 2003): 71–84.

53. Congressional Budget Office, "Medicare—March 2012 Baseline" (March 13, 2012), http://www.cbo.gov/sites/default/files/cbofiles/attachments/43060_Medicare.pdf.

54. Kaiser Family Foundation, "Total Number of Medicare Beneficiaries, 2011," http://www.statehealthfacts.org/comparemaptable.jsp?yr=200&typ=1&ind=290&cat=6&sub=74.

55. Ibid.

56. The Balanced Budget Act of 1997 implemented substantial cuts to Medicare reimbursement, some of which targeted the size of graduate medical education payments to hospitals. This created a significant financial challenge for many teaching hospitals, which depend on these payments to maintain physician training programs. *The Balanced Budget Act of 1997: A Look at the Current Impact on Providers and Patients: Hearing Before the Subcommittee on Health and Environment of the Committee on Commerce* (Washington, DC: US Government Printing Office, 2000).

57. Rick Mayes, "The Origins, Development, and Passage of Medicare's Revolutionary Prospective Payment System," *Journal of Medicine and Allied Sciences*, 21, no. 1 (2007): 21–55.

58. Shelah Leader and Marilyn Moon, "Medicare Tends in Ambulatory Surgery," *Health Affairs* 8, no.1 (1989): 158–70.

59. See William C. Hsiao et al., "Resource-Based Relative Values: An Overview," *Journal of the American Medical Association* 260, no. 16 (1988): 2347–53.

60. John D. Goodman, "Unintended Consequences of Resource-Based Relative Scale Reimbursement," *Journal of the American Medical Association* 298, no. 19 (2007): 2308–10.

61. Gregory C. Pope and John E. Schneider, "Trends in Physician Income," *Health Affairs* 11, no. 1 (Spring 1992): 181–93.

62. Congressional Budget Office, "Estimates for the Insurance Coverage Provisions of the Affordable Care Act Updated for the Recent Supreme Court Decision" (2012), 20.

63. The creation of early health insurance plans is described in Starr, *The Social Transformation*, 295–310.

64. Ibid., 297.

65. Ibid., 311.

66. 26 U.S.C. § 3121.

67. Kaiser Family Foundation, "Update on Individual Health Insurance" (August 2004), 1, http://www.kff.org/insurance/upload/Update-on-Individual-Health-Insurance.pdf.

68. For a discussion of the significance of the tax subsidy for employment-based insurance for overall health care finance, see Woolhandler and Himmelfarb, "Paying for National Health Insurance."

69. Thomas M. Selden and Bradley M. Gray, "Tax Subsidies for Employment-Related Health Insurance: Estimates for 2006," *Health Affairs* 25, no. 6 (2006): 1568–79.

70. Ibid.

71. Employee Retirement Income Security Act, 29 U.S.C. §1144.

72. See Jana K. Strain and Eleanor D. Kinney, "The Road Paved with Good Intentions: Problems and Potential for Employer-Sponsored Health Insurance Under ERISA," *Loyola University of Chicago Law Journal* 31, no. 1 (1999): 29–68.

73. For a discussion of the history and structure of HMOs, see Anthony R. Kovner, "Health Maintenance Organizations and Managed Care," in *Health Care Delivery in the United States*, 6th ed., eds. Anthony R. Kovner and Steven Jonas (New York: Springer, 1999), 280–300.

74. Field, *Health Care Regulation*, 78.

75. Starr, *The Social Transformation*, 393–405.

76. 42 U.S.C. §§280c, 300c, et seq.

77. See the discussion in Allen Dobson, Donald Moran, and Gary Young, "The Role of Federal Waivers in the Health Policy Process," *Health Affairs* 11, no. 4 (1992): 72–94. See also Field, *Health Care Regulation*, 105–06.

78. Balanced Budget Act of 1997, P.L. 105–33, 111 Stat. 251 (1997).

79. Medicare Prescription Drug, Improvement and Modernization Act of 2003, P.L. 108–173, 117 Stat. 2066, codified at 42 U.S.C. §1395.

80. Martin Markovich, "The Rise of HMOs" (Rand Corporation, March 2003), http://www.rand.org/publications/RGSD/RGSD172?index.html.

81. Jon B. Christianson et al., "The HMO Industry: Evolution in Population Demographics and Market Structure," *Medical Care Review* 48, no. 1 (1991): 3–46.

82. Gary Claxton et al., "Health Benefits in 2007: Premium Increases Fall to an Eight-Year Low, While Offer Rates and Enrollment Remain Stable," *Health Affairs* 26, no. 5 (September/October 2007): 1407–16.

83. Andrea Sisko et al., "Health Spending Projections Through 2018: Recession Effects Add Uncertainty to the Outlook," *Health Affairs*, web exclusive (February 24, 2009): w346–w357. http://content.healthaffairs.org/content/28/2/w346.full.

84. Sean P. Keehan et al., "National Health Expenditure Projections: Modest Annual Growth Until Coverage Expands and Economic Growth Accelerates," *Health Affairs* 31, no. 1 (July 2012): 1600–12.

85. Kaiser Family Foundation, "Trends and Indicators in the Changing Health Care Marketplace," February 8, 2006, Section 5—Structure of the Health Care Marketplace, exhibit 5.1—Health Care Employment and Share of Total Non-Farm Employment, 1990–2005p, http://www.kff.org/insurance/7031/ti2004-5-set.cfm.

86. National Institutes of Health, "NIH Awards by State of Recipient, Fiscal Year 2005," http://report.nih.gov/award/index.cfm?ot=&fy=2005&state=&ic=&fm=&orgid=&distr=&rfa=&om=n&pid=#tab1. Detailed data on NIH funding by state and by region within each state for fiscal years 2005–2011 are available at http://heart.org/HEARTORG/General/State-by-state-NIH-Allocations_UCM_440585_Article.jsp.

87. Michael Mandel and Joseph Weber, "What's Really Propping Up the Economy?" *BusinessWeek Online*, September 25, 2006, http://www.businessweek.com/magazine/content/06_39/b4002001.htm.

88. Michael E. Kanell, "During a Recession, Some Jobs Survive—and Thrive," *Atlanta Journal Constitution*, December 12, 2010, http://www.ajc.com/news/business/during-a-recession-some-jobs-survive-and-thrive/nQnqf/.

89. The relationship of the Obama health reform effort to past efforts is discussed in James A. Marone, "Presidents and Health Reform: From Franklin D. Roosevelt to Barack Obama," *Health Affairs* 29, no. 6 (2010): 1096–1100. The alliances that Obama forged with various industry groups to gain passage of his health reform plan are discussed in Jonathan Oberlander, "Long Time Coming: Why Health Reform Finally Passed," *Health Affairs* 29, no. 6 (2010): 1112–16.

90. The World Health Organization, *The World Health Report 2000*.

91. The Dartmouth Institute for Health Policy and Clinical Practice, "Dartmouth Atlas of Health Care," http://www.dartmouthatlas.org/.

92. Institute of Medicine, *To Err Is Human: Building a Safer Health System,* eds. Linda T. Kohn, Janet M. Corrigan, and Molla S. Donaldson (Washington, DC: National Academy Press, 1999).

93. The World Health Organization, *The World Health Report 2000*.

94. One of the few penalties that hospitals face is contained in a provision of the Affordable Care Act (sec. 3025) that discourages the premature discharge of patients. It authorizes the Medicare program to impose financial penalties on hospitals that readmit excessive numbers of patients for the same condition that caused the initial hospitalization. Although this provision applies to a limited range of quality lapses, advocates of more stringent quality control believe it could be used as a model for mechanisms to disincentivize other kinds of substandard care. The provision is discussed at Centers for Medicare & Medicaid Services, "Readmission Reduction Program" (2013), http://www.cms.gov/Medicare/Medicare-Fee-for-Service-Payment/AcuteInpatientPPS/Readmissions-Reduction-Program.html.

95. David M. Studdert, Michelle M. Mello, and Troyen A. Brennan, "Medical Malpractice," *New England Journal of Medicine* 350, no. 3 (January 2014): 283–92.

96. Patient Protection and Affordable Care Act, P.L. 111–148, 124 Stat. 119 through 124 Stat. 1025.

Chapter 3

1. Alan Rappeport, "Drug Companies and Scientists Ire Over Budget Cuts," *The Financial Times*, March 16, 2011, http://www.ft.com/intl/cms/s/0/7b3df6d2-4a4c-11e0-b802-00144feab49a.html#axzz2aoygXcoJ.

2. Ibid.

3. Benjamin Zycher, Joseph A. DiMasi, and Christopher-Paul Milne, "Private Sector Contributions to Pharmaceutical Science: Thirty-Five Summary Case Histories," *American Journal of Therapeutics* 17, no. 1 (2010): 101–20. In this study, the authors seek to demonstrate the value of industry research and development in bringing important new drugs to patients, but they begin their analysis by observing that, "the importance of government-funded research, particularly in terms of the science of disease processes and applications to pharmacologic advances, is not in dispute."

4. Ibid.

5. Iain M. Cockburn and Rebecca M. Henderson, "Absorptive Capacity, Coauthoring Behavior, and the Organization of Research in Drug Discovery," *The Journal of Industrial Economics* 46, no. 2 (1998): 157–82.

6. For information on Medicare Part D spending, see Kaiser Family Foundation, "Medicare Spending and Financing Fact Sheet" (August 2010), http://www.kff.org/medicare/upload/7305-05.pdf. For information on Medicare Part B, see Medicare Payment Advisory Commission, "A Data Book: Healthcare Spending and the Medicare Program" (June 2010), www.medpac.gov/documents/jun10databookentirereport.pdf.

7. John Holahan et al., "Medicaid Spending Growth over the Last Decade and the Great Recession 2000–2009" (Kaiser Family Foundation, February 2011), www.kff.org/medicaid/upload/8152.pdf.

8. Drug Price Competition and Patent Term Restoration Act, P.L. 98–417, 1984 Stat. 1538 (codified as amended in scattered sections of 21 and 35 U.S.C.).

9. Food and Drug Administration Modernization Act of 1997, P.L. 105–115, 111 Stat. 2296.

10. See, for example, Donald W. Light and Joel R. Lexchin, "Pharmaceutical Research and Development: What Do We Get for All That Money?," *British Medical Journal* 344 (August 7, 2012): e4348–e4353.

11. Matthew Herper, "The First Drug with a $1 Million Price Tag May Already Be on the Market," *Forbes*, May 1, 2012, http://www.forbes.com/sites/matthewherper/2012/05/01/the-first-drug-with-a-1-million-price-tag-is-already-on-the-market/.

12. Kaiser Family Foundation, "Trends and Indicators in the Changing Health Care Marketplace," February 8, 2006, http://www.kff.org/insurance/7031/ti2004-1-21.cfm.

13. IMS Health, "IMS Health Reports."

14. IMS Health, "IMS Forecasts."

15. The appropriate accounting for pharmaceutical profitability is somewhat controversial. Some analysts believe that the treatment of research and development costs in standard assessments is incorrect. They contend that it should be treated as an investment subject to depreciation rather than an expense. This approach generates much lower rates of profits in comparison to assets. Nevertheless, the resulting profitability is still consistently higher than the average for all American industries. F. M. Scherer, "The Pharmaceutical Industry— Prices and Progress," *New England Journal of Medicine* 351, no. 9 (August 26, 2004): 927–32.

16. Ibid.

17. Congressional Budget Office, "Research and Development in the Pharmaceutical Industry" (October 2006), http://www.cbo.gov/ftpdocs/76xx/doc7615/10-02-DrugR-D.pdf.

18. Ibid.

19. Ibid.

20. Pharmaceutical Research and Manufacturers of America, "About PhRMA," http://www.phrma.org/about/phrma.

21. Congressional Budget Office, "Research and Development," 7.

22. Ibid., 14.

23. National Institutes of Health, "NIH Budget," http://www.nih.gov/about/budget.htm.

24. Andrew A. Toole, *The Impact of Public Basic Research on Industrial Innovation: Evidence from the Pharmaceutical Industry* (Stanford, CA: Stanford Institute for Economic Policy Research, November 2000), http://www.stanford.edu/group/siepr/cgi-bin/siepr/?q=system/files/shared/pubs/papers/pdf/00-07.pdf.

25. Iain M. Cockburn and Rebecca M. Henderson, "Publicly Funded Science and the Productivity of the Pharmaceutical Industry," in *Innovation Policy and the Economy, vol. 1*, eds. Adam B. Jaffe, Josh Lerner, and Scott Stern, National Bureau of Economic Research (Cambridge, MA: MIT Press, 2001), http://www.nber.org/chapters/c10775.pdf.

26. Victoria A. Harding, "A Short History of the National Institutes of Health," National Institutes of Health Office of NIH History, 2005, http://history.nih.gov/exhibits/history/index.html.

27. Ibid.

28. Victoria A. Harding, *Inventing the NIH: Federal Biomedical Research Policy, 1887–1937* (Baltimore, MD: Johns Hopkins University Press, 1986), 3.

29. Victoria A. Harding, "A Short History of the National Institutes of Health: WW I and the Randsdell Act of 1930," National Institutes of Health Office of NIH History, 2005, http://history.nih.gov/exhibits/history/docs/page_04.html.

30. Ransdell Act, P.L. 71–251, 46 Stat. 379 (1930).

31. Harding, "A Short History of the National Institutes of Health."

32. Franklin D. Roosevelt, "The Dedication of the National Institutes of Health," *Clinical Research* 36, no. 1 (1988): 1–2.

33. Judith Robinson, *Noble Conspirators: Florence S. Mahoney and the Rise of the National Institutes of Health* (Washington, D.C.: Francis Press, 2001), 59.

34. Ibid.

35. Public Health Service Act, 42 U.S.C. §§ 201 et. seq.

36. National Institutes of Health, "NIH Almanac, Appropriations (Section 2)," 2012, http://www.nih.gov/about/almanac/appropriations/part2.htm.

37. James A. Shannon, "The Advancement of Medical Research: A Twenty-Year View of the Role of the National Institutes of Health," *Academic Medicine* 42, no. 2 (1967): 97–108, 103.

38. The growth of NIH in response to concerns about specific diseases is described in Field, *Health Care Regulation,* 213.

39. Richard B. Thompson, "Foundations for Blockbuster Drugs in Federally Sponsored Research," *The FASEB Journal* 15 (2001): 1671–76.

40. Ibid.

41. Gil Ben-Menachem, Steven M. Ferguson, and Krishna Balakrishnan, "Doing Business with the NIH," *National Biotechnology* 24, no. 1 (2006): 17–20.

42. *Diamond v. Chakrabarty,* 447 U.S. 303 (1980).

43. Patent and Trademark Law Amendment Act of 1980, P.L. 96-517.

44. Patents are occasionally used defensively to prevent competitors from manufacturing an invention while the inventor decides whether it is worthwhile to take it to market. To avoid such possible misuse of the Act's benefits, it contains a "march-in" provision that gives NIH the ability to circumvent a patent when a product is potentially life-saving. That provision has been rarely used, but it remains a check on potential abuses.

45. Stevenson-Wydler Technology Innovation Act of 1980, P.L. 96-480 (codified as amended at 15 U.S.C. §§ 3710 et seq.).

46. A description of the office can be found at NIH Office of Technology Transfer, "Science, Ideas, Breakthroughs," http://www.ott.nih.gov/licensing_royalties/royalties_administration.aspx.

47. Technology Transfer Act, P.L. 99-502.

48. *Diamond v. Chakrabarty,* 447 U.S. 303 (1980).

49. Although the patentability of artificially engineered genes was resolved by the *Chakrabarty* decision, the patentability of human genes had been unsettled since the early 1990s, when the US Patent and Trademark Office approved the first gene patent applications. Many observers attribute the rise of the genetic testing industry since then to the availability

of patents that grant companies the excusive right to use the genes involved for commercial purposes. Others contend that gene patents have stifled innovation by limiting access to genes for experimentation. The Supreme Court resolved the issue by invalidating patents on human genes in their natural form in its decision in *Association for Molecular Technology v. Myriad Genetics* (No. 12-398, US June 13, 2013). It is not clear whether the ruling will ultimately promote or constrict genomic research but it will nonetheless play a major role in determining the shape of all industries that rely on genetic technologies.

50. Richard H. Myers, "Huntington's Disease Genetics," *NeuroRx* 1, no. 2 (2004): 255–62.

51. Michael Abramowicz, "The Human Genome Project in Retrospect," *Advances in Genetics* 50 (2003): 231–61.

52. J. Craig Venter et al., "The Sequence of the Human Genome," *Science* 291, no. 5507 (2001): 1304–15.

53. National Human Genome Research Institute, "International Consortium Completes Human Genome Project," April 14, 2003, http://www.genome.gov/11006929.

54. Myriad's patents on the BRCA genes were invalidated along with all patents on naturally occurring human genes by the Supreme Court in the case of *Association for Molecular Pathology v. Myriad Genetics*, (No. 12-398, US June 13, 2013). However, Myriad is likely to continue to hold a dominant market position even without patent protection for the genes involved. As sole provider of the test for mutations in the genes, it has compiled a database with results for thousand of patients, which gives it a strong advantage over potential competitors.

55. J. J. Colao, "How a Breast Cancer Pioneer Finally Turned a Profit," *Forbes*, October 17, 2012, http://www.forbes.com/sites/jjcolao/2012/10/17/how-a-breast-cancer-pioneer-finally-turned-a-profit/.

56. Gautam Naik, "Report Touts Economic Impact of Gene Project," *Wall Street Journal*, May 11, 2011, http://online.wsj.com/article/SB10001424052748704681904576315253143162630.html.

57. Paul Basken, "Federal Spending on Science Pays Off, Analyses by Research Advocates Say," *The Chronicle of Higher Education*, May 10, 2011.

58. Margaret A. Hamburg and Frances S. Collins, "The Path to Personalized Medicine," *New England Journal of Medicine* 363 (2010): 301–304.

59. Kurt Samson, "New NIH Translational Research Center Plan Moves Forward: What It Could Mean for Neurology," *Neurology Today* 11, no. 7 (April 7, 2011): 39–43.

60. Francis S. Collins, "Reengineering Translational Science: The Time is Right," *Science Translational Medicine* 3, no. 90 (2011): 1–6, http://stm.sciencemag.org/content/3/90/90cm17.full?sid=73716974-dobf-49fc-af5e-1645f92e214f.

61. Elias A. Zerhouni, "Translational and Clinical Science—Time for a New Vision." *New England Journal of Medicine* 353, no. 15 (2005): 1621–23.

62. Francis Collins had previously served as director of the Human Genome Project.

63. Collins, "Reengineering Translational Science," 2.

64. National Center for Health Statistics, "Health, United States, 2010" (Washington, DC: US Government Printing Office, 2010), 372, Table 126, http://www.cdc.gov/nchs/data/hus/hus10.pdf.

65. Kaiser Family Foundation, "Health Care Costs: A Primer" (May 2012), 10–11 http://www.kff.org/insurance/upload/7670-03.pdf.

66. Kaiser Family Foundation, "Prescription Drug Trends, May 2010" (2010), http://www.kff.org/rxdrugs/upload/3057-08.pdf.

67. Ibid.

68. For example, Zaltrap, a prescription drug used to treat colorectal cancer after initial courses of treatment prove futile, initially cost $11,000 a month. "Incredible Prices for Cancer Drugs," *New York Times*, November 12, 2012, http://www.nytimes.com/2012/11/13/opinion/incredible-prices-for-cancer-drugs.html.

69. National Center for Health Statistics, "Health, United States, 2010," 372, table 126.

70. The regulation of health care professionals is described in Field, *Health Care Regulation*, 19–40.

71. Wallace Janssen, "The Story of the Law Behind the Labels," *FDA Consumer* 15, no. 5 (1981): 32–45.

72. Upton Sinclair, *The Jungle* (New York: Grosset & Dunlap, 1906).

73. The scandal involving elixir of sulfanilamide and its effect in promoting passage of enhanced drug safety legislation is described in Cynthia Crossen, "How Elixir Deaths Led U.S. to Require Proof of New Drugs' Safety," *Wall Street Journal*, October 3, 2005, B1. It is also chronicled in Carol Ballentine, "Taste of Raspberries, Taste of Death: The 1938 Elixir of Sulfanilamide Incident," *FDA Consumer* 31, no. 6 (1981), and Arthur Hull Hayes, "Food and Drug Regulation after 75 Years," *Journal of the American Medical Association* 246, no. 11 (1981): 1223–26.

74. Federal Food, Drug, and Cosmetic Act, 21 U.S.C. § 355c (1938).

75. The story of thalidomide and its effect in encouraging the passage of stricter drug safety legislation is told in Trent Stephens, *Dark Remedy: The Impact of Thalidomide and Its Revival as a Vital Medicine* (Cambridge, MA: Perseus, 2001).

76. Drug Amendments Act of 1962, P.L. 87-781, 76 Stat. 780 (1962).

77. A major incident in which the FDA failed to spot a serious drug safety hazard involved the arthritis drug Vioxx and attracted considerable attention in the media in 2004. Vioxx had been approved in 1999 based on an expedited review and was later found to increase the risk of heart attacks with long-term use. The episode is recounted in Alex Berenson, et al, "Despite Warnings, Drug Giant Took Long Path to Vioxx Recall," *New York Times*, November 14, 2004, http://www.nytimes.com/2004/11/14/business/14merck.html?_r=0. The public outcry that ensued led to passage of the Food and Drug Administration Amendments Act of 2007, P. L. 110-85, 121 Stat. 823, which strengthened FDA oversight of drugs after they reach the market.

78. Bara Vaida and Christopher Weaver, "Drug Lobby's Tax Filings Reveal Big Spending in Health Debate," *NPR.org, Shots* (2010), http://www.npr.org/blogs/health/2010/12/01/131731212/drug-lobby-s-tax-filings-reveal-big-spending-in-health-debate-role. The total amount of spending annually on lobbying by all pharmaceutical companies combined, including that of the industry's trade organization, Pharmaceutical Research & Manufacturers of America, exceeded $233 million in 2012, according to one estimate. See OpenSecrets.org, "Lobbying: Pharmaceuticals/Health Products" (2012), http://www.opensecrets.org/lobby/indusclient.php?id=H04&year=a.

79. See Peter Lurie et al., "Financial Conflicts of Interest Disclosure and Voting Patterns at Food and Drug Administration Drug Advisory Committee Meetings," *The Journal of the American Medical Association* 295, no. 16 (2006): 1921–28.

80. See Lynne Taylor, "FDA Processes 'Impede US Public Health, Investment, Innovation,'" *Pharma Times*, February 21, 2011, http://www.pharmatimes.com/article/11-02-21/FDA_processes_impede_US_public_health_investment_innovation.aspx.

81. See Daniel P. Carpenter, "The Political Economy of FDA Drug Review: Processing, Politics, and Lessons For Policy," *Health Affairs* 23, no. 1 (2004): 52–63.

82. Joshua M. Sharfstein, "The FDA—A Misunderstood Agency," *Journal of the American Medical Association* 306, no. 11 (2011): 1250–51.

83. Julie Appleby, "Poll: Confidence in FSA Still Strong Despite Blunders," *USA Today*, November 23, 2004, http://usatoday30.usatoday.com/news/health/2004-11-23-fda_x.htm.

84. See C.F. Larry Heimann, *Acceptable Risks: Politics, Policy, and Risky Technologies* (Ann Arbor, MI: University of Michigan Press, 1997), 63.

85. Drug Price Competition and Patent Term Restoration Act, P.L. 98-417, 1984 Stat. 1538 (codified as amended in scattered sections of 21 and 35 U.S.C.).

86. US Food and Drug Administration, "Facts About Generic Drugs," 2012, http://www.fda.gov/drugs/resourcesforyou/consumers/buyingusingmedicinesafely/understandinggenericdrugs/ucm167991.htm.

87. Orphan Drug Act, 21 U.S.C. §§ 360aa et seq. (1983).

88. US Food and Drug Administration, "Regulatory Information: Orphan Drug Act," 2011, http://www.fda.gov/RegulatoryInformation/Legislation/FederalFoodDrugandCosmeticActFDCAct/SignificantAmendmentstotheFDCAct/OrphanDrugAct/default.htm.

89. FDA Consumer Health Information, "Developing Orphan Products: FDA and Rare Disease Day," 1–2 (2009), http://www.fda.gov/downloads/ForConsumers/ConsumerUpdates/ucm107301.pdf.

90. Food and Drug Administration Modernization Act of 1997, P.L. 105-115, 111 Stat. 2296.

91. These laws are the Best Pharmaceuticals for Children Act of 2002, P.L. 107-109 and the Pediatric Research Equity Act of 2003, P.L. 108-155. FDA efforts to encourage the development and testing of pediatric drugs are described in Susan Thaul, "FDA's Authority to Ensure that Drugs Prescribed to Children Are Safe and Effective," Congressional Research Service, 7-5700, RL33986 (2012), http://www.fas.org/sgp/crs/misc/RL33986.pdf.

92. Robert Steinbrook, "Testing Medications in Children," *New England Journal of Medicine* 347, no. 18 (2002): 1462–70.

93. Hamburg and Collins, "The Path to Personalized Medicine."

94. Ibid., 304.

95. Kenneth C. Whang, "The Applicability of Tax Credits to Medial Research and Development," American Association for the Advancement of Science, http://www.aaas.org/spp/cstc/pne/pubs/fundscience/papers/whang.htm.

96. Laura Tyson and Greg Linden, "The Corporate R&D Tax Credit and U.S. Innovation and Competitiveness," Center for American Progress (2012), http://www.americanprogress.org/issues/2012/01/pdf/corporate_r_and_d.pdf.

97. Drug companies do not have the option, as do manufacturers in some other industries, of protecting product information as trade secrets because key data on drugs must be disclosed to the FDA during the approval process.

98. United States Constitution, The Patent Copyright Clause, article 1, section 8.

99. Roswell Quinn, "Rethinking Antibiotic Research and Development: World War II and the Penicillin Collaborative," *American Journal of Public Health* 103, no. 3 (2013): 426–34.

100. A second mainstay of cardiac care that has been even more widely prescribed, beta-blockers, also owes its existence to a government–industry partnership. (Zycher, DiMasi, and Milne, "Private Sector Contributions.") Their versatility and ubiquity have made them a staple of contemporary practice, and they are used to treat a range of conditions effectively, from high blood pressure to cardiac arrhythmias to angina pectoris to anxiety to migraine headaches, with relatively few side effects. The NIH funded the basic research that identified the chemical pathway behind high blood pressure at the University of Georgia in the 1940s. The first molecule to be synthesized to block it, which became known as a beta-blocker, was developed in 1957 at Eli Lilly and Company, and its effectiveness was confirmed by researchers at Emory University. Follow-up work was conducted at Imperial Chemical Industries, which today is part of AstraZeneca, leading to development of the first drug available for clinical use, which was known as pronethalol. An improved version with fewer side effects, propranolol, was introduced a few years later, in 1964. Over the years, several drug companies have introduced their own beta-blockers, and there are 17 different kinds on the market today. They are so varied that they now fall into subclasses with differing clinical effects. Twenty drug companies sell a beta-blocker product of some sort, and more than 2,000 patents have been issued related to them. In 2007, Americans received more than 132 million prescriptions for beta-blockers, making them the fifth most widely prescribed class of drugs. (IMS Health, "Top Therapeutic Classes by U.S. Dispenses Prescriptions," http://www.imshealth.com/deployed-files/ims/Global/Content/Corporate/Press%20Room/Top-Line%20Market%20Data%20&%20Trends/2011%20Top-line%20Market%20Data/Top_Therapy_Classes_by_RX.pdf.) In 2001, sales only to Medicare beneficiaries exceeded $2 billion. (John F. Moeller, G. Edward Miller, and Jessica S. Banthin, "Looking Inside the Nation's Medicine Cabinet: Trends in Outpatient Drug Spending by Medicare Beneficiaries, 1997 and 2001," *Health Affairs* 23, no. 5 [September/October 2004]: 217–25.) The large sales volume is even more remarkable when it is considered that over 73 percent of prescriptions are for relatively inexpensive generic versions. In the words of one observer, "The pharmaceutical industry would not be what it is today without beta-blockers, the knowledge and profit gained catapulted the industry to a new height." (Jie Jack Li, *Laughing Gas, Viagra, and Lipitor: The Human Stories Behind the Drugs We Use* [New York: Oxford University Press, 2006], 90–94.)

101. Philip A. Rea, "Statins: From Fungus to Pharma," *American Scientist* (2008), http://www.americanscientist.org/issues/pub/statins-from-fungus-to-pharma.

102. Consumers Union, "The Statin Drugs: Prescription and Price Trends October 2005 to December 2006" (February, 2007), http://www.consumerreports.org/health/resources/pdf/best-buy-drugs/Statins-RxTrend-FINAL-Feb2007.pdf.

103. Jonathan A. Tobert, "Lovastatin and Beyond: The History of the HMG-COA Reductase Inhibitors," *Nature Reviews Drug Discovery* 2 (2003): 517–26.

104. Richard B. Thompson, "Foundations for Blockbuster Drugs in Federally Sponsored Research," *The FASEB Journal* 15 (2001): 1671–76.

105. Ibid.

106. Ibid.

107. The full name of the enzyme is hydroxymethyl glutaryl coenzyme A reductase.

108. Tobert, "Lovastatin and Beyond."

109. Ibid.

110. Daniel Steinberg, "An Interpretive History of the Cholesterol Controversy, Part V: The Discovery of the Statins and the End of the Controversy," *Journal of Lipid Research* 47 (2006): 1339–51.

111. Ibid.

112. Suzanne White Junod, "Statins: A Success Story Involving FDA, Academia and Industry," Food and Drug Administration, http://www.fda.gov/AboutFDA/WhatWeDo/History/ProductRegulation/SelectionsFromFDLIUpdateSeriesonFDAHistory/ucm082054.htm.

113. Ibid.

114. American Heart Association, "Good vs. Bad Cholesterol," http://www.heart.org/HEARTORG/Conditions/Cholesterol/AboutCholesterol/Good-vs-Bad-Cholesterol_UCM_305561_Article.jsp.

115. Nobel Prize, "The Nobel Prize in Physiology or Medicine 1985," http://www.nobelprize.org/nobel_prizes/medicine/laureates/1985/.

116. Richard B. Thompson, "Foundations for Blockbuster Drugs in Federally Sponsored Research," *Federation of American Societies for Experimental Biology* 15, no. 10 (2001): 1673.

117. Ibid., 1671.

118. Ibid., 1674.

119. Alan Rappeport, "FDA Issues Warning on Cholesterol Drugs," *Financial Times*, February 28, 2012, http://www.ft.com/cms/s/0/aaa20352-624f-11e1-872e-00144feabdco.html#axzz10YoFdEw1.

120. Catherine Larkin, "Lipitor Topped Worldwide Drug Sales in 2010; Crestor Gains Most," *Bloomberg*, February 10, 2011, http://www.bloomberg.com/news/2011-02-10/lipitor-topped-worldwide-drug-sales-in-2010-crestor-gains-most.html.

121. Melanie Haiken, "The Latest Statin Scare: Are You at Risk?" *Forbes*, February 9, 2012, http://www.forbes.com/sites/melaniehaiken/2012/02/29/the-latest-statin-scare-are-you-at-risk/.

122. Frank Stephenson, "A Tale of Taxol," Office of Research, Florida State University, http://www.rinr.fsu.edu/fall2002/taxol.html.

123. United States Government Accountability Office, "Technology Transfer: NIH-Private Sector Partnership in the Development of Taxol" (June 2003), http://www.gao.gov/new.items/d03829.pdf.

124. Ibid. The drug was assigned the generic name taxol upon its discovery. In 1992, that name was trademarked, and the commercially available version became known by the brand name Taxol. The generic name was changed to paclitaxel. From that time, references to the compound have used the generic name, whereas those to the commercial product use the brand name.

125. Taxol inhibits mitosis in rapidly dividing cells, such as cancer cells. It interferes with the beta subunit of tubulin, an important part of the microtubules that facilitate cell division. It does this by promoting the polymerization of tubulin, which causes cell death by disrupting the normal microtubule dynamics required for cell division. See Stephenson, "A Tale of Taxol."

126. Zycher, DiMasi, and Milne, "Private Sector Contributions."

127. Stephenson, "A Tale of Taxol."

128. Ibid.

129. United States Government Accountability Office, "Technology Transfer."

130. Ibid., 5.

131. Stephenson, "A Tale of Taxol."

132. Ibid.

133. United States Government Accountability Office, "Technology Transfer," 3.

134. Stephenson, "A Tale of Taxol."

135. The size of BMS's income from Taxol has generated considerable controversy. In 1993, Senate Ron Wyden of Oregon led hearings into the drug's high price, although no Congressional action followed. After the CRADA expired, BMS was able to forestall the entry of generic competition by filing patent infringement lawsuits. This move enabled it to reap an additional $4 billion in sales. In 2001, it was sued by attorneys general in 29 states who charged that it committed fraud in its efforts to delay the entry of generic paclitaxel in the market. Ibid.

136. BMS's success in developing Taxol based on FSU's semisynthesis technique also led to an environmental benefit. Ibid. By 1993, the company no longer needed large supplies of yew bark and terminated a contract for wide-scale bark collection. Before this, the contest between protecting forests and treating cancer had developed into a sensitive conflict. Now, the goals no longer clashed. The company's accomplishment was recognized in 2004 with the Greener Synthetic Pathways Award from the Environmental Protection Agency. Zycher, DiMasi, and Milne, "Private Sector Contributions."

137. United States Government Accountability Office, "Technology Transfer."

138. Litigation in which BMS sought to further delay the sale of generic paclitaxel was ongoing at the time it first reached the market and was not finally resolved until 2002.

139. National Institutes of Health, "Paclitaxel-Coated Stents."

140. See Angioplasty.org, "TAXUS Express2: Paclitaxel-Eluting Coronary Stent System," http://www.ptca.org/articles/taxus_profileframe.html.

141. Rahul Sakhuja and Laura Mauri, "Controversies in the Use of Drug-Eluting Stents for Acute Myocardial Infarction: A Critical Appraisal of the Data," *Annual Review of Medicine* 61 (February 2010): 215–31.

142. Innovia, "History," http://innovia-llc.theinnoport.com/company/history/.

143. Other examples of CRADAs that have resulted in new medical technologies successfully reaching the market are described by the NIH at http://www.ott.nih.gov/about_nih/success_stories.aspx.

144. Biotechnology Information Institute, "FDA Approves Hepatitis A Virus Vaccine," *Antiviral Agents Bulletin*, March 1995, http://www.bioinfo.com/havrix.html.

145. National Institutes of Health Office of Technology Transfer, "Havrix Waging War Against a Common Enemy: A Case Study" (October 22, 2002), http://www.ott.nih.gov/pdfs/HavrixCS.pdf.

146. Centers for Disease Control and Prevention, "Hepatitis A FAQs for the Public," September 17, 2009, http://www.cdc.gov/hepatitis/a/afaq.htm.

147. World Health Organization, "Hepatitis A Vaccines, WHO Position Paper," *Weekly Epidemiological Record* 75, no. 5 (February 4, 2000): 37–44, http://www.who.int/docstore/wer/pdf/2000/wer7505.pdf.

148. National Institutes of Health, "Havrix Waging War."

149. Ibid.

150. Ibid.

151. Ibid; and Biotechnology Information Institute, "FDA Approves."

152. "SmithKline Beecham Biologicals Receives FDA License to Market Havrix, the World's First Hepatitis A Vaccine," *PR Newswire*, February 22, 1995, http://www.thefreelibrary.com/SMITHKLINE+BEECHAM+BIOLOGICALS+RECEIVES+FDA+LICENSE+TO+MARKET+HAVRIX,...-a016535483.

153. "Centers for Disease Control and Prevention Awards SmithKline Beecham 1997 Pediatric Hepatitis A Vaccine Contract," *PR Newswire*, Oct. 21, 1996, http://www.thefreelibrary.com/Centers+for+Disease+Control+and+Prevention+Awards+SmithKline+Beecham...-a018782951.

154. Andrew Humphreys, "Havrix," Med Ad News, May 1, 1998, http://business.highbeam.com/437048/article-1G1-50078232/havrix.

155. Cormac Sheridan, "Vaccine Market Boosters," *Nature Biotechnology* 27, no. 6 (2009): 499–501.

156. Ibid.

157. William T. Elliott and James Chan, "Twinrix—A New Vaccine for Hepatitis A and B," *Internal Medicine Alert*, August 15, 2001, http://www.highbeam.com/doc/1G1-77626152.html.

158. Biotechnology Information Institute, "FDA Approves."

159. Árpád Furka, "Combinatorial Chemistry: 20 Years on..." *Drug Discovery Today* 7, no. 1 (January 2002): 1–4.

160. Ibid.

161. Rosalie David, "The Art of Healing in Ancient Egypt: A Scientific Reappraisal," *The Lancet* 372, No. 9652 (2008): 1802–03.

162. Gregory J. Higby, "American Hospital Pharmacy from the Colonial Period to the 1930s," *American Journal of Hospital Pharmacy* 51, no. 22 (1994): 2817–23.

163. Gavin Yamey, "Dispute as Rival Groups Publish Details of Human Genome," *British Medical Journal* 322, no. 7283 (2001): 381.

164. One investigation described instances in which the FDA failed to take action against drugs for which the data submitted by the manufacturers were found to be missing or fraudulent. Rob Grover and Charles Seife, "FDA Let Drugs Approved on Fraudulent Research Stay on the Market," *Propublica*, April 15, 2012, http://www.propublica.org/article/fda-let-drugs-approved-on-fraudulent-research-stay-on-the-market.

165. The controversy surrounding Vioxx is discussed in note 77. See also US Food and Drug Administration, "Drugs: Vioxx (rofecoxib) Questions and Answers," 2009, http://www.fda.gov/Drugs/DrugSafety/PostmarketDrugSafetyInformationforPatientsandProviders/ucm106290.htm.

Chapter 4

1. Robert Martensen, "History of Medicine: How Medicare and Hospitals Have Shaped American Health Care," *American Medical Association Journal of Ethics* 13, no. 11 (2011): 808–12.

2. National Center for Health Statistics, "Health, United States, 2010," 354, table 113.

3. Ibid., 369, table 125.

4. National Center for Health Statistics, "Health, United States, 2006," 377, table 123.

5. Ibid., 362, table 119.

6. Public Broadcast Service, "Healthcare Crisis: Who's At Risk?" http://www.pbs.org/healthcarecrisis/medicare.html.

7. National Center for Health Statistics, "Health, United States, 2010," 354, table 113.

8. Ashok Selvam, "For-Profits Rising: Investor-owned Hospitals Add Market Share, Along with Growing Numbers of Ventures with Not-for-profit Counterparts," *Modern*

Healthcare,   March   3,   2012,   http://www.modernhealthcare.com/article/20120303/MAGAZINE/303039958#ix.

9. Ashok Selvam, "For-Profits Rising: Not-for-profits Still Dominate, but Rivals Advance," *Modern Healthcare,* December 15, 2012, http://www.modernhealthcare.com/article/20121215/SUPPLEMENT/312159997.

10. Rosemary Stevens, *In Sickness and in Wealth* (New York: Basic Books, 1989), 293.

11. Guenter B. Risse, *Mending Bodies, Saving Souls: A History of Hospitals* (New York: Oxford University Press, 1999).

12. Commonwealth Fund Commission on Hospital Care, *Hospital Care in the United States* (New York: The Commonwealth Fund, 1947), 519.

13. Penn Medicine, "About Pennsylvania Hospital: History & Overview," http://www.pennmedicine.org/pahosp/about.

14. Starr, *The Social Transformation,* 150 (describing almshouses as providing very minimal care so as to deter poverty and the use of public assistance).

15. Ibid. King George III chartered New York Hospital in 1771, but the Revolutionary War delayed the hospital's opening until 1791. Fabrizio Michelassi and Thomas J. Fahey III, "The Department of Surgery at New York-Presbyterian Hospital/Weill Cornell Medical Center: At the Forefront of Surgical Innovation," *American Surgeon* 75, no. 8 (2009): 643–48.

16. Ibid., 155–56.

17. Martensen, "History of Medicine," 808.

18. Commonwealth Fund, "Hospital Care," 519.

19. Ibid., 520. These figures may be underestimates, because some hospitals were uncounted. However, the trend in expansion of the number of hospitals and in nationwide hospital bed capacity are clear.

20. Flexner, *Medical Education.*

21. Starr, *The Social Transformation,* 118–21.

22. Ibid., 355.

23. Charles E. Rosenberg, *The Care of Strangers: The Rise of American's Hospital System* (New York: Basic Books, Inc., 1987), 341.

24. Martensen, "History of Medicine," 808.

25. Between 1960 and 2008, national spending on hospital care increased from $23.3 million to $1.952 billion. National Center for Health Statistics, "Health, United States, 2010," 369, table 125. During the 1970s, employment in hospitals in the United States increased by 37.6 percent. Edward S. Sekscenski, "The Health Services Industry: A Decade of Expansion," *Monthly Labor Review* 104, no. 5 (1981): 9–16, 9–10.

26. Starr, *The Social Transformation,* 147–62 (describing the transformation of US hospitals from institutions of social welfare into cutting-edge medical science institutions).

27. John Kastor, *Mergers of Teaching Hospitals in Boston, New York, and Northern California* (Ann Arbor, MI: University of Michigan Press, 2001).

28. Ibid.

29. Ibid.

30. Rosenberg, *The Care of Strangers,* 343.

31. The first marine hospital was established at the state level by Virginia in 1787, and the federal government followed its lead in creating the Marine Hospital Service. The agency's name was changed in 1902 to the US Public Health and Marine Hospital Service and in 1912 to the US Public Health Service. It now administers a range of different health care programs. Commonwealth Fund, "Hospital Care," 547.

32. Ibid., 530.

33. Ibid., 538.

34. Ibid., 551–54.

35. Ibid., 548–51.

36. Ibid., 558–60.

37. Ibid., 520–21.

38. Hill-Burton Act, 42 U.S.C. § 291 (2006).

39. The law's formal name is the Hospital Survey and Construction Act of 1946, P.L. 79-725, 60 Stat. 1040 (1946).

40. Ibid. § 601, 60 Stat. at 1041.

41. Starr, *The Social Transformation*, 350.

42. Roger K. Newman, *Hill-Burton Act (1946)*, in *Major Acts of Congress*, ed. Brian K. Landsberg (New York: Macmillan Reference USA, 2004), 166–67.

43. Ibid.

44. "Hill-Burton Facilities Compliance & Recovery," U.S. Department of Health and Human Services, Health Resources & Services Administration, http://www.hrsa.gov/gethealthcare/affordable/hillburton/compliance.html. For a discussion of the role of federal funding in facilitating the growth of rural health facilities in the United States, see Mary K. Zimmerman and Rodney McAdams, *Public Support for Rural Health Care: Federal Programs and Local Hospital Subsidies*, in *Chronic Care, Health Systems and Services Integration* 25, ed. Jennie Jacobs Kronenfeld (Bingley, UK: Emerald Group Publishing Limited, 2004), 27–29.

45. US Department of Health and Human Services, "Medical Treatment in Hill-Burton Funded Healthcare Facilities," http://www.hhs.gov/ocr/civilrights/understanding/Medical%20Treatment%20at%20Hill%20Burton%20Funded%20Medical%20Facilities/index.html. These requirements are embodied in regulations published at 42 C.F.R. § 124 (2010). The indigent-care obligation varied with the nature of the funding received, lasting either for 20 years, until federal loans were repaid, or in perpetuity. Sharon Kearney Coleman, "The Hill-Burton Uncompensated Services Program" (Congressional Research Service, 2005), http://www.policyarchive.org/handle/10207/bitstreams/719.pdf.

46. Although the Hill-Burton Act outlawed racial discrimination by hospitals that received funds, until 1963, hospitals were permitted to provide racially segregated services that were of equal quality. Starr, *The Social Transformation*, 350. See also David Barton Smith, *Health Care Divided* (Ann Arbor, MI: University of Michigan Press, 1999), 46–47.

47. The requirements are contained in regulations of the Department of Health and Human Services (HHS). *See* 42 C.F.R. § 124 (2010).

48. Comprehensive Health Planning and Services Act, 42 U.S.C. § 246 (1966).

49. Ibid.

50. The states without certificate-of-need programs include Arizona, California, Colorado, Idaho, Indiana, Kansas, Minnesota, New Mexico, North Dakota, Pennsylvania, South Dakota, Texas, Utah, Wisconsin, and Wyoming. National Conference of State Legislatures, "Certificate of Need: State Health Laws and Programs," http://www.ncsl.org/issues-research/health/con-certificate-of-need-state-laws.aspx.

51. Ololade Olakanmi, "Report on Historical Links Between the American Medical Association and the 'Hill-Burton Act,'" http://www.ama-assn.org/resources/doc/ethics/hillburton.pdf.

52. Dennis W. Johnson, *The Laws That Shaped America: Fifteen Acts of Congress and Their Lasting Impact* (New York: Routledge, 2009), 342.

53. Corning, "Social Security History," chapter 4.

54. Ibid.

55. The passage of Medicare is described in David Blumenthal and James A. Morone, *The Heart of Power: Health and Politics in the Oval Office* (Berkeley, CA: University of California Press, 2009), 133.

56. The history of Medicare's reimbursement system is described in Mayes, "The Origins, Development, and Passage."

57. US Social Security Administration Office of Retirement and Disability Policy, "Medicaid Program Description and Legislative History," http://www.ssa.gov/policy/docs/statcomps/supplement/2011/medicaid.html.

58. Rick Mayes and Robert A. Berenson, *Medicare Prospective Payment and the Shaping of U.S. Health Care* (Baltimore, MD: Johns Hopkins University Press, 2006), 131.

59. Ibid.

60. As of May 2010, the total number of Medicare beneficiaries was nearly 46.6 million. Henry J. Kaiser Family Foundation, "Total Number of Medicare Beneficiaries, 2010," http://www.statehealthfacts.org/comparemaptable.jsp?yr=138&typ=1&ind=290&cat=6&sub=74.

61. Kaiser Family Foundation, "State Health Facts: Medicare," 2013, http://kff.org/state-category/medicare/.

62. US Department of Health and Human Services, "Fiscal Year 2010 Budget in Brief" (May 7, 2009), 52, http://www.hhs.gov/about/budget/fy2010/fy2010bib.pdf.

63. Ibid.

64. Ibid.

65. Stevens, *In Sickness*, 291.

66. Rosenberg, *The Care of Strangers*, 349.

67. Martensen, "History of Medicine," 808.

68. Stevens, *In Sickness*, 284.

69. National Center for Health Statistics, "Health, United States, 2010," 371–72, table 126.

70. Ibid., 402–403, table 140.

71. National Center for Health Statistics, "Health, United States, 2006," 365, table 113, 410–411, table 141 and "Health, United States, 2010," 408, table 144.

72. Eli Ginzberg, *Tomorrow's Hospital* (New Haven, CT: Yale University Press, 1996), 13.

73. Julian Pettengill, "The Financial Position of Private Community Hospitals, 1961–77," *Social Security Bulletin* 36 no. 11 (November 1973): 3–19.

74. Martensen, "History of Medicine," 808.

75. Pettengill, "The Financial Position," 5.

76. Ginzberg, *Tomorrow's Hospital*, 13.

77. Ibid., 12.

78. Ibid., 13.

79. Ibid., 23.

80. Balanced Budget Act of 1997, P.L. 105–33, 111 Stat. 251 (1997).

81. Mayes and Berenson, "Medicare Prospective Payment," 115.

82. Ibid., 114.

83. See, generally, Mayes, "The Origins, Development, and Passage" (detailing the development of the Medicare reimbursement system).

84. National Center for Health Statistics, "Health, United States, 2010," 371, table 126.

85. Kinkead, "Medicare Payment," 49–74.

86. Ibid.

87. See ibid., 56.

88. Ibid.

89. In fact, the number of hospital beds decreased slightly between 1975 and 2004. National Center for Health Statistics, "Health, United States, 2006," 392, table 130.

90. See "Medical Technology and Costs of the Medicare Program," OTA-H-227 (Washington, DC: United States Office of Technology Assessment, 1984), http://www.fas.org/ota/reports/8419.pdf.

91. James C. Robinson, "The Changing Boundaries of the American Hospital," *Milbank Quarterly* 72, no. 2 (1994): 259–75, 260. ("Between 1972 and 1990, acute care facilities diversified rapidly, but significant areas of health care remain outside the boundaries of the hospital organization.").

92. The federal law mandating that states adopt certificate-of-need programs was the National Health Planning and Resources Development Act of 1974, P.L. 93-641, 88 Stat. 2225 (1975), codified at 42 U.S.C. subchapter XII sec. 300K et seq. and 42 U.S.C. subchapter XIV § 3000 et seq.

93. McGinley, "Beyond Health Care Reform."

94. "Health, 2011," table 143, 409.

95. Mayes and Berenson, "Medicare Prospective Payment," 135.

96. Graduate Medical Education payments under Medicare consist of two components. Direct payments reflect the cost of salaries of residents. Indirect payments reflect the burden of training on hospital productivity, most notably in the reduced productivity of supervising physicians.

97. Centers for Medicare and Medicaid Services, "Acute Inpatient PPS," http://www.cms.gov/Medicare/Medicare-Fee-for-Service-Payment/AcuteInpatientPPS/index.html?redirect=/acuteinpatientpps/.

98. Mayes and Berenson, "Medicare Prospective Payment," 148.

99. See for example Gale Scott, "Hospital Ads: They're Everywhere," *Crain's New York Business*, July 31, 2011, http://www.crainsnewyork.com/article/20110731/SUB/110739999.

100. James C. Robinson, "Hospital Market Concentration, Pricing, and Profitability in Orthopedic Surgery and Interventional Cardiology," *American Journal of Managed Care* 17, no. 6 (2011): e241–248.

101. The nature of hospital marketing is discussed in Patrick T. Buckley, *The Complete Guide to Hospital Marketing*, 2nd ed. (Marblehead, MA: HCPro, Inc., 2009).

102. See Bruce C. Vladeck, "Medicare Hospital Payment by Diagnosis-Related Groups," *Annals of Internal Medicine* 100, no. 4 (1984): 585–90.

103. Hospitals' selection of staff physicians based on the profitability of their specialty is known as "economic credentialing." Several courts have upheld this practice. See, e.g., *Mahan* v. *Avera St. Luke's*, 621 N.W.2d 150, 160 (S.D. 2001) (holding that Avera St. Luke's decision to close its facility for certain procedures was "reasonable" because the hospital had established that "the closures were necessary to insure the continued viability of the hospital," which provided "comprehensive medical services to the…community"); see also John D. Blum, "Beyond the Bylaws: Hospital-Physician Relationships, Economics, and

Conflicting Agendas," *Buffalo Law Review* 53 (2005): 459–74 (detailing the emergence of economic credentialing, the legal response, and its potential consequences).

104. See Elizabeth A. Weeks, "The New Economic Credentialing: Protecting Hospitals From Competition by Medical Staff Members," *Journal of Health Law* 36, no. 2 (2003): 247–300.

105. See Gerald L. Glandon and Michael A. Morrisey, "Redefining the Hospital-Physician Relationship Under Prospective Payment," *Inquiry* 23, no. 3 (1986): 166–75.

106. Employment arrangements for physicians have been criticized for going too far in reducing incentives for productivity and creating disincentives for it instead. When compensation is based on a set salary, there is little financial reward for seeing more patients. In response, many hospitals and health systems have devised more complex compensation structures that encourage desired levels of work effort.

107. Mayes and Berenson, "Medicare Prospective Payment," 147.

108. *Mahan v. Avera St. Luke's*, 621 N.W.2d 150 (S.D. 2001).

109. Centers for Medicare and Medicaid Services, "Specialty Hospital Issues," http://www.cms.gov/Medicare/Fraud-and-Abuse/PhysicianSelfReferral/specialty_hospital_issues.html.

110. Mayes and Berenson, "Medicare Prospective Payment," 148.

111. Physician-owned specialty hospitals may actually have an advantage over general hospitals in earning bonuses and avoiding penalties on quality measures under the Affordable Care Act. The hospitals claim this is because they focus more aggressively on quality; however critics claim this is because their physician-owners select the healthiest patients for treatment in them. See Jordan Rau, "Doctor-Owned Hospitals Prosper Under Health Law," *Kaiser Health News*, April 12, 2013, http://www.kaiserhealthnews.org/stories/2013/april/12/doctor-owned-hospitals-quality-bonuses.aspx.

112. David M. Cutler ed., *The Changing Hospital Industry: Comparing Not-for-Profit and For-Profit Institutions* (Chicago: University of Chicago Press, 2000), 197.

113. Ibid.

114. Ibid.

115. American Medical Association, "RBRVS: Resource-Based Relative Value Scale," https://www.ama-assn.org/ama/pub/physician-resources/solutions-managing-your-practice/coding-billing-insurance/medicare/the-resource-based-relative-value-scale.page.

116. Mayes and Berenson, "Medicare Prospective Payment," 100.

117. These operations are performed through a thin tube inserted into a small opening in the body instead of through a major surgical incision.

118. Robert Treuting, "Minimally Invasive Orthopedic Surgery: Arthroscopy," *Ochsner Journal* 2, no. 3 (July 2000): 158–63.

119. See for example, Andrew J. Pugely et al., "Outpatient Surgery Reduces Short-Term Complications in Lumbar Discectomy," *Spine* 38, no. 3 (2013): 264–71.

120. Gary N. Holland et al., "Results of Inpatient and Outpatient Cataract Surgery. A Historical Cohort Comparison," *Ophthalmology* 99, no. 6 (1992): 845–52.

121. See Centers for Medicare and Medicaid Services, "American Medical Group Association Compensation Survey Data 2009 Report" (2009), http://www.cms.gov/Medicare/Medicare-Fee-for-Service-Payment/AcuteInpatientPPS/Downloads/AMGA_08_template_to_09.pdf (estimating the median salary for physicians in orthopedic surgery and diagnostic radiology to be between $400,000 and $500,000 annually, varying upward for subspecialties).

122. See Tracy K. Johnson et al., "Ambulatory Surgery: Next-Generation Strategies for Physicians and Hospitals," *Healthcare Financial Management* 54, no. 1 (January 2000): 48–51.

123. Mayes and Berenson, "Medicare Prospective Payment," 102.

124. 42 U.S.C. §1320a-7b.

125. Mayes and Berenson, "Medicare Prospective Payment," 102.

126. "A number of legislative changes have altered the environment for Medicare beneficiaries, underscoring and strengthening the incentives for a shift from inpatient hospital care to outpatient sites such as hospital outpatient departments, ambulatory surgery centers, and physicians' offices." Leader and Moon, "Medicare Tends in Ambulatory Surgery."

127. Ibid., 163, exhibit 2.

128. Ibid., 167, exhibit 6.

129. Mayes and Berenson, "Medicare Prospective Payment," 100.

130. Ibid., 110.

131. Ibid., 121.

132. The impetus for the formation of these systems also lay in an effort to counteract the growing bargaining power of managed care companies, as discussed in Chapter 6. See ibid., 113.

133. Medicare Payment Advisory Commission (MedPAC), http://medpac.gov/.

134. Balanced Budget Act of 1997, P.L. 105-33, 111 Stat. 251.

135. Mayes and Berenson, "Medicare Prospective Payment," 140.

136. "About MedPAC," Medicare Payment Advisory Commission, http://www.medpac.gov/about.cfm.

137. National Association of Children's Hospitals and Related Institutions, http://www.childrenshospitals.net//AM/Template.cfm?Section=Home3.

138. National Center for Health Statistics, "Health, United States, 2010," 394, table 137.

139. Ibid., 408, table 144.

140. Ibid., 407, table 143.

141. Ibid., 394, table 137.

142. Genevieve M. Kenney et al., "Opting in to the Medicaid Expansion under the ACA: Who Are the Uninsured Adults Who Could Gain Health Insurance Coverage?" (Robert Wood Johnson Foundation, August 2012), http://www.urban.org/UploadedPDF/412630-opting-in-medicaid.pdf.

143. Kaiser Family Foundation, "Medicaid Matters: Understanding Medicaid's Role in Our Health Care System" (2011), http://www.kff.org/medicaid/upload/8165.pdf.

144. March of Dimes, "National Child Health Advocates Urge Congress to Reject Harmful Cuts to Medicaid in Administration's Budget Proposal," February 7, 2005, http://www.marchofdimes.com/24497_25619.asp.

145. Ibid.

146. National Association of Children's Hospitals and Related Institutions, http://www.childrenshospitals.net//AM/Template.cfm?Section=Home3.

147. Ibid.

148. Medicaid.gov, "Children's Health Insurance Program (CHIP)," http://www.medicaid.gov/Medicaid-CHIP-Program-Information/By-Topics/Childrens-Health-Insurance-Program-CHIP/Childrens-Health-Insurance-Program-CHIP.html.

149. Medicare standards for hospitals are described at Centers for Medicare & Medicaid Services, "Conditions for Coverage (CfCs) and Conditions of Participation (CoPs)," May 11, 2012, http://www.cms.gov/Regulations-and-Guidance/Legislation/CFCsAndCoPs/index.html?redirect=/cfcsandcops/.

150. See Emergency Treatment and Labor Act, 42 U.S.C. § 1395dd(a)–(c) (2006).

151. Ibid.

152. See Laurence C. Baker and Linda Schuurman Baker, "Excess Cost of Emergency Department Visits for Non-Urgent Care," *Health Affairs* 13, no. 5 (1994): 162–71, 170 (finding "significant excess expenditures associated with the use of emergency departments for nonurgent care").

153. Omnibus Budget Reconciliation Act, P.L. 101-508 (1991).

154. High Information Technology for Economic and Clinical Health Ac, P.L. 11-5, 123 Stat. 227 (2009).

155. Patient Protection and Affordable Care Act, P.L. 111-148, 124 Stat. 119, §§1401- 1421 (2010) (to be codified in scattered sections of Titles 21, 25, 26, 29, & 42 U.S.C.).

156. 26 U.S.C. sec. 501(c)(3).

157. In some states, such as Pennsylvania and Utah, extension of the federal tax exemption to state and local taxes, such as real estate and sales taxes, is not automatic. Hospitals must prove that they actually serve a charitable function in their communities. However, most nonprofit hospitals continue to qualify for tax-exempt status. See, for example, Institutions of Purely Public Charity Act, 10 P.S. § 371. et seq. (laying out specific criteria for determining whether an institution is a "purely public charity" and therefore exempt from state taxation).

158. I.R.C. § 145(a) (2006). Tax-exempt bonds represent an important government subsidy that reduces borrowing costs for hospitals. See American Health Lawyers Association, "Tax Exempt Bonds," http://www.healthlawyers.org/hlresources/Health%20Law%20Wiki/Tax%20Exempt%20Bonds.aspx.

159. I.R.C. § 501(c)(3); see also "Exemption Requirements: 501(c)(3) Organizations," Internal revenue Service, http://www.irs.gov/Charities-&-Non-Profits/Charitable-Organizations/Exemption-Requirements-Section-501(c)(3)-Organizations (providing an overview of exemption requirements); Field, *Health Care Regulation*, 189–94 (outlining the regulation of tax-exempt status, including the process of gaining and maintaining it, and penalties for violating its restrictions).

160. See Internal Revenue Service General Counsel Memo 39,862 (November 21, 1991) (concluding that a hospital can lose its section 501(c)(3) tax-exempt status if it enters into certain hospital–physician joint ventures that involve the sale of part of the hospital's net revenue stream).

161. The IRS first articulated the community-benefit standard for assessing the charitable operations of hospitals in 1969. See Revenue Ruling 69-545, 1969-2 C.B. 117 (using examples to illustrate under what circumstances a nonprofit hospital would meet the public-interest standard required to receive tax-exempt status); see also John D. Columbo, "The Role of Tax Exemption in a Competitive Health Care Market," *Journal of Health Politics, Policy and Law* 31, no. 3 (2006): 623–42, 629–35 (analyzing whether the community-benefit requirement leads to better performance according to several identified criteria).

162. Congressional Budget Office, "Nonprofit Hospitals," 3.

163. See generally Jill R. Horwitz, "Why We Need the Independent Sector: The Behavior, Law, and Ethics of Not-for-Profit Hospitals," *UCLA Law Review* 50, no. 6 (2003): 1345–411.

164. Starr, *The Social Transformation*, 170.

165. Ibid., 219.

166. Some examples of for-profit academic medical centers include Hahnemann University Hospital, http://www.hahnemannhospital.com/en-US/Pages/default.aspx; St. Christopher's Hospital for Children, http://www.stchristophershospital.com/; and Palmetto General Hospital, http://www.palmettogeneral.com/en-US/Pages/default.aspx.

167. For information on six major for-profit hospital chains in the United States, see Fitch Ratings, "Hospitals Credit Diagnosis: Operating Trends Remain Weak but Solid Liquidity Supports Credit Profiles" (September 18, 2012), http://www.beckersasc.com/media/FitchRatingsForProfit92012.pdf.

168. Hospital Corporation of America, "Our History," http://hcahealthcare.com/about/our-history.dot. The company's founder, Dr. Thomas Frist, was the father of Tennessee Senator Bill Frist, who served from 1995 to 2007.

169. Ibid.

170. Ibid.

171. Ibid.

172. Ibid.

173. Hospital Corporation of America, "About Our Company," http://hcahealthcare.com/about/.

174. Hospital Corporation of America, "Pricing and Financial Information," http://hcahealthcare.com/pricing-financing/.

175. Hospital Corporation of America, "About Our Company," http://hcahealthcare.com/about/.

176. Community Health Services, "History," http://www.chs.net/company_overview/history.html.

177. Community Health Systems, "About Us," http://www.chs.net/company_overview/index.html.

178. Ibid.

179. Tenet Health, "About," http://www.tenethealth.com/about/pages/default.aspx.

180. "Tenet Healthcare," *CNN Money*, May 23, 2011, http://money.cnn.com/magazines/fortune/fortune500/2011/snapshots/2176.html.

181. Several states passed laws that clarified the oversight process for the conversion of hospitals from nonprofit to for-profit status. Some of these are described in Patricia A. Butler, "State Policy Issues in Nonprofit Conversion," *Health Affairs* 16, no. 2 (1997): 71–72. Growth of for-profit facilities was also aided by the repeal in several states of certificate-of-need laws that require approval of hospital expansion. This is discussed in Fred J. Hellinger, "The Effect of Certificate-of-Need Laws on Hospital Beds and Healthcare Expenditures: An Empirical Analysis," *American Journal of Managed Care* 15, no. 10 (2009): 737–44, http://www.ajmc.com/publications/issue/2009/2009-10-vol15-n10/AJMC_09Oct_Hellinger_737to744/.

182. Stevens, *In Sickness*, 297.

183. Ibid., 299.

184. Mayes and Berenson, "Medicare Prospective Payment," 102.

185. David M. Cutler, ed., *The Changing Hospital Industry*, 55.

186. Ibid.

187. Association of American Medical Colleges, "About the AAMC," https://www.aamc.org/about/.

188. Association of American Medical Colleges, "Teaching Hospital Press Kit," https://www.aamc.org/newsroom/presskits/teaching_hospitals/.

189. Don Detmer and Elaine Steen eds., *The Academic Health Center: Leadership and Performance* (Cambridge, UK: Cambridge University Press, 2005).

190. Association of Academic Health Centers, "Academic Health Centers: Providing Health Care Services and Expanding Access," http://www.aahcdc.org/Portals/0/pdf/FG_AHC_Providing_Health%20Care_Services_Expanding_Access.pdf.

191. Association of American Medical Colleges, "What Does Medicare Have to Do with Graduate Medical Education?," https://www.aamc.org/download/253380/data/medi-care-gme.pdf.

192. Association of Academic Health Centers, "Academic Health Centers: Creating the Knowledge Economy," http://aahcdc.org/Portals/0/pdf/FG_AHC_Creating_the_Knowlege_Economy_04-09.pdf.

193. Association of American Medical Colleges, "What Does Medicare."

194. Association of Academic Health Centers, "Academic Health Centers."

195. Ibid.

196. John K. Iglehart, "The Uncertain Future of Medicare and Graduate Medical Education," *New England Journal of Medicine* 365, no. 14 (2011): 1340–45.

197. Association of American Medical Colleges, "What Does Medicare."

198. Erika Steinmetz and Christopher B. Morse, "Hospital Transfers of Medicare Patients," *American Association of Medical Colleges Analysis in Brief* 9, no. 1 (February 2009), https://www.aamc.org/download/82440/data/aibvol9no1.pdf.

199. American Association of Medical Colleges, "Teaching Hospitals Press Kits," https://www.aamc.org/newsroom/presskits/teaching_hospitals/.

200. Ibid.

201. Tripp Umbach Co., "Even Small Cuts Have Major Impacts: The National and State Economic Impacts of Proposed Reductions in Medicare IME Payments to AAMC Teaching Hospitals" (June 2011), https://www.aamc.org/download/255072/data/cutimpa-ctreport2011.pdf.

202. Charles E. Burbridge, "The Historical Background of the Teaching Hospital in the United States," *Journal of the National Medical Association* 49, no. 3 (1957): 176–79.

203. Ibid.

204. Ibid.

205. Ibid.

206. Ibid., Starr, *The Social Transformation*, 150.

207. The Institutional Records of The Johns Hopkins Hospital, "Brief History of the Johns Hopkins Hospital," http://www.medicalarchives.jhmi.edu/hospitalrecords.html.

208. Starr, *The Social Transformation*, 120.

209. Burbridge, *The Historical Background*.

210. New York-Presbyterian Hospital, "2010 Annual Report," http://nyp.org/pdf/annual_report_2010.pdf.

211. Montefiore Medical Center, "Advancing the Front Lines of Health, 2010–2011 Annual Report," http://www.myvirtualpaper.com/doc/montefiore/montefiore-annual-report-2010-2011/2011083101/#42.

212. Partners HealthCare, "Company Information," http://www.partners.org/About/Company-Information/Default.aspx.

213. Robert Weisman, "Partners HealthCare Posts $195 Million Gain," *Boston Globe*, December 3, 2010, http://www.boston.com/business/ticker/2010/12/partners_health_5.html.

214. Penn Medicine, "Facts & Figures 2012," http://www.uphs.upenn.edu/news/facts/PennMedicineFacts2012.pdf

215. University of Pittsburgh Medical Center, "Why UPMC?," http://www.upmc.com/aboutupmc/TheUPMCStory/Pages/default.aspx.

216. University of Pittsburgh Medical Center, "By the Numbers: UPMC Facts and Figures," http://www.upmc.com/aboutupmc/fast-facts/Pages/FactsandFigures.aspx.

217. University of Pittsburgh Medical Center, "Financial Information," http://www.upmc.com/aboutupmc/FinancialInformation/Pages/Default.aspx.

218. Detmer and Steen, *The Academic Health Center*, 13.

219. Commonwealth Fund Task Force on Academic Health Centers, "Envisioning the Future of Academic Health Centers" (The Commonwealth Fund, 2004), http://www.commonwealthfund.org/Publications/Fund-Reports/2003/Feb/Envisioning-the-Future-of-Academic-Health-Centers.aspx.

220. Detmer and Steen, *The Academic Health Center*.

221. Commonwealth Fund Task Force on Academic Health Centers, *Leveling the Playing Field: Financing the Missions of Academic Health Centers* (New York: The Commonwealth Fund, 199): 13–16.

222. Association of American Medical Colleges, "What Does Medicare."

223. John K. Iglehart, "The Uncertain Future of Medicare and Graduate Medical Education," 1340.

224. Tripp Umbach Co., "Even Small Cuts Have Major Impacts."

225. Iglehart, "The Uncertain Future."

226. Ibid.

227. Kastor, *Mergers of Teaching Hospitals in Boston*.

228. Ibid.

229. Mayes and Berenson, "Medicare Prospective Payment," 110.

230. Ibid., 140–42.

231. See discussion in Ibid.

232. *Fisher v. United States,* 529 U.S. 667 (2000).

233. Ibid., 718.

234. Significant reductions in Medicare reimbursement rates could put many hospitals out of business, as well as many other kinds of health care providers, like home health agencies, inpatient rehabilitation hospitals, and skilled nursing facilities. See Mayes and Berenson, "Medicare Prospective Payment," 142.

235. Ibid., 142.

236. Robert Berenson and Stephen Zuckerman, "How Will Hospitals Be Affected by Health Care Reform?" (Robert Wood Johnson Foundation, July 2010), http://www.rwjf.org/content/dam/farm/reports/issue_briefs/2010/rwjf62544.

237. Martensen, "History of Medicine," 811.

238. Mayes and Berenson, "Medicare Prospective Payment," 156.

Chapter 5

1. W. Bruce Fye, *American Cardiology* (Baltimore, MD: Johns Hopkins University Press, 1996), 225–26.

2. "Medscape Physician Compensation Report: 2011 Results," http://www.staging.medscape.com/features/slideshow/compensation/2011/#.

3. Ellyn R. Boukus, Alwyn Cassil, and Ann S. O'Malley, "A Snapshot of U.S. Physicians: Key Findings From the 2008 Health Tracking Physician Survey," Center For Studying Health System Change, *Data Bulletin* 35 (September 2009), http://hschange.org/CONTENT/1078/1078.pdf.

4. "Medscape Physician Compensation Report: 2011: Who Makes the Most Money?," http://www.medscape.com/viewarticle/740086_2.

5. US Census Bureau, "State and Country Quick Facts," http://quickfacts.census.gov/qfd/states/00000.html.

6. Chris L. Peterson and Rachel Burton, "U.S. Health Care Spending: Comparison with Other OECD Countries," RL34175 (Washington, DC: Congressional Research Service, September 17, 2007): 18, http://digitalcommons.ilr.cornell.edu/key_workplace/311/.

7. Catherine Rampell, "How Much Do Doctors in Other Countries Make?" *New York Times, Economix*, July 14, 2009, http://economix.blogs.nytimes.com/2009/07/15/how-much-do-doctors-in-other-countries-make/#.

8. Ibid.

9. Starr, *The Social Transformation*, 141–44.

10. Ibid., 40.

11. Ibid., 128.

12. Ibid., 112–16.

13. Ibid., 63.

14. Karen E. Lasser, Steffie Woolhandler, and David U. Himmelstein, "Sources of U.S. Physician Income: The Contribution of Government Payments to the Specialist-Generalist Income Gap," *Journal of General Internal Medicine* 23, no. 9 (2008): 1477–81.

15. Douglas Starr, "Early Practices: Leeches," http://www.pbs.org/wnet/redgold/basics/leeches.html.

16. Starr, *The Social Transformation*, 99–102.

17. Ibid., 78.

18. American Medical Association, "The Founding of the AMA," Public Broadcasting Service, http://www.ama-assn.org/ama/pub/about-ama/our-history/the-founding-of-ama.page?.

19. Starr, *The Social Transformation*, 117–18.

20. Deborah Haas-Wilson, *Managed Care and Monopoly Power: The Antitrust Challenge* (Cambridge, MA: Harvard University Press, 2003), 12–15.

21. Royal College of Physicians, "History of the RCP," http://www.rcplondon.ac.uk/about/history.

22. Starr, *The Social Transformation*, 102–12.

23. Ibid., 102–04.

24. Kenneth C. Yohn, "The History and Role of the Federation of State Medical Boards of the United States," *Federation Bulletin* 75, no. 9 (1988): 275–77.

25. In most states, the regulation of osteopathic practice has remained separate and is overseen by a distinct board of osteopathic medicine that operates in parallel with the board of medicine that oversees allopathic practice.

26. "Regulating the Practice of Medicine," *New York Times*, March 6, 1903, http://query.nytimes.com/mem/archive-free/pdf?res=F00716F93F5F12738DDDAF0894DB405B838CF1D3.

27. Osteopathic medical training is overseen by a separate accreditation process governed by the Commission on Osteopathic College Accreditation of the American

Osteopathic Association. However, the vast majority of American physicians are governed by the AMA-sanctioned process, as osteopaths represent less than 10 percent of the total.

28. Starr, *The Social Transformation*, 117.

29. Ibid.

30. Ibid.

31. Flexner, *Medical Education*.

32. Starr, *The Social Transformation*, 117.

33. Liaison Committee on Medical Education, "Overview: Accreditation and the LCME," http://www.lcme.org/overview.htm.

34. Yohn, "The History and Role," 275–77.

35. American Medical Association, "Our History," http://www.ama-assn.org/ama/pub/about-ama/our-history.page.

36. American Board of Internal Medicine, "Exam Administration History," http://www.abim.org/about/examInfo/year.aspx.

37. American Board of Medical Specialties, "About ABMS Member Boards," http://www.abms.org/About_ABMS/member_boards.aspx.

38. Starr, *The Social Transformation*, 355.

39. Boukus, Cassil, and O'Malley, "A Snapshot of U.S. Physicians."

40. Lynne Peeples, "Do Specialist Doctors Make Too Much Money?" *Reuters*, October 25, 2010, http://www.reuters.com/article/2010/10/25/us-specialist-doctors-idUSTRE69O4RW20101025.

41. Starr, *The Social Transformation*, 148.

42. Martensen, "History of Medicine," 808–12.

43. Ibid.

44. Starr, *The Social Transformation*, 156–57.

45. Gerald M. Eisenberg, "The Medical Staff Structure—Its Role in the 21st Century," *Annals of Health Law* 12, no. 2 (2003): 249–64.

46. Boukus, Cassil, and O'Malley, "A Snapshot of U.S. Physicians."

47. Jonathan P. Weiner, "A Shortage of Physicians or a Surplus of Assumptions?" *Health Affairs* 21, no. 1 (January 2002): 160–62.

48. Thomas C. Ricketts, III, ed., *Rural Health in the United States* (New York: Oxford University Press, 1999), 47.

49. Health Professions Educational Assistance Act of 1963, P.L. 88-129, 77 Stat. 164 (1963).

50. Health Professions Educational Assistance Amendments, P.L. 89-290, 79 Stat. 1052 (1965).

51. David Blumenthal, "New Steam from an Old Cauldron—The Physician-Supply Debate," *New England Journal of Medicine* 350, no. 17 (2004): 1780–87.

52. Aaron Young et al., "A Census of Actively Licensed Physicians in the United States, 2010," *Journal of Medical Regulation* 96, no. 4 (2011): 10–20, http://www.fsmb.org/pdf/fpdc-physician-census.pdf.

53. Council on Graduate Medical Education, "Physician Workforce Policy Guidelines for the United States, 2000–2020," US Health Resources and Services Administration (January 2005), http://www.hrsa.gov/advisorycommittees/bhpradvisory/cogme/Reports/sixteenthreport.pdf.

54. Jessica Townsend, "Financing Medical Education," in Institute of Medicine, *Medical Education and Societal Needs: A Planning Report for the Health Professions* 243–60,

254–88 (Washington, DC: National Academy Press, 1983), http://www.nap.edu/openbook. php?record_id=729&page=243.

55. National Institutes of Health, "The NIH Almanac, Appropriations," http://www. nih.gov/about/almanac/appropriations/index.htm.

56. Ibid.

57. Kenneth G. Manton, Xi-Liang Gu, Gene Lowrimore, Arthur Ullian, and H. Dennis Tolley, "NIH Funding Trajectories and Their Correlations with US Health Dynamics From 1950 to 2004," *Proceedings of the National Academy of Sciences* 106, no. 27 (2009): 10981– 86, http://www.pnas.org/content/106/27/10981.full.

58. Ibid.

59. US Department of Health and Human Services, "Health Resources and Services Administration," http://www.hrsa.gov/index.html.

60. American Medical Association, "International Medical Graduates in American Medicine: Contemporary Challenges and Opportunities" (January 2010): 10, www.ama-assn.org/resources/doc/img/img-workforce-paper.pdf.

61. Council on Graduate Medical Education, "Summary of Eleventh Report: International Medical Graduates, the Physician Workforce, and GME Payment Reform" (March 1998), http://www.hrsa.gov/advisorycommittees/bhpradvisory/cogme/Reports/ eleventhreport.html.

62. Edward S. Salsberg and Gaetano J. Forte, "Trends in the Physician Workforce, 1980–2000," *Health Affairs* 21, no. 5 (2002): 165–73.

63. Ibid.

64. Rosemary Stevens, "Health Care in the Early 1960s," *Health Care Financing Review* 18, no. 2 (Winter 1996): 11, http://www.ssa.gov/history/pdf/HealthCareEarly1960s.pdf.

65. Centers for Medicare & Medicaid Services, "Fact Sheet: Medicare End-stage Renal Disease (ESRD) Network Organization Program" (2012), http://www.cms. gov/Medicare/End-Stage-Renal-Disease/ESRDNetworkOrganizations/Downloads/ ESRDNWBackgrounder-Jun12.pdf.

66. Robin Fields, "Dialysis: An Experiment in Universal Health Care," *National Public Radio*, November 9, 2010, http://www.npr.org/templates/story/story.php?storyId= 131167638.

67. Medicare Prescription Drug, Improvement and Modernization Act of 2003, P.L. 108-173, 117 Stat. 2066, codified at 42 U.S.C. §1395.

68. Martensen, "History of Medicine."

69. Robert Mechanic, Kevin Coleman, and Allen Dobson, "Teaching Hospital Costs: Implications for Academic Mission in a Competitive Market," *Journal of the American Medical Association* 280, no. 11 (1998): 1015–19, 1017.

70. Richard Verville and Joel A. DeLisa, "The Evolution of Medicare Financing Policy for Graduate Medical Education and Implications for PM&R: A Commentary," *Archives of Physical Medicine and Rehabilitation* 82, no. 4 (2001): 558–62.

71. Martensen, "History of Medicine," 809.

72. Centers for Medicare & Medicaid Services, "Acute Inpatient PPS."

73. Joseph P. Newhouse and Gail R. Wilensky, "Paying for Graduate Medical Education: The Debate Goes On," *Health Affairs* 20, no. 2 (2001): 136–47.

74. Catherine Dower, "Graduate Medical Education," *Health Affairs*, Health Policy Briefs, August 31, 2012, http://www.healthaffairs.org/healthpolicybriefs/brief. php?brief_id=75.

75. Ibid.

76. Ibid.

77. Although there are generally enough residency slots to accommodate all graduates of American medical schools, the number of slots in many specialties is often less than the demand.

78. Medicare Payment Advisory Commission, "Report to Congress: Aligning Incentives in Medicare" (June 2010), http://www.medpac.gov/documents/jun10_entirereport.pdf.

79. Ibid.

80. George Weisz, *Divide and Conquer: A Comparative History of Medical Specialization* (New York: Oxford University Press, 2006), xxi.

81. Fred G. Donini-Lenhoff and Hannah L. Hedrick, "Growth of Specialization in Graduate Medical Education," *Journal of the American Medical Association* 284, no. 10 (2000): 1284–89.

82. Ibid.

83. Ibid.

84. Lewis G. Sandy et al., "The Political Economy of U.S. Primary Care," *Health Affairs* 28, no. 4 (July/August 2009): 1136–44.

85. Donini-Lenhoff and Hedrick, "Growth of Specialization."

86. Dower, "Health Policy Brief."

87. Sandy et al., "The Political Economy."

88. Ibid.

89. George Weisz, *Divide and Conquer*, 142–43.

90. Hill-Burton Act, 42 U.S.C. §§ 291 et seq. (1946). The Act is described in more detail in chapter 4 with relation to its effects on the hospital industry.

91. Weisz, *Divide and Conquer*, 227–28.

92. Starr, *The Social Transformation*, 358.

93. John K. Iglehart, "The American Health Care System—Medicare," *New England Journal of Medicine* 327, no. 20 (1992): 1467–72, 1470.

94. Mayes and Berenson, "Medicare Prospective Payment," 83.

95. Sandy and others, "The Political Economy."

96. Ibid.

97. American Medical Association, "RVS Update Process" (2007), www.ama-assn. org/ama1/pub/upload/mm/380/rvs_booklet_07.pdf.

98. American Medical Association, "Overview of the RBRVS," http://www.ama-assn. org/ama/pub/physician-resources/solutions-managing-your-practice/coding-billing-insurance/medicare/the-resource-based-relative-value-scale/overview-of-rbrvs.page.

99. Uwe E. Reinhardt, "The Little-Known Decision-Makers for Medicare Physician Fees," *New York Times, Economix*, December 10, 2010, http://economix.blogs.nytimes. com/2010/12/10/the-little-known-decision-makers-for-medicare-physicans-fees/?gwh=6 E1E316DC549F5BBC93D1DE7E4D29B8D.

100. Robert Lowes, "Lawsuit Targets Medicare Pay 'Bias' Toward Specialists," *Medscape*, August 10, 2011, http://www.medscape.com/viewarticle/747847.

101. Mayes and Berenson, "Medicare Prospective Payment," 148.

102. John D. Goodson, "Unintended Consequences of Resourced-Based Relative Value Scale Reimbursement," *Journal of the American Medical Association* 298, no. 19 (2007): 2308–10.

103. Joe Eaton, "Little-Known AMA Group Has Outsized Influence on Medicare Payments," Center for Public Integrity, November 7, 2010, http://www.publicintegrity.org/2010/11/07/2333/little-known-ama-group-has-outsized-influence-medicare-payments.

104. Anna Wilde Mathews and Tom McGinty, "Physician Panel Prescribes the Fees Paid by Medicare," *Wall Street Journal*, October 26, 2010, http://online.wsj.com/article/SB10001424052748704657304575540440173772102.html?KEYWORDS=ruc.

105. American Medical Association, "RVS Update Process."

106. American Medical Association, "The RVS Update Committee," http://www.ama-assn.org/ama/pub/physician-resources/solutions-managing-your-practice/coding-billing-insurance/medicare/the-resource-based-relative-value-scale/the-rvs-update-committee.page.

107. Lowes, "Lawsuit Targets Medicare."

108. Pauline W. Chen, "How One Small Group Sets Doctors' Pay," *New York Times, Well Blog*, September 22, 2011, http://well.blogs.nytimes.com/2011/09/22/how-one-small-group-sets-doctors-pay.

109. Ibid.

110. Ibid.

111. Ibid.

112. American Medical Association, "RVS Update Process."

113. Reinhardt, "The Little-Known Decision-Makers."

114. Kent J. Moore et al., "What Every Physician Should Know About the RUC," *Family Practice Management* 15, no. 2 (2008): 36–39, http://www.aafp.org/fpm/2008/0200/p36.html.

115. Lowes, "Lawsuit Targets Medicare."

116. Mathews and McGinty, "Physician Panel Prescribes."

117. Anna Wilde Mathews, "Dividing the Medicare Pie Pits Doctor Against Doctor," *Wall Street Journal*, April 7, 2011, http://online.wsj.com/article/SB10001424052702303341904575576480649488148.html?KEYWORDS=ruc.

118. Mathews and McGinty, "Physician Panel Prescribes."

119. Mark D. Schwartz et al., "Changes in Medical Students' Views of Internal Medicine Careers from 1990 to 2007," *Annals of Internal Medicine* 171, no. 8 (2011): 744–49.

120. Anna Wilde Mathews, "Primary-Care Doctors Push for Raise," *Wall Street Journal*, September 8, 2011, http://online.wsj.com/article/SB10001424053111903648204576554903022884780.html?KEYWORDS=ruc.

121. Lasser, Woolhandler, and Himmelstein, "Sources of U.S. Physician Income."

122. Ibid.

123. Ibid

124. Ibid.

125. Martensen, "History of Medicine."

126. Ibid., 812.

127. National Center for Health Statistics, "Health, United States, 2010," 347, table 107.

128. Donini-Lenhoff and Hedrick, "Growth of Specialization."

129. Some government-created incentives for physician entrepreneurship may not have been deliberate, but observers have noted a conscious attempt in various public policies to promote it. See Mark A. Rodwin, *Conflicts of Interest and the Future of Medicine: The United States, France and Japan* (New York: Oxford University Press, 2011), 139.

130. Mayes and Berenson, "Medicare Prospective Payment," 146.

131. Ibid., 147.

132. Because of the potential to inflict financial harm on traditional hospitals, the Medicare program imposed a moratorium on reimbursement for these facilities. However, a number of them continue to operate, and they could proliferate if Medicare were to change its policy.

133. Ibid., 147–48.

134. Ibid., 148.

135. Louis J. Acierno, *The History of Cardiology* (New York: Parthenon Publishing Group, 1994), 4.

136. Ibid., 7.

137. Ibid., 3.

138. James B. Herrick, *A Short History of Cardiology* (Baltimore, MD: Charles C. Thomas, 1942), 25.

139. Fye, *American Cardiology* 13.

140. Ibid., 8.

141. Ibid., 59.

142. Ibid., 67.

143. American College of Cardiology, "History," http://www.cardiosource.org/ACC/About-ACC/Who-We-Are/History.aspx.

144. Fye, *American Cardiology,* 346.

145. Ibid.

146. Ibid., 225.

147. Ibid., 225–26.

148. Ibid., 226.

149. Ibid., 227.

150. Ibid.

151. Ibid.

152. Ibid., 228.

153. Ibid., 229.

154. Ibid., 234.

155. Ibid., 243.

156. Ibid., 300.

157. Kristina Fiore, "ACC Sues HHS Over Medicare Rate Cuts," *Medpage Today,* December 29, 2009, http://www.medpagetoday.com/PublicHealthPolicy/Medicare/17729.

158. The role of the NIH generally in advancing the treatment of cardiac conditions is discussed in National Institutes of Health, "Turning Discovery into Health," NIH Pub. No. 11-7634 (January 2011), http://www.nih.gov/about/discovery/viewbook_2011.pdf. The development of statins is discussed in Daniel Steinberg, "The Statins in Preventive Cardiology," *New England Journal of Medicine* 359, no. 14 (2008): 1426–27. The development of beta-blockers is discussed in Benjamin Zycher, Joseph A. DiMasi, and Christopher-Paul Milne, "Private Sector Contributions to Pharmaceutical Science: Thirty-Five Summary Case Histories," *American Journal of Therapeutics* 17, no. 1 (2010): 101–20. The development of catheterization and valve repair are discussed in Gretchen A. Case, "National Cancer Institute Oral History Project: Interview with Alan S. Rabson, MD" (July 11, 1997),

http://history.nih.gov/archives/downloads/rabsontranscript.pdf. The development of cardiac stents is discussed in National Institutes of Health Office of Technology Transfer,
"Paclitaxel-Coated Stents: A Way to Bypass By-Pass Surgery," June 2003, http://www.ott.
nih.gov/pdfs/TaxusCS.pdf. The development of defibrillators is discussed in William M.
Smith and Raymond E. Ideker, "Automatic Implantable Cardioverter-Defibrillators," *Annual
Review of Biomedical Engineering* 1, no. 1 (1999): 331–46. The development of cardiac
bypass surgery is discussed in William S. Stoney, "Historical Perspectives in Cardiology,"
Circulation 119, no. 21 (2009): 2844–53. See also National Heart, Lung, and Blood Institute,
"2012 Fact Book: Important Events," May 13, 2013, http://www.nhlbi.nih.gov/about/fact-
book/chapter3.htm.

159. Fye, *American Cardiology*, 254.

160. Ibid., 113.

161. Lemelson-MIT, "Thomas Fogarty: Embolectomy Balloon Catheter, Inventor of
the Week Archive," http://web.mit.edu/invent/iow/fogarty.html.

162. Fye, *American Cardiology*, 301.

163. Lemels Ni-MIT, "Thomas Fogarty."

164. Fye, *American Cardiology*, 304.

165. Ibid., 305.

166. The Society for Cardiovascular Angiography and Interventions, "Salary
Survey Results for Invasive Cardiologists" (2004), http://www.scai.org/asset.
axd?id=6e562027-34d2-49af-9476-954852b0695c&t=633958630135230000.

167. Fye, *American Cardiology*, 319.

168. Medscape News, "Cardiologist Compensation Report 2012."

169. Harris Meyer, "How Much Should Doctors Really Make?" *Medscape*, September
25, 2012, http://www.medscape.com/viewarticle/771433.

170. Victoria Stagg Elliott, "Doctors Describe Pressures Driving Them From
Independent Practice," American Medical Association, November 19, 2012. http://www.
ama-assn.org/amednews/2012/11/19/bil21119.htm.

171. Allison Liebhaber and Joy M. Grossman, *Tracking Report: Physicians Moving to
Mid-Sized, Single-Specialty Practices* (Washington, DC: Center for Studying Health System
Change, August 2007), http://www.hschange.com/CONTENT/941/941.pdf.

172. Gardiner Harris, "More Doctors Giving Up Private Practices," *New York
Times*, March 25, 2010, http://www.nytimes.com/2010/03/26/health/policy/26docs.
html?pagewanted=all.

173. Ibid.

174. Stephen L. Isaacs, Paul S. Jellinek, and Walker K. Ray, "The Independent
Physician—Going, Going..." *New England Journal of Medicine* 360, no. 7 (2009): 655–57.

175. Ibid.

176. Victoria Stagg Elliott, "Ownership Loses Its Luster: Physicians Less Likely to
Go Solo," *American Medical News*, October 19, 2009, http://www.ama-assn.org/amed-
news/2009/10/19/bisa1019.htm.

177. Isaacs, Jellinek, and Ray, "The Independent Physician."

178. *Arizona v. Maricopa County Medical Society*, 457 U.S. 332 (1982).

179. American Medical Association, "Opinion 6.03—Fee Splitting: Referrals to
Health Care Facilities," American Medical Association Code of Medical Ethics, http://www.
ama-assn.org/ama/pub/physician-resources/medical-ethics/code-medical-ethics/opin-
ion603.page?.

180. 42 U.S.C. § 1320a-7B.

181. *United States v. Greber*, 760 F.2d 68, cert. denied, 474 U.S. 988, 106 S.Ct. 396, 88 L.Ed. 2d 348 (3rd Cir. 1985).

182. 42 CFR § 1001.952.

183. 42 U.S.C. § 1395nn.

184. The Ethics in Patient Referrals Act, commonly known as the Stark Amendments, contains an exception to its prohibition against referrals between providers who have a financial relationship for referrals between physicians in a group practice. 42 U.S.C. sec. 1395nn.

185. Patient Protection and Affordable Care Act, P.L. 111-148, 124 Stat. 119, § 3022 (2010); 42 C.F.R 425.

186. Staff of the Washington Post, *Landmark: The Inside Story of America's New Health-Care Law and What It Means for Us All* (New York: Public Affairs, 2010), 131.

187. Health Information Technology for Economic and Clinical Health Act, P.L. 111-5, 123 Stat. 226, 2009.

188. US Department of Health & Human Services. "HITECH Act Enforcement Interim Final Rule," http://www.hhs.gov/ocr/privacy/hipaa/administrative/enforcementrule/hitechenforcementifr.html.

189. Richard Hillestad, "Can Electronic Medical Record Systems Transform Health Care? Potential Health Benefits, Savings, and Costs," *Health Affairs* 24, no. 5 (September 2005): 1103–17.

190. Harris, "More Doctors Giving."

191. "Ronald Reagan Speaks Out on Socialized Medicine" (1961), http://www.youtube.com/watch?v=AYrlDlrLDSQ.

192. John Colombotos, "Physicians and Medicare: A Before-After Study of the Effects of Legislation on Attitudes," *American Sociological Review* 34, no. 3 (1969): 318–34.

193. Ibid.

194. Physicians were active in ancient Greece. James E. Bailey, "Asklepios: Ancient Hero of Medical Caring," *Annals of Internal Medicine* 124, no. 2 (1996): 257–63.

195. Starr, *The Social Transformation*, 68–69.

196. Rampell, "How Much Do Doctors."

Chapter 6

1. Congressional Budget Office, *Tax Subsidies for Medical Care: Current Policies and Possible Alternatives* (Washington, DC: US Government Printing Office, 1980), 2, http://www.cbo.gov/sites/default/files/cbofiles/ftpdocs/91xx/doc9180/80doc01b.pdf.

2. Milton Friedman, "How to Cure Health Care," *The Public Interest* no. 142 (Winter 2001): 6–7.

3. "Fortune 500, Our Annual Ranking of America's Largest Corporations, Health Care: Insurance and Managed Care" *CNN Money*, http://money.cnn.com/magazines/fortune/fortune500/2012/industries/223/.

4. Ibid.

5. "Fortune 500, Our Annual Ranking of America's Largest Corporations, Top Industries: Fast Grower," *CNN Money*, http://money.cnn.com/magazines/fortune/fortune500/2009/performers/industries/profits/assets.html.

6. National Center for Health Statistics, "Health, United States, 2011," 368–69, table 124.

7. Ibid.

8. Centers for Medicare & Medicaid Services, "National Health Expenditures 2011 Highlights," 1, https://www.cms.gov/Research-Statistics-Data-and-Systems/Statistics-Trends-and-Reports/NationalHealthExpendData/Downloads/highlights.pdf.

9. Kaiser Family Foundation, "Health Care Costs: A Primer."

10. Kaiser Family Foundation, "Health Care Spending in the United States and Selected OECD Countries April 2011," exhibit 12, http://www.kff.org/insurance/snapshot/oecd042111.cfm.

11. Organisation for Economic Co-operation and Development, "Policy Brief— Private Health Insurance in OECD Countries" (September 2004), figure 1, www.oecd.org/dataoecd/42/6/33820355.pdf.

12. Centers for Medicare & Medicaid Services, "National Health Expenditures," 2.

13. Sean P. Keehan et al., "National Health Spending Projections Through 2020: Economic Recovery and Reform Drive Faster Spending Growth," *Health Affairs* 30, no. 8 (2011): 1594–605.

14. National Center for Health Statistics, "Health, United States, 2011," 376–78, table 129.

15. Field, *Health Care Regulation*, 75.

16. Commonwealth Fund, *"Hospital Care,"* 572–73.

17. Starr, *The Social Transformation*, 237–38.

18. Price V. Fishback and Shawn Everett Kantor, *A Prelude to the Welfare State: The Origins of Workers' Compensation* (Chicago: University of Chicago Press, 2000).

19. Patient Protection and Affordable Care Act, P.L. 111-148, 124 Stat. 119, §§1401-1421 (2010) (to be codified in scattered sections of Titles 21, 25, 26, 29, & 42 U.S.C.).

20. Robert Cunningham III and Robert M. Cunningham Jr., *The Blues: A History of the Blue Cross and Blue Shield System* (DeKalb, IL: Northern Illinois University Press, 1997). See also Sallyanne Payton and Rhoda M. Powsner, "Regulation Through the Looking Glass: Hospitals, Blue Cross, and Certificate-of-Need," *University of Michigan Law Review* 79, no. 2 (1980): 214–28, and Starr, *The Social Transformation*, 295–98.

21. Starr, *The Social Transformation*, 295–98.

22. Commonwealth Fund, "Hospital Care," 575–76.

23. Starr, *The Social Transformation*, 295–98.

24. Ibid.

25. Starr, *The Social Transformation*, 306–308.

26. Ibid.

27. Executive Order 9328 of April 8, 1943, Relating to the Stabilization of Wages, Prices, and Salaries.

28. Starr, *The Social Transformation*, 311.

29. Ibid.

30. Commonwealth Fund, "Hospital Care," 574.

31. Melissa Thomasson, "Health Insurance in the United States," Economic History Association, January 1, 2010, http://eh.net/encyclopedia/article/thomasson.insurance.health.us.

32. Internal Revenue Code of 1954, P.L. 83–591.

33. Thomas M. Selden and Bradley M. Grey, "Tax Subsidies for Employment-Related Health Insurance: Estimates for 2006," *Health Affairs* 25, no. 6 (2006): 1568–79, http://content.healthaffairs.org/cgi/reprint/25/6/1568.

34. Ibid.

35. Kaiser Family Foundation, "Tax Subsidies for Health Insurance: An Issue Brief" (July 2008), http://www.kff.org/insurance/upload/7779.pdf.

36. Executive Office of the President Council of Economic Advisers, "The Economic Effects of Health Care Reform on Small Businesses and Their Employees" (July 25, 2009), http://www.whitehouse.gov/assets/documents/CEA-smallbusiness-july24.pdf.

37. American Academy of Actuaries, *Critical Issues in Health Reform: Risk Pooling* (Washington, DC: American Academy of Actuaries, 2009), http://www.actuary.org/pdf/health/pool_july09.pdf.

38. US Government Accountability Office, "Private Health Insurance: Estimates of Individuals with Pre-Existing Conditions Range from 36 Million to 122 Million," GAO-12-346 (March 2012), http://gao.gov/assets/590/589618.pdf.

39. A limited tax exemption is available for health insurance purchased by some self-employed workers, but its value is considerably less than that enjoyed by those who obtain health coverage from an employer.

40. US Census Bureau, "Health Insurance, Highlights 2010," http://www.census.gov/hhes/www/hlthins/data/incpovhlth/2010/highlights.html.

41. Jane Hiebert-White, "52 Million Uninsured Americans by 2010," *Health Affairs Blog*, June 2, 2009, http://healthaffairs.org/blog/2009/06/02/52-million-uninsured-americans-by-2010/.

42. Comprehensive Omnibus Budget Reconciliation Act, 26 U.S.C. § 9801 (1986). The amount of time during which former employees can maintain health coverage with a firm is 18 months for those whose employment terminated because of a layoff and 36 months for those who lost coverage because of divorce or separation from the covered worker.

43. Health Insurance Portability and Accountability Act, 42 U.S.C. §§ 300gg, et seq. (1996).

44. D. Andrew Austin and Thomas L. Hungerford, "The Market Structure of the Health Insurance Industry, Congressional Research Service," 7.5700 (November 17, 2009), 5–6, http://www.fas.org/sgp/crs/misc/R40834.pdf.

45. Commonwealth Fund, "Hospital Care," 573–74.

46. Starr, *The Social Transformation*, 329–30.

47. Lisa Jackson Conwell, "The Role of Health Insurance Brokers: Providing Small Employers with a Helping Hand, Center for Studying Health System Change," Issue Brief No. 57, October 2002, http://hschange.org/CONTENT/480/.

48. "What Is NAHU?" National Association of Health Underwriters, 2012, http://www.nahu.org/about/index.cfm.

49. McCarran-Ferguson Act, 15 U.S.C. §§ 1011–1014.

50. Employee Retirement Income Security Act of 1974, 29 USC § 1144(b)(2), et seq. (1974).

51. Ibid.

52. Larry J. Pittman, "ERISA's Preemption Clause: Progress Towards a More Equitable Preemption of State Laws," *Indiana Law Review* 34, no. 2 (2001): 207–94.

53. Carlos Zarabozo, "Milestones in Medicare Managed Care," *Health Care Financing Review* 22, no. 1 (2002), http://www.cms.gov/Research-Statistics-Data-and-Systems/Research/HealthCareFinancingReview/downloads/00fallpg61.pdf.

54. Kovner, "Health Maintenance Organizations."

55. Commonwealth Fund, "Hospital Care," 572.

56. Neva Deardorff, "The Health Insurance Plan of Greater New York Begins Service," *The Social Service Review* 21, no. 2 (1947).

57. K. Scott, "Case Study. Group Health Association: Can Humana Resuscitate the Moribund HMO?" *Health Systems Lead* 2, no. 4 (May 1995): 12–18.

58. Anthony R. Kovner and James R. Knickman, eds., *Health Care Delivery in the United States*, 10th ed. (New York: Springer Publishing Co., 2011), 57.

59. Starr, *The Social Transformation*, 327.

60. Health Maintenance Organization Act, 42 U.S.C. §280c, 300c, et seq. (1973).

61. Joseph L. Dorsey, "The Health Maintenance Organization Act of 1973 (P.L. 93-222) and Prepaid Group Practice Plan," *Medical Care* 13, no. 1 (January, 1975): 6–7.

62. Arnold J. Rosoff, "The Business of Medicine: Problems with the Corporate Practice of Medicine Doctrine," *Specialty Law Digest—Health Care Monthly* 9, no. 14 (1988) 7–25.

63. Martin Markovich, "The Rise of HMOs" (Rand Corporation, March 2003), http://www.rand.org/pubs/rgs_dissertations/RGSD172.html.

64. Joseph Weber, "In This Corner, It's U.S. Healthcare." *BusinessWeek*, March 22, 1992, http://www.businessweek.com/stories/1992-03-22/in-this-corner-its-u-dot-s-dot-healthcare-dot-dot-dot.

65. Kaiser Family Foundation, "Employer Health Benefits 2012 Annual Survey, 2012," 67, exhibit 5.1, http://ehbs.kff.org/pdf/2012/8345.pdf.

66. Health Maintenance Organization Amendments of 1976, P.L. 94–460; Health Maintenance Organization Amendments of 1978, P.L. 95–559.

67. Starr, *The Social Transformation*, 415.

68. Ibid., 415.

69. Alvin R. Tarlov, "HMO Enrollment Growth and Physicians: The Third Compartment," *Health Affairs* 5, no. 1 (Spring 1986): 23, 30, exhibit 2.

70. Gary Claxton et al., "Health Benefits in 2007: Premium Increases Fall to an Eight-Year Low, While Offer Rates and Enrollment Remain Stable," *Health Affairs* 26, no. 5 (2007): 1407, 1413 exhibit 4 (September/October 2007).

71. Ibid.

72. Alain C. Enthoven, "Why Managed Care Has Failed to Contain Health Costs," *Health Affairs* 12, no. 3 (1993): 27–43.

73. Starr, *The Social Transformation*, 439.

74. Martin Gaynor & Deborah Haas-Wilson, "Change, Consolidation, and Competition in Health Care Markets," *Journal of Economic Perspectives* 13, no. 1 (1999): 141– 64, 142–44 (describing the 1990s horizontal consolidation of health care organizations via mergers and acquisitions).

75. Tim Smart and Keith H. Hammonds, "Aetna's Booster Shot: An $8.9 Billion Merger Makes it No. 1 in Managed Care," *BusinessWeek*, April 14, 1996, http://www.businessweek.com/stories/1996-04-14/aetnas-booster-shot.

76. Larger provider networks and better prices for services also gave larger national HMOs a significant advantage over smaller regional ones in attracting employers as customers. Weber, "In This Corner."

77. Mayes and Berenson, "Medicare Prospective Payment," 113.

78. New York-Presbyterian, "History," http://nyp.org/about/history.html; Partners Healthcare, "History of Partners," http://www.partners.org/About/Company-Information/

History-of-Partners.aspx; John A. Kastor, *Governance of Teaching Hospitals: Turmoil at Penn and Hopkins* (Baltimore, MD: Johns Hopkins University Press, 2004), 28–76.

79. Francis J. Crosson, "21st-Century Health Care—the Case for Integrated Delivery Systems," *New England Journal of Medicine* 361 (2009): 1324–25.

80. Mayes and Berenson, "Medicare Prospective Payment," 121.

81. Ibid.

82. Carey Goldberg, "A Behind-the-Ledger Look at Partners HealthCare's Billions," *CommonHealth Reform and Reality*, August 19, 2011, http://commonhealth.wbur.org/2011/08/partners-healthcare-billions.

83. The consolidation on the provider side that managed care wrought may have changed the structure of the managed care market, as well. The large provider networks that formed to gain negotiating strength succeeded in extracting higher prices. The consequent higher cost to plans led many of them to merge to enhance their own bargaining clout. With the mergers reducing the amount of competition in the market, many plans raised premiums, which led some employers to shift workers from HMOs, which no longer held a price advantage, to other forms of managed care with fewer restrictions, such as PPOs and POS plans. The result was an industry that had fewer companies but that offered a broader range of products. Mayes and Berenson, "Medicare Prospective Payment," 113.

84. Kaiser Family Foundation, "Medicare Spending and Financing," November 2012, http://www.kff.org/medicare/upload/7305-07.pdf.

85. Robert J. Myers, *Medicare* (Bryn Mawr, PA: McCahan Foundation, 1970), 307.

86. Susan Bartlett Foote, "Focus on Locus: Evolution of Medicare's Local Coverage Policy," *Health Affairs* 22, no. 4 (2003): 137–46, http://content.healthaffairs.org/content/22/4/137.full.

87. The role and history of intermediaries in Medicare is discussed in Susan Bartlett Foote, "Focus on Locus."

88. Coverage for outpatient prescription drugs was added in 2003 by the Medicare Prescription Drug, Improvement and Modernization Act of 2003, P.L. 108-173, 117 Stat. 2066, codified at 42 U.S.C. §1395. Coverage for some preventive care was added in 2010 by the Patient Protection and Affordable Care Act, P.L. 111-148, 124 Stat. 119, §§1401–1421 (2010) (to be codified in scattered sections of Titles 21, 25, 26, 29, & 42 U.S.C.).

89. Myers, *Medicare*, 308–11.

90. Omnibus Reconciliation Act of 1981, P.L. 97-35. The development and early experience with waivers that permitted states to use managed care to deliver Medicaid services is discussed in Dobson, Moran, and Young, "The Role of Federal Waivers."

91. Michael Sparer, "Medicaid Managed Care: Costs, Access, and Quality of Care," Synthesis Report No. 23, Robert Wood Johnson Foundation, September 2012, 3, http://www.rwjf.org/content/dam/farm/reports/reports/2012/rwjf401106.

92. Ibid.

93. Ibid., 1.

94. Ibid.

95. John Holahan et al., "Medicaid Managed Care in Thirteen States," *Heath Affairs* 17, no. 3 (1998): 43–63.

96. Michael Gluck and Virginia Reno, "Reflections on Implementing Medicare," National Academy of Social Insurance (January 2001), http://www.nasi.org/research/2001/reflections-implementing-medicare-second-edition.

97. Thomas G. McGuire, Joseph P. Newhouse, and Anna D. Sinaiko, "An Economic History of Medicare Part C," *Milbank Quarterly* 89, no. 2 (2011): 289–332.

98. Balanced Budget Act of 1997, P.L. 105–33, 111 Stat. 251 (1997).

99. Ibid., § 4001.

100. Medicare Prescription Drug, Improvement and Modernization Act of 2003, P.L. 108-173, 117 Stat. 2066, codified at 42 U.S.C. §1395.

101. Mayes and Berenson, "Medicare Prospective Payment," 131.

102. Medicare Prescription Drug, Improvement and Modernization Act of 2003, P.L. 108-173, 117 Stat. 2066, codified at 42 U.S.C. §1395.

103. Mark Merlis, "The Value of Extra Benefits Offered by Medicare Advantage Plans in 2006" (Kaiser Family Foundation, 2008), 1, http://www.kff.org/medicare/upload/7744.pdf.

104. See discussion in Thomas R. Oliver, Philip R. Lee, and Helene L. Lipton, "A Political History of Medicare and Prescription Drug Coverage," *Milbank Quarterly* 82, no. 2 (2004): 283–354.

105. Medpac, "Part D Payment System: Payment Basics," October 2011, http://www.medpac.gov/documents/MedPAC_Payment_Basics_11_PartD.pdf.

106. Marsha Gold et al., "Medicare Advantage 2012 Data Spotlight: Enrollment Market Update" (Kaiser Family Foundation), http://www.kff.org/medicare/upload/8323.pdf.

107. Jennifer O'Sullivan, "Medicare Part D Prescription Drug Benefit: A Primer" (Congressional Research Service, 2008), 28, 39, http://www.aging.senate.gov/crs/medicare12.pdf.

108. The Boards of Trustees of the Federal Hospital Insurance and Federal Supplementary Medical Insurance Trust Funds, "2012 Annual Report" (2012), 117, table III.D1, http://www.cms.gov/Research-Statistics-Data-and-Systems/Statistics-Trends-and-Reports/ReportsTrustFunds/downloads/tr2012.pdf.

109. Kaiser Family Foundation, "Analysis of Medicare Prescription Drug Plans in 2012 and Key Trends Since 2006" (2012), 20, Exhibit 19, http://www.kff.org/medicare/upload/8357.pdf.

110. US House of Representatives, "New Report Highlights Medicare Advantage Insurers' Higher Administrative Spending," Committee on Energy and Commerce, http://democrats.energycommerce.house.gov/index.php?q=news/new-report-highlights-medicare-advantage-insurers-higher-administrative-spending.

111. Sarah Kliff, "Does Medicare Advantage Cost Less? Or Does It Cost More?" *The Washington Post*, August 22, 2012, http://www.washingtonpost.com/blogs/wonkblog/wp/2012/08/22/does-medicare-advantage-cost-less-or-does-it-cost-more/.

112. Jordan Rau, "Do Medicare Advantage Plans Skim Off the Healthiest?" *AARP Blog*, February 4, 2013, http://blog.aarp.org/2013/02/04/do-medicare-advantage-plans-skim-off-the-healthiest-customers/.

113. Karen Davis and Kristof Stremikis, "Medicare Works: Public Program Continues to Outperform Private Insurance in Ensuring Access to Care and Providing Financial Protection," The Commonwealth Fund, July 24, 2012, http://www.commonwealthfund.org/Blog/2012/Jul/Medicare-Works-Continues-to-Outperform-Private-Insurance.aspx.

114. See Mark V. Pauly, "Competition and New Technology," *New England Journal of Medicine* 24, no. 6 (2005): 1523–35.

115. National Commission on Fiscal Responsibility and Reform, "About the National Commission on Fiscal Responsibility and Reform," http://www.fiscalcommission.gov/about/.

116. Trudy Lieberman, "Medicare Vouchers Explained," *Columbia Journalism Review*, January 18, 2012, http://www.cjr.org/campaign_desk/medicare_vouchers_explained.php?page=all.

117. For a description of such a plan, see Gretchen Jacobson, Tricia Neuman, and Anthony Damico, "Transformation of Medicare into a Premium Support System: Implications for Beneficiary Premiums" (Kaiser Family Foundation, October 2012), http://kaiserfamilyfoundation.files.wordpress.com/2013/01/8373.pdf.

118. Pew Research Center for the People and the Press, "Medicare Voucher Plan Remains Unpopular," August 21, 2012, http://www.people-press.org/2012/08/21/medicare-voucher-plan-remains-unpopular/1/.

119. See Mayes and Berenson, "Medicare Prospective Payment," 131. Medicare managed care, both in the form of Medicare + Choice and of Medicare Advantage, has proved more expensive than traditional Medicare. In 2003, its coverage cost about 4 percent more. In 2004, the first year that private plans operated under the MMA, the difference was 8.4 percent. It would have reached 15 percent if account were taken of the fact that many of the plans insured healthier patient populations than traditional Medicare. In 2005, the difference was 6.6 percent.

120. Aetna, "Aetna History," http://www.aetna.com/about-aetna-insurance/aetna-corporate-profile/aetna-history/index.html.

121. Ibid.

122. Smart and Hammonds, "Aetna's Booster Shot."

123. Ibid.

124. Gilbert S. Gaul, "U.S. Healthcare's Abramson: Dedicated, Perhaps Ruthless," *Philadelphia Inquirer*, April 2, 1996, http://articles.philly.com/1996-04-02/news/25661373_1_leonard-abramson-hospitals-health-care.

125. Funding Universe, "U.S. Healthcare, Inc. History," http://www.fundinguniverse.com/company-histories/u-s-healthcare-inc-history/.

126. Carpenter, *BusinessWeek*.

127. Fay Rice, "America's Hottest HMO: U.S. Healthcare Shows that Medical Bills Can Be Managed with Disease Prevention Programs and Cost Controls," *Fortune*, July 15, 1991, http://money.cnn.com/magazines/fortune/fortune_archive/1991/07/15/75259/index.htm.

128. Kimberly Carpenter, "Can a Pioneering HMO Crack the Tough Markets?" *Business Week*, February 10 1986.

129. Gilbert M. Gaul, "U.S. Healthcare's Abramson: Dedicated, Perhaps Ruthless."

130. Funding Universe, "U.S. Healthcare, Inc. History," http://www.fundinguniverse.com/company-histories/u-s-healthcare-inc-history/.

131. Rice, *Fortune*.

132. Ibid.

133. Carpenter, "Can a Pioneering HMO."

134. Ibid.

135. Carpenter, "Can a Pioneering HMO."

136. Ibid.

137. Mandel and Weber, "What's Really Propping."

138. David R. Olmos, "Aetna Will Buy U.S. Healthcare for $8.6 Billion," *Los Angeles Times*, April 2, 1996, http://articles.latimes.com/1996-04-02/news/mn-53913_1_health-care.

139. Ibid.

140. Aetna, "Aetna History," http://www.aetna.com/about-aetna-insurance/aetna-corporate-profile/aetna-history/index.html.

141. Ibid.

142. Ibid.

143. James C. Robinson, "From Managed Care to Consumer Health Insurance: The Rise and Fall of Aetna," *Health Affairs* 23, no. 2 (2004): 43–55, at 51.

144. Aetna, "Aetna Facts," http://www.aetna.com/about-aetna-insurance/aetna-corporate-profile/facts.html.

145. Ibid.

146. U.S. News, "The Top 25 Health Insurance Companies," http://health.usnews.com/health-plans/national-insurance-companies.

147. Kaiser Permanente, "Fast Facts About Kaiser Permanente," http://xnet.kp.org/newscenter/aboutkp/fastfacts.html.

148. Ibid.

149. Kaiser Permanente, "Kaiser Permanente—More than 60 Years of Quality," http://xnet.kp.org/newscenter/aboutkp/historyofkp.html.

150. Ibid.

151. Ibid.

152. Ibid.

153. Ibid.

154. Ibid.

155. Starr, *The Social Transformation*, 322.

156. Ibid., 322.

157. Commonwealth Fund, "Hospital Care," 573.

158. Kaiser Permanente, "Kaiser Permanente—More Than 60 Years of Quality," 2013, http://xnet.kp.org/newscenter/aboutkp/historyofkp.html.

159. Rickey Hendricks, "Medical Practice Embattled: Kaiser Permanente, the American Medical Association, and Henry J. Kaiser on the West Coast, 1945–1955," *Pacific Historical Review* 60, no.4 (1991): 439–73; see also Starr, *The Social Transformation*, 324–27.

160. Ibid., 395.

161. Funding Universe, "Kaiser Foundation Health Plan, Inc. History," http://www.fundinguniverse.com/company-histories/kaiser-foundation-health-plan-inc-history/.

162. Richey Hendricks, *A Model for National Health Care: The History of Kaiser Permanente* (New Brunswick, NJ: Rutgers University Press, 1993), 205.

163. Funding Universe, "Kaiser Foundation Health."

164. Ibid.

165. Starr, *The Social Transformation*, 322.

166. Tom Murphy, "Report: Overhaul Offers Key Insurer Growth Chance," *Boston.com*, October 2, 2012, http://www.boston.com/business/news/2012/10/02/report-overhaul-offers-key-insurer-growth-chance/YmPU4fXgk4CojdErArJWNO/story.html.

Chapter 7

1. Bruce C. Vladeck and Thomas Rice, "Market Failure and the Failure of Discourse: Facing up to the Power of Sellers," *Health Affairs* 28, no. 5 (2009): 1305–15, 1306.

2. World Health Organization, "World Health Statistics 2012" (2012), 140, http://www.who.int/gho/publications/world_health_statistics/EN_WHS2012_Full.pdf.

3. Kaiser Family Foundation, *Health Care Costs*, 4.

4. Ezra Klein, "Two Charts That Should Be in Every Health-Care Discussion," *Washington Post*, January 25, 2013, http://www.washingtonpost.com/blogs/wonkblog/wp/2013/01/25/the-charts-that-should-dominate-the-health-care-discussion/.

5. David A. Squires, "Explaining High Health Care Spending in the United States: An International Comparison of Supply, Utilization, Prices, and Quality," *The Commonwealth Fund* 10, http://www.commonwealthfund.org/Publications/Issue-Briefs/2012/May/High-Health-Care-Spending.aspx.

6. Ibid.

7. "Top Industries: Most Profitable," *CNN Money*, http://money.cnn.com/magazines/fortune/fortune500/2009/performers/industries/profits/.

8. Raymond Goldberg, *Drugs Across the Spectrum*, 6th ed. (Belmont, CA: Cengage Learning, 2010), 73.

9. National Institutes of Health, "NIH budget: Research for the People,"http://www.nih.gov/about/budget.htm.

10. Kaiser Family Foundation, "Total Hospitals," 2010, http://www.statehealthfacts.org/comparemaptable.jsp?cat=8&ind=382.

11. Hill-Burton Act, 42 U.S.C. §§ 291 et seq. (1946).

12. Peter Tyson, "The Hippocratic Oath Today," Public Broadcasting Service, March 27, 2001, http://www.pbs.org/wgbh/nova/body/hippocratic-oath-today.html.

13. Starr, *The Social Transformation*, 297.

14. Ibid.

15. Health Maintenance Organization Act, 42 U.S.C. § 280c, 300c, et seq. (1973).

16. Emily Walker, "Health Insurers Post Record Profits," *ABC News*, http://abcnews.go.com/Health/HealthCare/health-insurers-post-record-profits/story?id=9818699#.UEptg2hSTVQ.

17. Christopher J. Conover, "Health Care Regulation: A $169 Billion Hidden Tax," CATO Institute, 2004, http://www.cato.org/pubs/pas/pa527.pdf.

18. Health Insurance Portability and Accountability Act of 1996, P.L. 104-91.

19. Alan G. Williams, "The Cure for What Ails: A Realistic Remedy for the Medical Malpractice 'Crisis,'" *Stanford Law & Policy Review* 23 (2012): 478–79, 483.

20. David M. Studdert and others, "Claims, Errors, and Compensation Payments in Medical Malpractice Litigation," *The New England Journal of Medicine* 354, no. 19 (2006): 2024–33.

21. Conover, *Health Care Regulation*.

22. Most notably, the Cato Institute's estimate of the costs of health care regulation takes limited account of its full range of benefits. It gives minimal or no consideration to factors such as the facilitation of innovation, the expansion of the health system's size and accessibility, and the generation of public trust in health care goods and services.

23. FDA budgets, http://www.fda.gov/downloads/AboutFDA/ReportsManualsForms/Reports/BudgetReports/UCM301719.pdf.

24. Grant Newton, "The Private Sector—Alternative to Federal Funding of Biomedical Research," *Developmental Psychobiology* 2, no. 2 (1969): 55. Other examples of nonprofit foundations that provide funding for biomedical research include the Howard Hughes Medical Institute, http://www.hhmi.org/, and the Lucille P. Markey Charitable Trust, http://www.nap.edu/catalog.php?record_id=11627. Over the course of 15 years, the Lucille P. Markey Charitable Trust spent more than $500 million on four programs in the basic biomedical sciences.

25. E. Ray Dorsey et al., "Funding of US Biomedical Research, 2003–2008," *Journal of the American Medical Association* 303, no. 2 (2010): 137–43, 140.

26. Jeff Raikes, "Progress and Partnerships: 2010 Annual Report, CEO Letter" (Bill & Melinda Gates Foundation: 2010), http://www.gatesfoundation.org/annualreport/2010/Pages/grants-paid-summary.aspx.

27. Paul A. Samuelson, "The Pure Theory of Public Expenditure," *Review of Economics and Statistics* 36, no. 4 (1954): 387–89.

28. William L. Kissick, *Medicine's Dilemmas: Infinite Needs Versus Finite Resources* (New Haven, CT: Yale University Press, 1994).

29. National Institutes of Health, "The NIH Almanac: Nobel Laureates," http://www.nih.gov/about/almanac/nobel/index.htm.

30. National Institutes of Health, "Human Genome Project," http://report.nih.gov/nihfactsheets/ViewFactSheet.aspx?csid=45.

31. A poll conducted by the Kaiser Family Foundation in 2009 found that 51 percent of Medicare beneficiaries rate their coverage as excellent, compared with 32 percent of those below the age of 65 with private insurance. Kaiser Family Foundation, "Data Note: Americans' Satisfaction with Insurance Coverage" (2009), 5, http://www.kff.org/kaiserpolls/upload/7979.pdf.

32. David M. Studdert, Michelle M. Mello, and Troyen A. Brennan, "Medical Malpractice," *New England Journal of Medicine* 350, no. 3 (January 2014): 283–92.

33. One study found that higher rates of surgical complications at one hospital were associated with higher financial margins under Medicare and private insurance. Sunil Eappen and others, "Relationship Between Occurrence of Surgical Complications and Hospital Finances," *Journal of the American Medical Association* 309, no. 15 (2013): 1599–606. See also Christopher Weaver, "Treatment Woes Can Bolster Hospitals' Profit," *The Wall Street Journal*, April 16, 2013, http://online.wsj.com/article/SB10001424127887324345804578426693303833964.html?mod=djemHL_t.

34. Institute of Medicine, *To Err Is Human*.

35. The popularity of Medicare and the difficulty that it poses for efforts to reform the program are discussed in Robert Blendon and John M. Benson, "The Public's Views About Medicare and the Budget Deficit," *New England Journal of Medicine* 365, no. 4 (2011): e8(1)-e8(4).

36. Kaiser Family Foundation, "Health Care Costs," 18.

37. Kaiser Family Foundation, "Health Care Costs," 1.

38. World Health Organization, *The World Health Report 2000—Health Systems: Improving Performance* (2000), Geneva: World Health Organization. http://www.who.int/whr/2000/en/.

39. Ibid.

40. Dana P. Goldman, Mary Vaiana, and John A. Romley, "The Emerging Importance of Patient Amenities in Hospital Care," *New England Journal of Medicine* 363, no. 23 (December 2, 2010): 2185–87.

41. George Stigler, "The Theory of Economic Regulation," *The Bell Journal of Economics and Management Science* 2, no. 1 (1971): 3–21.

42. OpenSecrets.org, "Lobbying: Health, Sector Profile, 2012", http://www.opensecrets.org/lobby/indus.php?id=H.

43. OpenSecrets.org, "Lobbying: Top Spenders," http://www.opensecrets.org/lobby/top.php?indexType=s.

44. Robert E. Moffit, "Talking Points: A Guide to the Clinton Health Plan," The Heritage Foundation (1993), http://thf_media.s3.amazonaws.com/1993/pdf/tp_00.pdf.

45. Maggie E. Astor, "The Fine Line of Health-Care Politicking: A Comparative Analysis of Reform Efforts from Clinton to Obama," *Center for the Study of the Presidency & Congress* (2011), http://www.thepresidency.org/storage/Fellows2011/Astor-_Final_Paper.pdf.

46. Prescription Drug User Free Act, P.L. 102-571.

47. Medicare Prescription Drug, Improvement and Modernization Act of 2003, P.L. 108-173, 117 Stat. 2066, codified at 42 U.S.C. §1395.

48. See for example, Sam Baker and Elise Viebeck, "Overnight Health: Medicare Advantage Lobbying Heats Up," *The Hill*, March 18, 2013, http://thehill.com/blogs/health-watch/medicare/288853-overnight-health; Sam Baker, "Insurers Launch New TV Ads Against Medicare Advantage Cuts," *The Hill*, March 18, 2013, http://thehill.com/blogs/healthwatch/medicare/288771-insurers-launch-new-tv-ads-against-medicare-advantage-cuts.

49. Heather Perlberg, "Doctor Shortage Looms Amid Hospital Funding Gap," *Bloomberg*, October 5, 2011, http://www.bloomberg.com/news/2011-10-05/doctor-shortage-looms-as-teaching-hospitals-fight-for-funding.html.

50. American Association of American Medical Colleges, "Washington Highlights: Legislators Urge Increased NIH Funding," March 23, 2012, https://www.aamc.org/advocacy/washhigh/highlights2012/277490/legislatorsurgeincreasednihfunding.html.

51. RenalWeb, "Legislation Watch for Dialysis-related Issues," http://www.renalweb.com/legislation/bills.htm.

52. Peter Frost, "AMA Wants Higher Medicare Payments," *Chicago Tribune*, June 17, 2012, http://articles.chicagotribune.com/2012-06-17/news/ct-met-ama-0617-20120617_1_new-medicare-patients-health-care-law-ama-delegate.

53. Carpenter, "The Political Economy," 52.

54. Stephen N. Keith, "Prospective Payment for Hospital Costs Using Diagnosis-Related Groups: Will Cost Inflation Be Reduced?" *Journal of the National Medical Association* 75, no. 6 (1983): 609–23, 614.

55. Volume-and-Intensity Response Team, Office of the Actuary, HCFA, "Memorandum: Physician Volume & Intensity Response," Centers for Medicare & Medicaid Services (1998), http://www.cms.gov/Research-Statistics-Data-and-Systems/Research/ActuarialStudies/downloads/PhysicianResponse.pdf.

56. Ed Silverman, "Rare Opportunities: Orphan Drugs & Big Bucks," *Pharmalot*, August 23, 2012, http://www.pharmalot.com/2012/08/rare-opportunities-orphan-drugs-big-bucks/.

57. Katie Thomas, "In Documents on Pain Drug, Signs of Doubt and Deception," *New York Times*, June 24, 2012, http://www.nytimes.com/2012/06/25/health/in-documents-on-pain-drug-celebrex-signs-of-doubt-and-deception.html?pagewanted=all.

58. Organisation for Economic Co-operation and Development, "OECD Health Data 2012: How Does the United States Compare" (2012), http://www.oecd.org/unitedstates/BriefingNoteUSA2012.pdf.

59. Department of Health, NHS, http://www.dh.gov.uk/health/category/policy-areas/nhs/.

60. Yvonne Doyle and Adrian Bull, "Role of Private Sector in United Kingdom Healthcare System," *British Medical Journal* 321, no. 7260 (2000): 563–65.

61. Ibid.

62. The Commonwealth Fund, "International Profiles of Health Care Systems, 2011," 21–31, http://www.commonwealthfund.org/~/media/Files/Publications/Fund%20 Report/2011/Nov/1562_Squires_Intl_Profiles_2011_11_10.pdf.

63. Ibid., 78–85, 106–12.

64. In Switzerland, citizens who do not obtain insurance are not subject to a financial penalty, as they are under the ACA. Instead, the government assigns them to a plan. Ibid.

65. The Commonwealth Fund, "International Profiles," 78, 106.

66. Timothy Stoltzfus Jost, "The Experience of Switzerland and the Netherlands with Individual Health Insurance Mandates: A Model for the United States?" Washington and Lee University, http://law.wlu.edu/deptimages/Faculty/Jost%20The%20Experience%20 of%20Switzerland%20and%20the%20Netherlands.pdf.

67. Carol Propper and Katherine Green, "A Larger Role for the Private Sector in Financing UK Health Care: The Arguments and the Evidence," *Journal of Social Policy* 30, no. 4 (2001): 685–704.

68. The Commonwealth Fund, "International Profiles," 45–64, 73–77.

69. The term "medical-industrial complex" was first used in the early 1980s to describe the growing commercialization of various facets of health care that was becoming evident at that time. See Arnold S. Relman, "The New Medical-Industrial Complex," *New England Journal of Medicine* 303, no. 17 (October 1980): 963–70.

70. For a discussion of ways in which for-profit health care inflates America's spending, see Eduardo Porter, "Health Care and Profits, a Poor Mix," *New York Times*, January 8, 2013, B1, http://www.nytimes.com/2013/01/09/business/health-care-and-pursuit-of-profit-make-a-poor-mix.html?pagewanted=all&_r=0.

Chapter 8

1. Starr, *The Social Transformation*, 419.

2. Robert I. Field, "Regulation, Reform and the Creation of Free Market Health Care," *Hamline Journal of Public Law and Policy* 35 (2010): 301–31.

3. Starr, *The Social Transformation*, 244–57.

4. Theodore R. Marmor, *The Politics of Medicare* (Hawthorne, NY: Aldine Publishing Company, 1973), 8.

5. Ibid., 9.

6. Kaiser Family Foundation, "National Health Insurance—A Brief History of Reform Efforts in the U.S." (March 2009), 3, http://www.kff.org/healthreform/upload/7871.pdf.

7. Hill-Burton Act, 42 U.S.C. §§ 291 et seq. (1946).

8. Marmor, *The Politics of Medicare*, 11.

9. Ibid., 12.

10. Ibid.

11. Kerr-Mills Act, 86 P.L. 778, 74 Stat. 924 (1960). For a discussion on the Kerr-Mills Act, see Marmor, *The Politics of Medicare*, 35–36.

12. Health Insurance Benefits Act, 1961 H.R. 4222.

13. Peter A. Corning, "Social Security History, Chapter 4: The Fourth Round—1957 to 1965," http://www.ssa.gov/history/corningchap4.html.

14. US House of Representatives, "Party Divisions of the House of Representatives: 1789– Present," http://artandhistory.house.gov/house_history/partyDiv.aspx.

15. Public Broadcasting Service, "The Great Society," http://www.pbs.org/johngard-ner/chapters/4c.html.

16. David Blumenthal and James A. Morone, *The Heart of Power: Health and Politics in the Oval Office* (Berkeley: University of California Press 2009), 163.

17. Corning, "Social Security History, Chapter 4."

18. Starr, *The Social Transformation,* 375. See also Foote, "Focus on Locus."

19. Starr, *The Social Transformation,* 244–57.

20. Health Maintenance Organization Act, 42 U.S.C. §280c, 300c, et seq. (1973).

21. Paul Starr, *Remedy and Reaction: The Peculiar American Struggle over Health Care Reform* (New Haven, CT: Yale University Press, 2011), 55–56.

22. Carroll Kilpatrick, "Nixon Resigns," *Washington Post,* August 9, 1974, http://www.washingtonpost.com/wp-srv/national/longterm/watergate/articles/080974-3.htm.

23. The Washington Post, "The Watergate Story: Timeline," http://www.washington-post.com/wp-srv/politics/special/watergate/timeline.html.

24. Barry R. Furrow, "Health Reform and Ted Kennedy: The Art of Politics…and Persistence," *New York University Journal of Legislation and Public Policy* 14, no. 2 (2011): 445–76.

25. Ibid.

26. For a description of the Clinton plan, see James C. Robinson, *The Corporate Practice of Medicine* (Berkeley, CA: University of California Press, 1999), 45–48.

27. Starr, *Remedy and Reaction,* 81–82.

28. Lawton R. Burns, Gloria J. Bazzoli, Linda Dynan, and Douglas R. Wholey, "Managed Care, Market Stages, and Integrated Delivery Systems: Is There a Relationship?," *Health Affairs* 16, no. 6 (1997): 204–18.

29. Starr, *Remedy and Reaction,* 112–19.

30. George J. Annas, "Health Care Reform in America: Beyond Ideology," *Indiana Health Law Review* 5 (2008): 441–61, 443 (specifically discussing Harry & Louise ads).

31. Michele L. Procino, "Note: The Death of Health Care Reform in 1994: Another example of Congress' Inability to Enact Major Reform," *Widener Law Symposium Journal* 1 (1996): 547–86.

32. Comprehensive Omnibus Budget Reconciliation Act, 26 U.S.C. § 9801 (1986). COBRA also covers those who lose insurance because of separation or divorce from the covered employee. Coverage can be retained for up to 18 months in the case of a terminated employee and up to 36 months for a spouse. However, the beneficiary must continue to pay his or her share of the premium and the share that the employer had been contributing.

33. Health Insurance Portability and Accountability Act, 42 U.S.C. §§ 300gg, et seq. (1996). HIPAA also requires insurance companies to offer individual policies to terminated employees, although there are no limits on the prices that may be charged for them. A separate set of provisions in the law regulates the privacy of patient medical records.

34. Some states established CHIP plans that extended coverage to parents of eligible children.

35. Medicare Prescription Drug, Improvement and Modernization Act of 2003, P.L. 108-173, 117 Stat. 2066, codified at 42 U.S.C. §1395.

36. Stuart M., "Using Tax Credits to Create an Affordable Health System," The Heritage Foundation, July 20, 1990, http://www.heritage.org/research/reports/1990/07/using-tax-credits-to-create-an-affordable-health-system; Robert H. Blank, "Regulatory

Rationing: A Solution to Health Care Resource Allocation," *University of Pennsylvania Law Review* 140, no. 5(1992): 1573–96, 1588.

37. Starr, *Remedy and Reaction*, 107–08.

38. Avik Roy, "The Tortuous History of Conservatives and the Individual Mandate," *Forbes*, February 7, 2012, http://www.forbes.com/sites/aroy/2012/02/07/the-tortuous-conservative-history-of-the-individual-mandate/.

39. Starr, *Remedy and Reaction*, 167–74.

40. Edmund F. Haislmaier, "Massachusetts Health Reform: What the Doctor Ordered," The Heritage Foundation, May 6, 2006, http://www.heritage.org/research/commentary/2006/05/massachusetts-health-reform-what-the-doctor-ordered.

41. Kaiser Family Foundation, "Massachusetts Health Reform: Six Years Later" (2012), http://www.kff.org/healthreform/upload/8311.pdf; Michael J. Zinner and Edward H. Livingston, "JAMA Forum — The Massachusetts Health Care Reform Experiment: A Success," *news@JAMA*, October 31, 2012, http://newsatjama.jama.com/2012/10/31/the-massachusetts-health-care-reform-experiment-a-success/.

42. Leighton Ku et al., *How Is the Primary Care Safety Net Faring in Massachusetts? Community Health Centers in the Midst of Health Reform* (Washington, DC: Kaiser Commission on Medicaid and the Uninsured: 2009), 9, http://www.kff.org/healthreform/upload/7878.pdf.

43. Martha Bebinger, "WBUR Poll: Most Mass. Residents Support State Health Care Law," *WBUR: Boston's NPR News Station*, February 15, 2012, http://www.wbur.org/2012/02/15/health-care-wbur-poll.

44. Ku and others, *How Is the Primary Care*, 9.

45. Ibid.

46. Change.gov: The Office of the President-Elect, "The Obama-Biden Plan," http://change.gov/agenda/health_care_agenda/.

47. Patient Protection and Affordable Care Act, P.L. 111-148, 124 Stat. 119, §§1401-1421 (2010) (to be codified in scattered sections of Titles 21, 25, 26, 29, & 42 U.S.C.).

48. Peter Baker, "Democrats Embrace Once Pejorative 'Obamacare' Tag," *New York Times*, August 3, 2012, http://www.nytimes.com/2012/08/04/health/policy/democrats-embrace-once-pejorative-obamacare-tag.html.

49. The Supreme Court decision that upheld the constitutionality of the Obama health reform plan included a ruling that changed the expansion of Medicaid from a requirement that all states participate to an option. *National Federation of Independent Business v. Sebelius*, 567 U.S. __, 132 S.Ct. 2566 (2012). Just prior to implementation of the expansion, only about half of the states had accepted the option and chosen to participate. The Advisory Board Company, "Where Each State Stands on ACA's Medicaid Expansion," (June 14, 2013), http://www.advisory.com/Daily-Briefing/2012/11/09/MedicaidMap#lightbox/o/.

50. Patient Protection and Affordable Care Act, P.L. 111-148, 124 Stat. 119, §§1401-1421 (2010) (to be codified in scattered sections of Titles 21, 25, 26, 29, & 42 U.S.C.).

51. Oberlander, "Long Time Coming," 1113.

52. James A. Morone, "Presidents and Health Reform: From Franklin D. Roosevelt to Barack Obama," *Health Affairs* 29, no. 6 (2010): 1096–100.

53. Starr, *Remedy and Reaction*, 23–24.

54. Troyen A. Brennan and David M. Studdert, "How Will Health Insurers Respond to New Rules Under Health Reform?" *Health Affairs* 29, no. 6 (2010): 1147–51.

55. Oberlander, "Long Time Coming," 1115.

56. Centers for Medicare & Medicaid Services, "Affordable Care Act Update: Implementing Medicare Cost Savings," http://www.cms.gov/apps/docs/ACA-Update-Implementing-Medicare-Costs-Savings.pdf.

57. Jeremy A. Lazarus, "AMA to Wall Street Journal: AMA Support of Affordable Care Act," American Medical Association, July 6, 2012, http://www.ama-assn.org/ama/pub/news/letters-editor/2012-07-06-wsj-ama-support-of-affordable-care-act.page.

58. Patient Protection and Affordable Care Act, P.L. 111-148, 124 Stat. 119, §§1401-1421 (2010) (to be codified in scattered sections of Titles 21, 25, 26, 29, & 42 U.S.C.).

59. Jennifer DePinto, "Public Opinion of the Health Care Law," CBS News, June 28, 2012, http://www.cbsnews.com/8301-250_162-57462689/public-opinion-of-the-health-care-law/.

60. Tom Cohen, "House Republicans Vote, Again, to Repeal Health Care Law," CNN, July 11, 2012, http://www.cnn.com/2012/07/11/politics/house-health-care/index.html.

61. National Federation of Independent Business v. Sebelius, 567 U.S. __, 132 S.Ct. 2566 (2012). This decision addressed several novel constitutional issues regarding the power of Congress to regulate commercial activity and to impose restrictions on the use of funds it grants to the states. Part of the ruling held that Congress exceeded its constitutional powers in mandating as part of the ACA that all Americans must have health insurance. However, it upheld that provision by characterizing the mandate as a tax on those who fail to maintain coverage rather than as a regulation requiring that they engage in commerce. The Court held that the law's expansion of Medicaid violated the Constitution as it was written because it imposed a major new condition on states in order to continue to receive funding for their programs. However, Congress could offer funds to states for expanding Medicaid as an option. This left the basic structure of the law intact, but added a complication to its implementation, since national consistency in eligibility for Medicaid was no longer assured. Nevertheless, the overall effect of the ruling was to permit the ACA to take effect.

62. Congressional Budget Office, "Updated Estimates for the Insurance Coverage Provisions of the Affordable Care Act" (March 2012), http://www.cbo.gov/sites/default/files/cbofiles/attachments/03-13-Coverage%20Estimates.pdf.

63. PricewaterhouseCoopers, "Top Health Industry Issues of 2013: Picking Up the Pace on Health Reform" (2013), 6, http://pwchealth.com/cgi-local/hregister.cgi/reg/pwc-hri-top-health-industry-issues-2013.pdf.

64. Sean Keehan and others, "Health Spending Projections Through 2017: The Baby-Boom Generation Is Coming to Medicare," Health Affairs 27, no. 2 (2008): 145–55.

65. Institute of Medicine, To Err Is Human.

66. Patient Protection and Affordable Care Act, P.L. 111-148, 124 Stat. 119, §§1401-1421 (2010) (to be codified in scattered sections of Titles 21, 25, 26, 29, & 42 U.S.C.).

67. National Center for Advancing Translational Sciences, National Institutes of Health, http://www.ncats.nih.gov/.

68. Health Information Technology for Economic and Clinical Health Act, P.L. 111-5, 123 Stat. 226, 2009.

69. The promotion of information technology under the HITECH Act has been described as a windfall that benefits large providers of computerized systems. Their newfound opportunities are attributed to sustained and skillful lobbying. See Julie Creswell, "A Digital Shift on Health Data Swells Profits in an Industry," New York Times, February 19,

2013, A1, http://www.nytimes.com/2013/02/20/business/a-digital-shift-on-health-data-swells-profits.html?pagewanted=all.

70. Robert I. Field, "Government as the Crucible for Free Market Health Care: Regulation, Reimbursement, and Reform," *University of Pennsylvania Law Review* 159, no. 6 (2011): 1669–726.

71. For a major analysis in the popular press of the relationship between the fee-for-service payment system and the high cost of health care in the United States, see Steven Brill, "Why Medical Bills Are Killing Us," *Time*, 2013, http://healthland.time.com/2013/02/20/bitter-pill-why-medical-bills-are-killing-us/.

72. Patient Protection and Affordable Care Act, P.L. 111-148, 124 Stat. 119 through 124 Stat. 1025.

73. At an approximate cost of $361 billion per year, administrative costs in the health care system consume 14 percent of all health care expenditures in the United States. Elizabeth Wikler, Peter Basch, and David Cutler, "Paper Cuts: Reducing Health Care Administrative Costs" (American Progress, 2012), 1, http://www.americanprogress.org/wp-content/uploads/issues/2012/06/pdf/papercuts_final.pdf.

74. Health Insurance Portability and Accountability Act, 42 U.S.C. §§ 300gg, et seq. (1996).

75. Patient Protection and Affordable Care Act, P.L. 111-148, 124 Stat. 119, §1302(a)-(d) (2010) (to be codified in scattered sections of Titles 21, 25, 26, 29, & 42 U.S.C.).

76. Atul Gawande, "The Cost Conundrum: What a Texas Town Can Teach Us About Healthcare," *The New Yorker*, June 1, 2009, http://www.newyorker.com/reporting/2009/06/01/090601fa_fact_gawande.

77. Richard Mark Kirkner, "The Enduring Temptation of Physician Self-Referral," *Managed Care*, October 2011, http://www.managedcaremag.com/content/enduring-temptation-physician-self-referral.

78. 42 U.S.C. §1320a-7b.

79. 42 USC § 1395nn.

80. Although the true costs of fraud and abuse are unknown, the Centers for Medicare and Medicaid estimated that, in 2010, the agency paid more than $65 billion in "improper federal payments," which are defined as "payments that should not have been made or were made in an incorrect amount." Improper payments made by state Medicaid programs adds $10 billion to that estimate for an estimated total of $75 billion in improper payments each year. T. R. Goldman, "Eliminating Fraud and Abuse," *Health Affairs*, Health Policy Briefs, July 31, 2012, http://www.healthaffairs.org/healthpolicy-briefs/brief.php?brief_id=72.

81. Affordable Care Act §6001. Ironically, although the ACA discourages the growth of specialty hospitals, it may actually reward those that were already in existence at the time of the law's enactment. One analysis has shown that these facilities are more likely than their general hospital counterparts to qualify for quality-based bonus payments under the Act. This is because their physician-owners tend to refer patients to them who are healthiest and therefore likely to have the best outcomes. Jordan Rau, "Doctor-Owned Hospitals Prosper Under Health Law," *Kaiser Health News*, April 12, 2012, http://www.kaiserhealthnews.org/Stories/2013/April/12/doctor-owned-hospitals-quality-bonuses.aspx.

82. Robert Lowes, "Number of Physicians Employed by Hospitals Snowballing," *Medscape*, January 24, 2012, http://www.medscape.com/viewarticle/757386.

83. The cost of Provenge is discussed in James D. Chambers and Peter J. Neumann, "Listening to Provenge—What a Costly Cancer Treatment Says About Future Medicare Policy," *New England Journal of Medicine* 364, no. 18 (2011): 1687–89. The high price of some oncology drugs led a group of oncologists to comment publicly on the detrimental effects this may have on care. See Experts on Chronic Myeloid Leukemia, "The Price of Drugs for Chronic Myeloid Leukemia (CML); A Reflection of the Unsustainable Prices of Cancer Drugs: From the Perspective of a Large Group of CML Experts," *Blood* doi:10.1182/blood-2013-03-490003 (2013), http://bloodjournal.hematologylibrary.org/content/early/2013/04/23/blood-2013-03-490003.full.pdf+html.

84. Robert Langreth, "Prostate Cancer Therapy Too Good to Be True Explodes Health Cost," *Bloomberg Businessweek*, March 26, 2012, http://www.businessweek.com/news/2012-03-26/prostate-cancer-therapy-too-good-to-be-true-explodes-health-cost.

85. See Ezekiel J. Emanuel and Steven D. Pearson, "It Costs More, But Is It Worth More?," *New York Times*, January 2, 2012, http://opinionator.blogs.nytimes.com/2012/01/02/it-costs-more-but-is-it-worth-more/ regarding the effectiveness of proton beam accelerators, and Sharon Begley, "Insight: New Doubts About Prostate-Cancer Vaccine Provenge," *Reuters*, March 30, 2012, http://www.reuters.com/article/2012/03/30/us-provenge-idUS-BRE82T07420120330 regarding the effectiveness of Provenge. Issues in weighing the costs and benefits of expensive medical technologies are discussed in Alan Garber, Dana P. Goldman, and Anupam B. Jena, "The Promise of Health Care Cost Containment," *Health Affairs* 26, no. 6 (2007): 1545–47.

SELECTED BIBLIOGRAPHY

Abbate, Janet. *Inventing the Internet.* Cambridge, MA: MIT Press, 2000.

Abramowicz, Michael. "The Human Genome Project in Retrospect." *Advances in Genetics* 50 (2003): 231–61.

Acierno, Louis J. *The History of Cardiology.* New York: Parthenon Publishing Group, 1994.

American Academy of Actuaries. "*Critical Issues in Health Reform: Risk Pooling,*" 2009. http://www.actuary.org/pdf/health/pool_july09.pdf.

Annas, George J. "Health Care Reform in America: Beyond Ideology." *Indiana Health Law Review* 5 (2008): 443–61.

Astor, Maggie E. "The Fine Line of Health-Care Politicking: A Comparative Analysis of Reform Efforts from Clinton to Obama." *Center for the Study of the Presidency & Congress* 2011. http://www.thepresidency.org/storage/Fellows2011/Astor-_Final_Paper.pdf.

Austin, D. Andrew, and Thomas L. Hungerford. "*The Market Structure of the Health Insurance Industry.*" *Congressional Research Service, 7-5700.* November 17, 2009. http://www.fas.org/sgp/crs/misc/R40834.pdf.

Baker, Laurence C., and Linda Schuurman Baker. "Excess Cost of Emergency Department Visits for Non-Urgent Care." *Health Affairs* 13, no. 5 (Winter 1994): 162–71.

Ben-Menachem, Gil, Steven M. Ferguson, and Krishna Balakrishnan. "Doing Business with the NIH." *National Biotechnology* 24, no. 1 (2006): 17–20.

Berenson, Robert, and Stephen Zuckerman. "*How Will Hospitals Be Affected by Health Care Reform?*" Robert Wood Johnson Foundation, July 2010. http://www.rwjf.org/content/dam/farm/reports/issue_briefs/2010/rwjf62544.

Blank, Robert H. "Models of Rationing: Regulatory Rationing: A Solution to Health Care Resource Allocation." *University of Pennsylvania Law Review* 140 (1992): 1573–96.

Blendon, Robert, and John Benson. "The Public's Views About Medicare and the Budget Deficit." *New England Journal of Medicine* 365, no. 4 (2011): e8(1)–8(4). http://www.nejm.org/doi/full/10.1056/NEJMp1107184.

Blum, John D. "Beyond the Bylaws: Hospital-Physician Relationships, Economics, and Conflicting Agendas." *Buffalo Law Review* 53 (2005): 470–74.

Blumenthal, David. "New Steam from an Old Cauldron—The Physician-Supply Debate." *New England Journal of Medicine* 350, no. 17 (2004): 1780–87.

Blumenthal, David, and James A. Morone. *The Heart of Power: Health and Politics in the Oval Office.* Berkeley: University of California Press, 2009.

Brennan, Troyen A., and David M. Studdert. "How Will Health Insurers Respond to New Rules Under Health Reform?" *Health Affairs* 29, no. 6 (2010): 1147–51.

Breyer, Stephen. *Regulation and Its Reform.* Cambridge, MA: Harvard University Press, 1984.

Burbridge, Charles E. "The Historical Background of the Teaching Hospital in the United States." *Journal of the National Medical Association* 176, no. 3 (1957): 176–79.

Burman, Leonard E., Sarah Goodell, and Surachai Khitatrakun. "*Tax Subsidies for Private Health Insurance: Who Benefits and at What Cost?*". Robert Wood Johnson Foundation, 2009. http://www.urban.org/UploadedPDF/1001297_tax_subsidies.pdf.

Burns, Lawton R., Gloria J. Bazzoli, Linda Dynan, and Douglas R. Wholey. "Managed Care, Market Stages, and Integrated Delivery Systems: Is There a Relationship?" *Health Affairs* 16, no. 6 (1997): 204–18.

Butler, Patricia A. "State Policy Issues in Nonprofit Conversion." *Health Affairs* 16, no. 2 (1997): 69–84.

Butler, Stuart M. "Using Tax Credits to Create an Affordable Health System." *The Heritage Foundation*. July 20, 1990. http://www.heritage.org/research/reports/1990/07/using-tax-credits-to-create-an-affordable-health-system.

Cannon, Michael F. *Health Competition: What's Holding Back Health Care and How to Free It*. Washington, DC: Cato Institute, 2005.

Carpenter, Daniel. *Reputation and Power: Organizational Image and Pharmaceutical Regulation at the FDA*. Princeton, NJ: Princeton University Press, 2010.

——. "The Political Economy of FDA Drug Review: Processing, Politics, and Lessons for Policy." *Health Affairs* 23, no. 1 (2004): 52–63.

Case, Gretchen A. "*National Cancer Institute Oral History Project, Interview with Alan S. Rabson, M.D.*" July 11, 1997. http://history.nih.gov/archives/downloads/rabsontranscript.pdf.

Case, Karl E., Ray C. Fair, and Sharon C. Oster. *Principles of Economics*. 10th ed. New York: Prentice Hall, 2011.

Centers for Medicare & Medicaid Services. "*American Medical Group Association Compensation Survey Data 2009 Report*." 2009. http://www.cms.gov/Medicare/Medicare-Fee-for-Service-Payment/AcuteInpatientPPS/Downloads/AMGA_08_template_to_09.pdf.

——. "*National Health Expenditure Projections 2011–2021: Forecast Summary*." http://www.cms.gov/Research-Statistics-Data-and-Systems/Statistics-Trends-and-Reports/NationalHealthExpendData/Downloads/Proj2011PDF.pdf.

Chambers, James D., and Peter J. Neumann. "Listening to Provenge—What a Costly Cancer Treatment Says about Future Medicare Policy." *New England Journal of Medicine* 364, no. 18 (2011): 1687–89.

Christianson, Jon B., S. M. Sanchez, D. R. Wholey, and M. Shadle. "The HMO Industry: Evolution in Population Demographics and Market Structure." *Medical Care Review* 48, no. 1 (1991): 3–46.

Claxton, Gary, Jon Gabel, Bianca DiJulio, Jeremy Pickreign, Heidi Whitmore, Benjamin Finder, Paul Jacobs, and Samantha Hawkins. "Health Benefits in 2007: Premium Increases Fall to an Eight-Year Low, While Offer Rates and Enrollment Remain Stable." *Health Affairs* 26, no. 5 (2007): 1407–16.

Cockburn, Iain M., and Rebecca M. Henderson. "Publicly Funded Science and the Productivity of the Pharmaceutical Industry." In *Innovation Policy and the Economy, volume 1*, edited by Adam B. Jaffe, Josh Lerner and Scott Stern, National Bureau of Economic Research. Cambridge, MA: MIT Press, 2001: 1–34.

——. "Absorptive Capacity, Coauthoring Behavior, and the Organization of Research in Drug Discovery." *The Journal of Industrial Economics* 46, no. 2 (1998): 157–82.

Coleman, Sharon Kearney. *"The Hill-Burton Uncompensated Services Program."* Congressional Research Service, 2005. http://www.policyarchive.org/handle/10207/bitstreams/719.pdf.

Collins, Francis S. "Reengineering Translational Science: The Time Is Right." *Science Translational Medicine* 3, no. 90 (2011): 1–6.

Colombotos, John. "Physicians and Medicare: A Before-After Study of the Effects of Legislation on Attitudes." *American Sociological Review* 34, no. 3 (1969): 318–34.

Columbo, John D. "The Role of Tax Exemption in a Competitive Health Care Market." *Journal of Health Politics, Policy and Law* 31, no. 3 (2006): 623–42.

Commonwealth Fund. *"International Profiles of Health Care Systems, 2011."* http://www.commonwealthfund.org/~/media/Files/Publications/Fund%20Report/2011/Nov/1562_Squires_Intl_Profiles_2011_11_10.pdf.

Commonwealth Fund Commission on Hospital Care. *Hospital Care in the United States.* New York: The Commonwealth Fund, 1947.

Commonwealth Fund Task Force on Academic Health Centers. *"Envisioning the Future of Academic Health Centers,"* The Commonwealth Fund, 2004. http://www.commonwealthfund.org/Publications/Fund-Reports/2003/Feb/Envisioning-the-Future-of-Academic-Health-Centers.aspx.

___. *"Leveling the Playing Field: Financing the Missions of Academic Health Centers,"* The Commonwealth Fund, 1999.

Compaine, Benjamin M. *"Size and Growth Trends of the Information Industry, 1970–1983,"* Program on Information Resources Policy, Center for Information Policy Research, Harvard University, 1986. http://www.pirp.harvard.edu/pubs_pdf/compain/compain-i86-2.pdf.

Congressional Budget Office. *"Estimates for the Insurance Coverage Provisions of the Affordable Care Act Updated for the Recent Supreme Court Decision."* July 24, 2012. http://www.cbo.gov/sites/default/files/cbofiles/attachments/43472-07-24-2012-CoverageEstimates.pdf.

___. *"Nonprofit Hospitals and the Provision of Community Benefits."* December 6, 2006. http://www.cbo.gov/ftpdocs/76xx/doc7695/12-06-Nonprofit.pdf.

___. *"Research and Development in the Pharmaceutical Industry."* October 2006. http://www.cbo.gov/ftpdocs/76xx/doc7615/10-02-DrugR-D.pdf.

___. *"Tax Subsidies for Medical Care: Current Policies and Possible Alternatives."* January 1980. http://www.cbo.gov/sites/default/files/cbofiles/ftpdocs/91xx/doc9180/80doco1b.pdf.

___. *"The Health Care System for Veterans: An Interim Report."* December 21, 2007. http://www.cbo.gov/sites/default/files/cbofiles/ftpdocs/88xx/doc8892/12-21-va_healthcare.pdf.

Conover, Christopher J. *"Health Care Regulation: A $169 Billion Hidden Tax."* CATO Institute, 2004. http://www.cato.org/pubs/pas/pa527.pdf.

Cooper, Richard A. "Medical Schools and Their Applicants: An Analysis." *Health Affairs* 22, no. 4 (July 2003): 71–84.

Council on Graduate Medical Education. *"Physician Workforce Policy Guidelines for the United States, 2000–2020,"* US Health Resources and Services Administration, January 2005. http://www.hrsa.gov/advisorycommittees/bhpradvisory/cogme/Reports/sixteenthreport.pdf.

___. *"Summary of Eleventh Report: International Medical Graduates, the Physician Workforce, and GME Payment Reform."* March 1998. http://www.hrsa.gov/advisory-committees/bhpradvisory/cogme/Reports/eleventhreport.html.

Crosson, Francis J. "21st-Century Health Care—the Case for Integrated Delivery Systems." *New England Journal of Medicine* 361 (2009): 1324–25.

Cunningham, Robert, III, and Robert M. Cunningham Jr. *The Blues: A History of the Blue Cross and Blue Shield System.* DeKalb: Northern Illinois University Press, 1997.

Cutler, David M., ed. *The Changing Hospital Industry: Comparing Not-for-Profit and For-Profit Institutions.* Chicago: University of Chicago Press, 2000.

Davis, Karen, and Kristof Stremikis. "Medicare Works: Public Program Continues to Outperform Private Insurance in Ensuring Access to Care and Providing Financial Protection." *The Commonwealth Fund.* July 24, 2012. http://www.commonwealthfund.org/Blog/2012/Jul/Medicare-Works-Continues-to-Outperform-Private-Insurance.aspx.

Davis, Karen, Cathy Schoen, Stuart Guterman, Tony Shih, Stephen C. Schoenbaum, and Ilana Weinbaum. *"Slowing the Growth of U.S. Health Care Expenditures: What are the Options?"* The Commonwealth Fund, January 29, 2007. http://www.cmwf.org/publications/publications_show.htm?doc_id=449510.

Detmer, Don, and Elaine Steen, eds., *The Academic Health Center: Leadership and Performance.* Cambridge, UK: Cambridge University Press, 2005.

Dobson, Allen, Donald Moran, and Gary Young. "The Role of Federal Waivers in the Health Policy Process." *Health Affairs* 11, no. 4 (1992): 72–94.

Dorsey, E. Ray. "Funding of US Biomedical Research, 2003–2008." *Journal of the American Medical Association* 303, no. 2 (2010): 137–43.

Dorsey, Joseph L. "The Health Maintenance Organization Act of 1973 (P.L. 93-222) and Prepaid Group Practice Plan." *Medical Care* 13, no. 1 (January, 1975): 6–7.

Dower, Catherine. "Graduate Medical Education," *Health Affairs.* Health Policy Brief, August 31, 2012. http://www.healthaffairs.org/healthpolicybriefs/brief.php?brief_id=75.

Doyle, Yvonne, and Adrian Bull. "Role of Private Sector in United Kingdom Healthcare System." *British Medical Journal* 321, no. 7260 (2000): 563–65.

Eappen, Sunil, Bennett H. Lane, Barry Rosenberg, Stuart A. Lipsitz, David Sadoff, Dave Matheson, William R. Berry, Mark Lester, and Atul A. Gawande. "Relationship Between Occurrence of Surgical Complications and Hospital Finances." *Journal of the American Medical Association* 309, no. 15 (2013): 1599–606.

Eisenberg, Gerald M. "The Medical Staff Structure—Its Role in the 21st Century." *Annals of Health Law* 12, no. 2 (2003): 249–64.

Ekelund, Robert B., Rand W. Ressler, and Robert D. Tollison. *Economics: Private Markets and Public Choice.* New York: Pearson, 2006.

Enthoven, Alain C. "Why Managed Care Has Failed to Contain Health Costs." *Health Affairs* 12, no. 3 (1993): 27–43.

Epstein, Richard A. *Overdose: How Excessive Government Regulation Stifles Pharmaceutical Innovation.* New Haven, CT: Yale University Press, 2008.

Field, Robert I. "Government as the Crucible for Free Market Health Care: Regulation, Reimbursement, and Reform." *University of Pennsylvania Law Review* 159 (2011): 1669–726.

___. "Regulation, Reform and the Creation of Free Market Health Care." *Hamline Journal of Public Law and Policy* 35 (2010): 306–31.

___. *Health Care Regulation in America: Complexity, Confrontation and Compromise.* New York: Oxford University Press, 2007.

Fishback, Price V., and Shawn Everett Kantor. *A Prelude to the Welfare State: The Origins of Workers' Compensation.* Chicago: University of Chicago Press, 2000.

Flexner, Abraham. *Medical Education in the United States and Canada: A Report to the Carnegie Foundation for the Advancement of Teaching.* New York: Carnegie Foundation for the Advancement of Teaching, 1910.

Foote, Susan Bartlett. "Focus on Locus: Evolution of Medicare's Local Coverage Policy." *Health Affairs* 22, no. 4 (2003): 137–46.

Friedman, Milton. *Capitalism and Freedom.* Chicago: University of Chicago Press, 2002.

Furrow, Barry R. "Health Reform and Ted Kennedy: The Art of Politics . . . and Persistence." *New York University Journal of Legislation and Public Policy* 14 (2011): 445–76.

Fye, W. Bruce. *American Cardiology.* Baltimore, MD: Johns Hopkins University Press, 1996.

Ganim, Louis J. "Baby Boomers and Medicare." *Health Affairs* 23, no. 2 (2004): 282–83.

Garber, Alan, Dana P. Goldman, and Anupam B. Jena. "The Promise of Health Care Cost Containment." *Health Affairs* 26, no. 6 (2007): 1545–47.

Gaynor, Martin, and Deborah Haas-Wilson. "Change, Consolidation, and Competition in Health Care Markets." *Journal of Economic Perspectives* 13, no. 1 (1999): 141–64.

Glandon, Gerald L., and Michael A. Morrisey. "Redefining the Hospital-Physician Relationship Under Prospective Payment." *Inquiry* 23, no. 3 (1986): 166–75.

Gold, Marsha, Gretchen Jacobson, Anthony Damico, and Tricia Neuman. "*Medicare Advantage 2012 Data Spotlight: Enrollment Market Update.*" Kaiser Family Foundation, May 31, 2012. http://www.kff.org/medicare/upload/8323.pdf.

Goldberg, Raymond. *Drugs Across the Spectrum.* 6th ed. Belmont, CA: Cengage Learning, 2010.

Goldman, Dana P., Mary Vaiana, and John A. Romley. "The Emerging Importance of Patient Amenities in Hospital Care." *New England Journal of Medicine* 363, no. 23 (2010): 2185–87.

Goldman, T. R. "Eliminating Fraud and Abuse." *Health Affairs.* Policy Briefs, July 31, 2012. http://www.healthaffairs.org/healthpolicybriefs/brief.php?brief_id=72.

Goodson, John D. "Unintended Consequences of Resourced-Based Relative Value Scale Reimbursement." *Journal of the American Medical Association* 298, no. 19 (2007): 2308–10.

Haas-Wilson, Deborah. *Managed Care and Monopoly Power: The Antitrust Challenge.* Cambridge, MA: Harvard University Press, 2003.

Haislmaier, Edmund F. "Massachusetts Health Reform: What the Doctor Ordered." *The Heritage Foundation.* May 6, 2006. http://www.heritage.org/research/commentary/2006/05/massachusetts-health-reform-what-the-doctor-ordered.

Hamburg, Margaret A., and Frances S. Collins. "The Path to Personalized Medicine." *New England Journal of Medicine* 363 (2010): 301–04.

Harding, Victoria A. "A Short History of the National Institutes of Health." *National Institutes of Health Office of NIH History,* 2005. http://history.nih.gov/exhibits/history/index.html.

___. *Inventing the NIH: Federal Biomedical Research Policy, 1887–1937.* Baltimore, MD: Johns Hopkins University Press, 1986.

Hayes, Arthur Hull. "Food and Drug Regulation after 75 Years." *Journal of the American Medical Association* 246, no. 11 (1981): 1223–26.

Heimann, C. F. Larry. *Acceptable Risks: Politics, Policy, and Risky Technologies*. Ann Arbor, MI: University of Michigan Press, 1997.

Hellinger, Fred J. "The Effect of Certificate-of-Need Laws on Hospital Beds and Healthcare Expenditures: An Empirical Analysis." *American Journal of Managed Care* 15, no. 10 (2009): 737–44.

Hendricks, Richey. *A Model for National Health Care: The History of Kaiser Permanente*. New Brunswick, NJ: Rutgers University Press, 1993.

Herrick, James B. *A Short History of Cardiology*. Baltimore, MD: Charles C. Thomas, 1942.

Higby, Gregory J. "American Hospital Pharmacy from the Colonial Period to the 1930s." *American Journal of Hospital Pharmacy* 51, no. 22 (1994): 2817–23.

Hillestad, Richard. "Can Electronic Medical Record Systems Transform Health Care? Potential Health Benefits, Savings, and Costs." *Health Affairs* 24, no. 5 (2005): 1103–17.

Holahan, John, Lisa Clemans-Cope, Emily Lawton, and David Rousseau. *"Medicaid Spending Growth over the Last Decade and the Great Recession 2000–2009."* Kaiser Family Foundation, February 2011. www.kff.org/medicaid/upload/8152.pdf.

Holahan, John, Stephen Zuckerman, Alison Evans, and Suresh Rangarajan. "Medicaid Managed Care in Thirteen States." *Heath Affairs* 17, no. 3 (1998): 43–63.

Holland, Gary N., D. T. Earl, N. C. Wheeler, B. R. Straatsma, T. H. Pettit, R. S. Hepler, R. E. Christensen, and R. K. Oye. "Results of Inpatient and Outpatient Cataract Surgery. A Historical Cohort Comparison." *Ophthalmology* 99, no. 6 (1992): 845–52.

Horwitz, Jill R. "Why We Need the Independent Sector: The Behavior, Law, and Ethics of Not-for-Profit Hospitals." *UCLA Law Review* 50, no. 6 (2003): 1345–411.

Hsiao, William C., Peter Braun, Daniel Dunn, and Edmund R. Becker. "Resource-Based Relative Values: An Overview." *Journal of the American Medical Association* 260, no. 16 (1988): 2347–53.

Iglehart, John K. "The Uncertain Future of Medicare and Graduate Medical Education." *New England Journal of Medicine* 365, no. 14 (2011): 1340–45.

———. "The American Health Care System: Medicare." *New England Journal of Medicine* 327, no. 20 (1992): 1467–72.

Institute of Medicine. *To Err Is Human: Building a Safer Health System*. Edited by Linda T. Kohn, Janet M. Corrigan, and Molla S. Donaldson. Washington, DC: National Academy Press, 1999.

Isaacs, Stephen L., Paul S. Jellinek, and Walker K. Ray. "The Independent Physician—Going, Going . . . " *New England Journal of Medicine* 360, no. 7 (2009): 655–57.

Jacobson, Gretchen, Tricia Neuman, and Anthony Damico. *"Transformation of Medicare into a Premium Support System: Implications for Beneficiary Premiums."* Kaiser Family Foundation, October 2012. http://kaiserfamilyfoundation.files.wordpress.com/2013/01/8373.pdf.

Janssen, Wallace. "The Story of the Law Behind the Labels." *FDA Consumer* 15, no. 5 (1981): 32–45.

Jenson, Jennifer. *"Government Spending on Health Care Benefits and Programs: A Data Brief,"* Congressional Research Service, 2008. http://www.aging.senate.gov/crs/medicaid7.pdf.

Johnson, Tracy K., Craig E. Holm, and Scott Goodshall. "Ambulatory Surgery: Next-Generation Strategies for Physicians and Hospitals." *Healthcare Financial Management* 54, no. 1 (January 2000), 48–51.

Jost, Timothy Stoltzfus. "The Experience of Switzerland and the Netherlands with Individual Health Insurance Mandates: A Model for the United States?" Washington and Lee

University.   http://law.wlu.edu/deptimages/Faculty/Jost%20The%20Experience%20 of%20Switzerland%20and%20the%20Netherlands.pdf.

Kaiser Family Foundation. *"Health Care Spending in the United States and Selected OECD Countries."* April 12, 2011. http://www.kff.org/insurance/snapshot/oecd042111.cfm.

___. *"Health Care Costs: A Primer."* May 1, 2012. http://www.kff.org/insurance/ upload/7670-03.pdf.

___. *"Massachusetts Health Reform: Six Years Later."* May 1, 2012. http://www.kff.org/ healthreform/upload/8311.pdf.

___. *"Medicaid Matters: Understanding Medicaid's Role in Our Health Care System."* March 1, 2011. http://www.kff.org/medicaid/upload/8165.pdf.

___. *"Medicare Spending and Financing."* November 14, 2012. http://www.kff.org/medi-care/upload/7305-07.pdf.

___. *"National Health Insurance—A Brief History of Reform Efforts in the U.S."* February 28, 2009. http://www.kff.org/healthreform/upload/7871.pdf.

___. *"Tax Subsidies for Health Insurance: An Issue Brief."* June 30, 2008. http://www.kff.org/ insurance/upload/7779.pdf.

Kastor, John A. *Governance of Teaching Hospitals: Turmoil at Penn and Hopkins.* Baltimore, MD: The Johns Hopkins University Press, 2004.

___. *Mergers of Teaching Hospitals in Boston, New York, and Northern California.* Ann Arbor, MI: University of Michigan Press, 2001.

Keehan, Sean P., Andrea M. Sisko, Christopher J. Truffer, John A. Poisal, Gigi A. Cuckler, Andrew J. Madison, Joseph M. Lizonitz, and Sheila D. Smith. "National Health Spending Projections Through 2020: Economic Recovery and Reform Drive Faster Spending Growth." *Health Affairs* 30, no. 8 (2011): 1594–605.

Keehan, Sean P., Gigi A. Cuckler, Andrea M. Sisko, Andrew J. Madison, Sheila D. Smith, Joseph M. Lizonitz, John A. Poisal, and Christian J. Wolfe. "National Health Expenditure Projections: Modest Annual Growth Until Coverage Expands and Economic Growth Accelerates." *Health Affairs* 31, no. 1 (July 2012): 1600–12.

Keith, Stephen N. "Prospective Payment for Hospital Costs Using Diagnosis-Related Groups: Will Cost Inflation Be Reduced?" *Journal of the National Medical Association* 75, no. 6 (1983): 609–23.

Kenney, Genevieve M., Stephen Zuckerman, Lisa Dubay, Michael Huntress, Victoria Lynch, Jennifer M. Haley, and Nathaniel Anderson. *"Opting in to the Medicaid Expansion under the ACA: Who Are the Uninsured Adults Who Could Gain Health Insurance Coverage?"* Robert Wood Johnson Foundation, August 2012. http://www.urban.org/ UploadedPDF/412630-opting-in-medicaid.pdf.

Kinkead, Brian M. "Medicare Payment and Hospital Capital: The Evolution of Policy." *Health Affairs* 3, no. 3 (Fall 1984): 49–74.

Kirkner, Richard Mark. "The Enduring Temptation of Physician Self-Referral." *Managed Care.* October 2011. http://www.managedcaremag.com/content/enduring-temptation-physician-self-referral.

Kissick, William L. *Medicine's Dilemmas: Infinite Needs Versus Finite Resources.* New Haven, CT: Yale University Press, 1994.

Kovner, Anthony R., and James R. Knickman, eds. *Health Care Delivery in the United States.* 10th ed. New York: Springer Publishing Co., 2011.

Krugman, Paul, and Robin Wells. *Microeconomics.* 3rd ed. New York: Worth Publishers, Inc., 2012.

Ku, Leighton, Emily Jones, Brad Finnegan, Peter Shin, and Sara Rosenbaum. *"How Is the Primary Care Safety Net Faring in Massachusetts? Community Health Centers in the Midst of Health Reform,"*.Kaiser Commission on Medicaid and the Uninsured, May 1, 2009. http://www.kff.org/healthreform/upload/7878.pdf.

Lasser, Karen E., Steffie Woolhandler, and David U. Himmelstein. "Sources of U.S. Physician Income: The Contribution of Government Payments to the Specialist-Generalist Income Gap." *Journal of General Internal Medicine* 23, no. 9 (2008): 1477–81.

Leader, Shelah, and Marilyn Moon. "Medicare Trends in Ambulatory Surgery." *Health Affairs* 8, no. 1 (1989): 158–70.

Li, Jie Jack. *Laughing Gas, Viagra, and Lipitor: the Human Stories Behind the Drugs We Use.* New York: Oxford University Press, 2006.

Lieberman, Trudy. "Medicare Vouchers Explained." *Columbia Journalism Review.* January 18, 2012.

Light, Donald W., and Joel R. Lexchin. "Pharmaceutical Research and Development: What Do We Get for All That Money?" *British Medical Journal* 344 (2012): e4348–53.

Lundy, Janet. *"Prescription Drug Trends."* Kaiser Family Foundation, 2010. http://www.kff.org/rxdrugs/upload/3057-08.pdf.

Lurie, Peter, Cristina M. Almeida, Nicholas Stine, Alexander R. Stine, and Sidney M. Wolfe. "Financial Conflicts of Interest Disclosure and Voting Patterns at Food and Drug Administration Drug Advisory Committee Meetings." *Journal of the American Medical Association* 295, no. 16 (2006): 1921–28.

Mankiw, N. Gregory. *Principles of Economics.* 6th ed. Mason, OH: South-Western Cengage Learning, 2011.

Manton, Kenneth G., Xi-Liang Gu, Gene Lowrimore, Arthur Ullian, and H. Dennis Tolley. "NIH Funding Trajectories and Their Correlations with US Health Dynamics from 1950 to 2004." *Proceedings of the National Academy of Sciences* 106, no. 27 (2009): 10981–86. http://www.pnas.org/content/106/27/10981.full.

Markovich, Martin. *"The Rise of HMOs."* Rand Corporation, March 2003. http://www.rand.org/pubs/rgs_dissertations/RGSD172.html.

Marmor, Theodore R. *Politics of Medicare.* Hawthorne, NY: Aldine Publishing Company, 1973.

Martensen, Robert. "History of Medicine: How Medicare and Hospitals Have Shaped American Health Care." *American Medical Association Journal of Ethics* 13, no. 11 (2011): 808–12.

Mayes, Rick. "The Origins, Development, and Passage of Medicare's Revolutionary Prospective Payment System." *Journal of the History of Medicine and Allied Sciences* 62, no. 1 (2007): 21–55.

Mayes, Rick, and Robert A. Berenson. *Medicare Prospective Payment and the Shaping of U.S. Health Care.* Baltimore, MD: Johns Hopkins University Press, 2006.

McGinley, Patrick John. "Beyond Health Care Reform: Reconsidering Certificate of Need Laws in a Managed Competition System." *Florida State University Law Review* 23 (1995): 141–88.

McGuire, Thomas G., Joseph P. Newhouse, and Anna D. Sinaiko. "An Economic History of Medicare Part C." *Milbank Quarterly* 89, no. 2 (June 2011): 289–332.

Mechanic, Robert, Kevin Coleman, and Allen Dobson. "Teaching Hospital Costs: Implications for Academic Mission in a Competitive Market." *Journal of the American Medical Association* 280, no. 11 (1998): 1015–19.

Medicare Payment Advisory Commission. "*A Data Book: Healthcare Spending and the Medicare Program.*" June 2010. www.medpac.gov/documents/jun10databookentirereport.pdf.

Mercer, Lloyd J. *Railroads and Land Grant Policy: A Study in Government Intervention.* Washington, DC: Beard Books 1982.

Merlis, Mark. "*The Value of Extra Benefits Offered by Medicare Advantage Plans in 2006.*" Kaiser Family Foundation, January 2, 2008. http://www.kff.org/medicare/upload/7744. pdf.

Michelassi, Fabrizio, and Thomas J. Fahey III. "The Department of Surgery at New York-Presbyterian Hospital/Weill Cornell Medical Center: At the Forefront of Surgical Innovation." *American Surgeon* 75, no. 8 (2009): 643–48.

Moeller, John F., G. Edward Miller, and Jessica S. Banthin. "Looking Inside the Nation's Medicine Cabinet: Trends in Outpatient Drug Spending by Medicare Beneficiaries, 1997 and 2001." *Health Affairs* 23, no. 5 (2004): 217–25.

Moore, Kent J., Thomas A. Felger, Walter L. Larimore, and Terry L. Mills Jr. "What Every Physician Should Know About the RUC." *Family Practice Management* 15, no. 2 (2008): 36–39.

Morone, James A. "Presidents and Health Reform: From Franklin D. Roosevelt to Barack Obama." *Health Affairs* 29, no. 6 (2010): 1096–100.

Myers, Robert J. *Medicare.* Bryn Mawr, PA: McCahan Foundation, 1970.

National Center for Health Statistics. *Health, United States, 2011.* Hyattsville, MD: United States Government Printing Office, 2012. http://www.cdc.gov/nchs/data/hus/hus11. pdf.

National Institutes of Health Office of Technology Transfer. "*Havrix Waging War Against a Common Enemy: A Case Study.*" October 22, 2002. http://www.ott.nih.gov/pdfs/ HavrixCS.pdf.

——."*Paclitaxel-Coated Stents: A Way to Bypass By-Pass Surgery.*" June 2005. http://www.ott. nih.gov/pdfs/TaxusCS.pdf.

Newhouse, Joseph P., and Gail R. Wilensky. "Paying for Graduate Medical Education: The Debate Goes On." *Health Affairs* 20, no. 2 (2001): 136–47.

O'Sullivan, Jennifer. "*Medicare Part D Prescription Drug Benefit: A Primer.*" Congressional Research Service, August 20, 2008. http://www.aging.senate.gov/crs/medicare12.pdf.

Oberlander, Jonathan. "Long Time Coming: Why Health Reform Finally Passed." *Health Affairs* 29, no. 6 (2010): 1112–16.

Oliver, Thomas R., Philip R. Lee, and Helene L. Lipton. "A Political History of Medicare and Prescription Drug Coverage." *Milbank Quarterly* 82, no. 2 (2004): 283–354.

Pauly, Mark V. "Competition and New Technology," *New England Journal of Medicine* 24, no. 6 (2005): 1523–35.

Payton, Sallyanne, and Rhoda M. Powsner. "Regulation Through the Looking Glass: Hospitals, Blue Cross, and Certificate-of-Need." *University of Michigan Law Review* 79, no. 2 (1980): 203–77.

Peterson, Chris L., and Rachel Burton. "*U.S. Health Care Spending: Comparison with Other OECD Countries,*" Congressional Research Service, September 17, 2007. http://digitalcommons.ilr.cornell.edu/key_workplace/311/.

Phillips, Jr., Robert L., Martey Dodoo, Carlos R Jaén, and Larry A Green. "COGME's 16th Report to Congress: Too Many Physicians Could be Worse Than Wasted." *Annals of Family Medicine* 3 (2005): 268–70.

Pittman, Larry J. "ERISA's Preemption Clause: Progress Towards a More Equitable Preemption of State Laws." *Indiana Law Review* 34 (2001): 207–94.

Pope, Gregory C., and John E. Schneider. "Trends in Physician Income." *Health Affairs* 11, no. 1 (1992): 181–93.

Procino, Michele L. "Note: The Death of Health Care Reform in 1994: Another example of Congress' Inability to Enact Major Reform." *Widener Law Symposium Journal* 1 (1996): 547–86.

Propper, Carol. "A Larger Role for the Private Sector in Health Care? A Review of the Arguments." *Journal of Social Policy* 30, no. 4 (2001): 685–704.

Quinn, Roswell. "Rethinking Antibiotic Research and Development: World War II and the Penicillin Collaborative." *American Journal of Public Health* 103, no. 3 (2013): 426–34.

Reinhardt, Uwe E. "Perspectives on the Pharmaceutical Industry." *Health Affairs* 20, no. 5 (2001): 136–49.

Relman, Arnold S. "The New Medical-Industrial Complex." *New England Journal of Medicine* 303, no. 17 (1980): 963–70.

Ricketts, Thomas C., III, ed. *Rural Health in the United States.* New York: Oxford University Press, 1999.

Risse, Guenter B. *Mending Bodies, Saving Souls: A History of Hospitals.* New York: Oxford University Press, 1999.

Robinson, James C. "Hospital Market Concentration, Pricing, and Profitability in Orthopedic Surgery and Interventional Cardiology." *American Journal of Managed Care* 17, no. 6 (2011): e241–48. http://www.ajmc.com/publications/issue/2011/2011-6-vol17-n6/ajmc_11jun_robinson_e241_248/1.

___. "From Managed Care to Consumer Health Insurance: The Rise and Fall of Aetna." *Health Affairs* 23, no. 2 (2004): 43–55.

___. "The Changing Boundaries of the American Hospital." *Milbank Quarterly* 72, no. 2 (1994): 259–75.

___. *The Corporate Practice of Medicine.* Berkeley, CA: University of California Press, 1999.

Robinson, Judith. *Noble Conspirators: Florence S. Mahoney and the Rise of the National Institutes of Health.* Washington, DC: Francis Press, 2001.

Rodgers, George. "Cardiology Workforce Crisis: Shortage or Surplus? Reply." *Journal of the American College of Cardiology* 55, no. 8 (2010): 834–88.

Rodwin, Mark A. *Conflicts of Interest and the Future of Medicine: The United States, France and Japan.* New York: Oxford University Press, 2011.

Rosenberg, Charles E. *The Care of Strangers: The Rise of American's Hospital System.* New York: Basic Books, Inc., 1987.

Rosoff, Arnold J. "The Business of Medicine: Problems with the Corporate Practice of Medicine Doctrine." *Specialty Law Digest—Health Care Monthly* 9, no. 14 (1988): 7–25.

Samson, Kurt. "New NIH Translational Research Center Plan Moves Forward: What It Could Mean for Neurology." *Neurology Today* 11, no. 7 (April 7, 2011): 39–43.

Samuelson, Paul A. "The Pure Theory of Public Expenditure." *The Review of Economics and Statistics* 36, no. 4 (1954): 387–89.

Sandy, Lewis G., Thomas Bodenheimer, L. Gregory Pawlson, and Barbara Starfield. "The Political Economy of U.S. Primary Care." *Health Affairs* 28, no. 4 (2009): 1136–44.

Scherer, F. M. "The Pharmaceutical Industry—Prices and Progress." *New England Journal of Medicine* 351, no. 9 (2004): 927–32.

Schwartz, Mark D., Steven Durning, Mark Linzer, and Karen E. Hauer. "Changes in Medical Students' Views of Internal Medicine Careers from 1990 to 2007." *Annals of Internal Medicine* 171, no. 8 (2011): 744–49.

Scott, K. "Case Study. Group Health Association: Can Humana Resuscitate the Moribund HMO?" *Health Systems Lead* 2, no. 4 (May 1995): 12–18.

Sean Keehan, Andrea Sisko, Christopher Truffer, Sheila Smith, Cathy Cowan, John Poisal, M. Kent Clemens, and the National Health Expenditure Accounts Projections Team. "Health Spending Projections Through 2017: The Baby-Boom Generation Is Coming To Medicare," *Health Affairs* 27, no. 2 (2008): 145–55.

Sekscenski, Edward S. "The Health Services Industry: A Decade of Expansion." *Monthly Labor Review* (May 1981): 9–16.

Selden, Thomas M., and Bradley M. Gray. "Tax Subsidies for Employment-Related Health Insurance: Estimates for 2006." *Health Affairs* 25, no. 6 (2006): 1568–79.

Shannon, James A. "The Advancement of Medical Research: A Twenty-Year View of the Role of the National Institutes of Health." *Journal of Medical Education* 42, no. 2 (1967): 97–108.

Sharfstein, Joshua M. "The FDA—A Misunderstood Agency." *Journal of the American Medical Association* 306, no. 11 (2011): 1250–51.

Sisko, Andrea, Christopher Truffer, Sheila Smith, Sean Keehan, Jonathan Cylus, John A. Poisal, M. Kent Clemens, and Joseph Lizonitz. "Health Spending Projections Through 2018: Recession Effects Add Uncertainty to the Outlook." *Health Affairs*, web exclusive (February 24, 2009): w346–57. http://content.healthaffairs.org/content/early/2009/02/24/hlthaff.28.2.w346.full.pdf+html.

Smith, Adam. *An Inquiry into the Nature and Causes of the Wealth of Nations.* New York: PF Collier & Son, 1909.

Smith, David Barton. *Health Care Divided.* Ann Arbor, MI: University of Michigan Press, 1999.

Sparer, Michael. "*Medicaid Managed Care: Costs, Access, and Quality of Care, Synthesis Report No. 23.*" Robert Wood Johnson Foundation. September 2012. http://www.rwjf.org/content/dam/farm/reports/reports/2012/rwjf401106.

Squires, David A. "*Explaining High Health Care Spending in the United States: An International Comparison of Supply, Utilization, Prices, and Quality.*" The Commonwealth Fund, May 3, 2012. http://www.commonwealthfund.org/~/media/Files/Publications/Issue%20Brief/2012/May/1595_Squires_explaining_high_hlt_care_spending_intl_brief.pdf.

Staff of the Washington Post. *Landmark: The Inside Story of America's New Health-Care Law and What It Means for Us All.* New York: Public Affairs, 2010.

Starr, Paul. *Remedy and Reaction: The Peculiar American Struggle Over Health Care Reform,* New Haven, CT: Yale University Press, 2011.

___. *The Creation of the Media.* New York: Basic Books, 2004.

___. *The Social Transformation of American Medicine.* New York: Basic Books, 1982.

Steinberg, Daniel. "The Statins in Preventive Cardiology." *New England Journal of Medicine* 359, no. 14 (2008): 1426–27.

Steinbrook, Robert. "Testing Medications in Children." *New England Journal of Medicine* 347, no. 18 (2002): 1462–70.

Steinmetz, Erika, and Christopher B. Morse. "*Hospital Transfers of Medicare Patients.*" American Association of Medical Colleges Analysis in Brief 9, no. 1 (February 2009). https://www.aamc.org/download/82440/data/aibvol9no1.pdf.

Stephens, Trent. *Dark Remedy: The Impact of Thalidomide and Its Revival as a Vital Medicine.* Cambridge, MA: Perseus, 2001.

Stevens, Rosemary. "Health Care in the Early 1960s." *Health Care Financing Review* 18, no. 2 (Winter 1996): 11–22.

___. *In Sickness and in Wealth.* New York: Basic Books, 1989.

Stigler, George. "The Theory of Economic Regulation." *The Bell Journal of Economics and Management Science* 2, no. 1 (1971): 3–21.

Stiglitz, Joseph E. *Globalization and Its Discontents.* New York: W. W. Norton and Company, Inc., 2003.

Stoney, William S. "Historical Perspectives in Cardiology." *Circulation* 119, no. 21 (2009): 2844–53.

Strain, Jana K., and Eleanor D. Kinney. "The Road Paved with Good Intentions: Problems and Potential for Employer-Sponsored Health Insurance Under ERISA." *Loyola University of Chicago Law Journal* 31, no. 1 (1999): 29–68.

Studdert, David M., Michelle M. Mello, Atul A. Gawande, Tejal K. Gandhi, Allen Kachalia, Catherine Yoon, Ann Louise Puopolo, and Troyen A. Brennan. "Claims, Errors, and Compensation Payments in Medical Malpractice Litigation." *The New England Journal of Medicine* 354, no. 19 (2006): 2024–33.

Studdert, David M., Michelle M. Mello, and Troyen A. Brennan. "Medical Malpractice." *New England Journal of Medicine* 350, no. 3 (January 2014): 283–92.

Tarlov, Alvin R. "HMO Enrollment Growth and Physicians: The Third Compartment." *Health Affairs* 5, no. 1 (1986): 23–35.

Thaul, Susan. "*FDA's Authority to Ensure That Drugs Prescribed to Children are Safe and Effective.*" Congressional Research Service, 7-5700, RL33986. 2012. http://www.fas.org/sgp/crs/misc/RL33986.pdf.

Thompson, Richard B. "Foundations for Blockbuster Drugs in Federally Sponsored Research." *The Federation of American Societies for Experimental Biology Journal* 15, no. 10 (2001): 1671–76.

Tobert, Jonathan A. "Lovastatin and Beyond: The History of the HMG-COA Reductase Inhibitors." *Nature Reviews Drug Discovery* 2 (2003): 517–26.

Toole, Andrew A. "*The Impact of Public Basic Research on Industrial Innovation: Evidence from the Pharmaceutical Industry,*" Stanford Institute for Economic Policy Research, November 1, 2000. http://www.stanford.edu/group/siepr/cgi-bin/siepr/?q=system/files/shared/pubs/papers/pdf/00-07.pdf.

Townsend, Jessica. "Financing Medical Education." In Institute of Medicine, *Medical Education and Societal Needs: A Planning Report for the Health Professions* 243–60. Washington, DC: National Academy Press, 1983.

US Census Bureau. *Statistical Abstract of the United States: 1999.* Washington, DC: US Government Printing Office, 1999.

US Government Accountability Office. "*New Drug Development: Science, Business, Regulatory, and Intellectual Property Issues Cited as Hampering Drug Development Efforts.*" GAO Report 07-49, 2006. http://www.gao.gov/new.items/d0749.pdf.

___. "*Private Health Insurance: Estimates of Individuals with Pre-Existing Conditions Range from 36 Million to 122 Million,*" GAO Report 12-346. March 2012. http://gao.gov/assets/590/589618.pdf.

Venter, J. Craig, Adams, Mark D., Myers, Eugene W., Li, Peter W., Mural, Richard J., and Sutton, Granger G. "The Sequence of the Human Genome," *Science* 291, no. 5507 (2001): 1304–15.

Verville, Richard, and Joel A. DeLisa. "The Evolution of Medicare Financing Policy for Graduate Medical Education and Implications for PM&R: A Commentary." *Archives of Physical Medicine and Rehabilitation* 82, no. 4 (2001): 558–62.

Vladeck, Bruce C. "Medicare Hospital Payment by Diagnosis-Related Groups." *Annals of Internal Medicine* 100, no. 4 (1984): 585–90.

Vladeck, Bruce C., and Thomas Rice, "Market Failure and the Failure of Discourse: Facing up to the Power of Sellers," *Health Affairs* 28, no. 5 (2009): 1305–15.

Weeks, Elizabeth A. "The New Economic Credentialing: Protecting Hospitals from Competition by Medical Staff Members." *Journal of Health Law* 36, no. 2 (2003): 247–300.

Weiner, Jonathan P. "A Shortage of Physicians or a Surplus of Assumptions?" *Health Affairs* 21, no. 1 (January 2002): 160–62.

Weisz, George. *Divide and Conquer: A Comparative History of Medical Specialization.* New York: Oxford University Press, 2006.

Whang, Kenneth C. "The Applicability of Tax Credits to Medial Research and Development." American Association for the Advancement of Science., 1999, http://www.aaas.org/spp/cstc/pne/pubs/fundscience/papers/whang.htm.

Williams, Alan G. "The Cure for What Ails: A Realistic Remedy for the Medical Malpractice 'Crisis.'" *Stanford Law & Policy Review* 23 (2012): 478.

Woolhandler, Steffie, and David U. Himmelstein. "Paying for National Health Insurance—And Not Getting It." *Health Affairs* 21, no. 4 (2002): 88–98.

World Health Organization. *World Health Statistics 2012.* Geneva: World Health Organization, 2012.

—. *World Health Report 2000—Health Systems: Improving Performance.* Geneva: World Health Organization, 2000.

Yamey, Gavin. "Dispute as Rival Groups Publish Details of Human Genome." *British Medical Journal* 322, no. 7283 (2001): 381.

Young, Aaron, Humayun J. Chaudhry, Janelle Rhyne, and Michael Dugan. "A Census of Actively Licensed Physicians in the United States, 2010." *Journal of Medical Regulation* 96, no. 4 (2011): 10–20.

Zarabozo, Carlos. "Milestones in Medicare Managed Care." *Health Care Financing Review* 22, no. 1 (2002): 61–67.

Zerhouni, Elias A. "Translational and Clinical Science—Time for a New Vision." *New England Journal of Medicine* 353, no. 15 (2005): 1621–23.

Zinner, Michael J., and Edward H. Livingston, "JAMA Forum—The Massachusetts Health Care Reform Experiment: A Success." *news@JAMA.* October 31, 2012. http://newsatjama.jama.com/2012/10/31/the-massachusetts-health-care-reform-experiment-a-success/.

Zycher, Benjamin, Joseph A. DiMasi, and Christopher-Paul Milne. "Private Sector Contributions to Pharmaceutical Science: Thirty-Five Summary Case Histories." *American Journal of Therapeutics* 17, no. 1 (2010): 101–20.

INDEX

AAMC (Association of American Medical Colleges), 126
ABIM (American Board of Internal Medicine), 127, 135
Abramson, Leonard, 180–181, 182
ACA. *See* Affordable Care Act
academic medical centers (AMCs)
  biomedical research at, 114–115, 119–120, 130
  graduate medical education payments for, 98, 116, 133–134, 253n96
  Medicare and Medicaid programs and, 116–117
  National Institutes of Health funding for, 119–120, 130
  organizational structure of, 113–114
  origins of, 114–115
  regional examples of, 115
ACC (American College of Cardiology), 145, 147
access to health care, xii, 46–47, 198
accountable care organizations (ACOs), 107, 153, 227
Accreditation Council for Graduate Medical Education (ACGME), 126
ACOs (accountable care organizations), 107, 153, 227
acute medical care, 101–104
administrative complexity of reimbursement procedures, 224–225
adverse selection phenomenon, 213
Aetna, Inc., 179–183
Affordable Care Act (ACA, 2010). *See also* health care reform; universal health care coverage
  accountable care organizations under, 107, 153, 227
  comparative effectiveness research, promotion of, 228
  development of, 216–223
  insurance exchanges under, x, xv, 218
  Medicaid population under, 104, 105
  objectives of, xiv–xv, 118, 159, 202
  opposition to, ix, xiv, 218, 220
  on premature discharge of hospital patients, 107, 240n94

public–private collaboration in, 158, 188, 218–219, 220–221
  reporting requirements of, 107
  specialty hospitals under, 227, 254n111
  uninsured populations under, 35, 43
Agriculture Department, United States, 75, 76
AHA (American Heart Association), 145
almshouses, 29, 87
AMA. *See* American Medical Association
ambulatory surgery centers (ASCs), 102, 103
AMCs. *See* academic medical centers
American Board of Internal Medicine (ABIM), 127, 135
American College of Cardiology (ACC), 145, 147
American Heart Association (AHA), 145
American Medical Association (AMA)
  Affordable Care Act, endorsement of, 202, 219
  on medical education, 31–32, 125–126
  Medicare, opposition to, 154, 211
  origins of, 31, 124
  on physician licensure, 31, 32, 124–125
  political influence of, 201
  prepaid care, opposition to, 186
  on referrals, 152
  socialized medicine concerns raised by, 210, 211
  on specialization, 127, 135
  standardization of medical profession by, 31–32, 88, 124–126, 193
American National Standards Institute (ANSI), 236n18
Anderson-King bill (1961), 92, 211
Angiotech, 78
ANSI (American National Standards Institute), 236n18
anti-kickback provisions, 142–143, 152, 226
antitrust laws, 151
Arizona v. Maricopa County Medical Society (1982), 151
ASCs (ambulatory surgery centers), 102, 103
Association for Molecular Pathology v. Myriad Genetics (2013), 243n49, 243n54
Association of American Medical Colleges (AAMC), 126
automobile industry, xi, 6, 8–10